AF413070

Progress in Atomic Medicine

VOLUME 4

Recent Advances in Nuclear Medicine

Progress in Atomic Medicine

Volume 4

Recent Advances in Nuclear Medicine

Edited by

John H. Lawrence, M.D., D.Sc.

Donner Laboratory and Donner Pavilion
Lawrence Radiation Laboratory
University of California, Berkeley, California

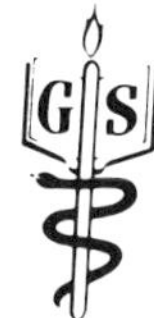

Grune & Stratton
A Subsidiary of Harcourt Brace Jovanovich, Publishers
New York • London

Contributors

Hal O. Anger, D.Sc., Donner Laboratory, Lawrence Berkeley Laboratory, University of California, Berkeley, California

William H. Blahd, M.D., Chief, Nuclear Medicine Service, Veterans Administration—Wadsworth Hospital Center, Los Angeles, California; and Professor of Medicine, University of California at Los Angeles, School of Medicine, Los Angeles, California

Thomas F. Budinger, M.D., Ph.D., Donner Laboratory, Lawrence Berkeley Laboratory, University of California, Berkeley, California

James McRae, F.R.A.C.P., Ph.D., Donner Laboratory, Lawrence Berkeley Laboratory, University of California, Berkeley, California

William G. Myers, M.D., Ph.D., Professor in Department of Radiology, Physiology & Medicine, Ohio State University Hospital, Columbus, Ohio; and Visiting Professor of Nuclear Medicine, Donner Laboratory—Division of Medical Physics, University of California, Berkeley, California

James H. Pritchard, M.D., Resident—Clinical Associate, Nuclear Medicine Service, Veterans Administration—Wadsworth Hospital Center, Los Angeles, California

Richard P. Spencer, M.D., Ph.D., Professor of Nuclear Medicine, Department of Radiology, Yale University School of Medicine, New Haven, Connecticut

Rainer Storb, M.D., Associate Professor of Medicine, Division of Oncology, Department of Medicine, University of Washington School of Medicine, Seattle, Washington; and United States Public Health Service Hospital, Seattle, Washington

E. Donnall Thomas, M.D., Professor of Medicine, Head, Division of Oncology, Department of Medicine, University of Washington School of Medicine, Seattle, Washington; and United States Public Health Service Hospital, Seattle, Washington

Arthur C. Upton, M.D., Dean, School of Basic Health Sciences, Health Sciences Center, State University of New York at Stony Brook, Stony Brook, New York

Martin A. Winston, M.D., Assistant Chief, Nuclear Medicine Service, Veterans Administration—Wadsworth Hospital Center, Los Angeles, California; and Assistant Professor of Medicine, University of California at Los Angeles, School of Medicine, Los Angeles, California

Preface

This is the fourth volume of this series, and looking at the present list of topics as well as previous ones, seeing the work being done today in Nuclear Medicine when visiting hospitals and laboratories of medical research, and hearing of the achievements and future possibilities in this field when attending medical meetings such as the Annual Meeting of the Society of Nuclear Medicine, one is impressed with the growth of the field of Nuclear Medicine and its many important applications to medical research, diagnosis, and therapy. Recently I reviewed some of the early studies with radioisotopes[1] as well as the more recent ones using today's very sophisticated instrumentation which allows us to use minute quantities of radioisotopes for accurate diagnostic evaluation of many medical problems. I feel the excitement of having been involved in this fast growing field from the pioneering days of the 1930's. In the first chapter of this volume, the very important subject of somatic and genetic hazards of radiation is presented by Dr. Arthur Upton, a distinguished leader in this field. Then Dr. Thomas Budinger, one of the leading young scientists on the frontiers of Nuclear Medicine discusses quantitative nuclear medicine which is so important in the analysis of metabolic processes with the aid of isotopes. Another pioneer, Dr. William Myers, a visiting Professor of Nuclear Medicine in the Donner Laboratory, brilliantly discusses Iodine-123 and its valuable applications and potential, especially in research and diagnosis. Irradiation and bone marrow transplantation is an important subject dis-

---

[1] George Von Hevesy Memorial Lecture, International Society of Nuclear Medicine, Athens, Greece, September 24, 1973.

cussed by the able and knowledgeable Dr. Donnall Thomas and his associate. Dr. James McRae and Hal Anger, pioneers in scanning, discuss the tomographic technique for diagnosis with isotopic compounds. Dr. William Blahd and associates discuss the correlation of ultrasonic and nuclear medicine techniques. And the last chapter by Dr. Richard Spencer, concerning the use of radioisotopes in studies of growth and development, should also be of interest to the reader of this volume. The future is bright for the contributions of Nuclear Medicine to the solution of problems in biology and medicine.

The Editor is grateful to the contributors for their willingness to undertake the task of writing the chapters, to the publishers for their helpfulness in assembling these chapters into this volume, and to Miss Janice DeMoor for her editorial assistance.

John H. Lawrence, M.D., D.Sc.

Contents

Arthur C. Upton

1

Somatic and Genetic Effects of Low-Level Radiation

INTRODUCTION

Expanding uses of ionizing radiation and radiation sources have prompted growing inquiry into the biological effects of low-level radiation. The extent of interest in this subject, within the public at large as well as the scientific community, is reflected by numerous articles in the popular press and by ongoing surveillance of the question by several national and international committees.[1-4]

Concern with the effects of small doses of radiation is an outgrowth of studies implying that some risk to human health might result from exposure to any appreciable increment above the natural background level. These studies have been reviewed extensively elsewhere,[3,4] along with findings from pertinent laboratory research; hence they are not considered again in detail here. Instead, the implications of the available human dose–effect data, analyzed in the light of cogent radiobiological research in other organisms, are surveyed in the sections to follow.

RADIOBIOLOGICAL AND BIOPHYSICAL CONSIDERATIONS

Man has evolved in the continuous presence of natural background radiation, from which he receives an average dose of about 0.1 rem per year.[3,4] Whether he or any other organisms experience biological effects attributable to irradiation at these low levels of exposure is a matter of speculation. Such effects, if present, would undoubtedly be too small to be feasibly detected. Hence their occurrence can only be predicted by extrapolation from observations at higher doses and higher dose rates, based on assumptions about the mathematical relationship between dose and effect, and about the biological mechanisms accounting for the effects in question.

The biological effects of radiation result from molecular alterations caused by the random absorption of radiation by atoms and molecules in cells. The molecular alterations are, in turn, amplified through biochemical and biological processes into functional and morphological changes, which may affect other cells, entire organs, individuals, or populations. Central to the biological effects of low-level irradiation, therefore, is the process by which otherwise minor changes at the molecular level become amplified biologically into significant forms of injury.

The relationship between dose and effect can fall into one of several major categories: (1) linear, in which case the effect is directly proportional to dose; (2) quadratic, in which case the effect varies as the square of the dose; (3) sigmoid, or other power functions of dose; and (4) threshold. In those instances where traversal of a cell by a single radiation track suffices to increase the probability of the effect in question, the dose–effect relation is linear. Conversely, where two or more tracks are required, the dose–effect relation is quadratic or of some other type. For induction of chromosomal aberrations and cell killing, which are thought to require the interaction of two or more alterations in a critical target (presumably DNA), the dose–effect curve for sparsely ionizing radiations, or radiations of low linear energy transfer (LET), such as x-rays, gamma rays, beta radiations, is characteristically linear at low doses and low dose rates, where the ionizing events from different tracks are so widely separated in space and time as to make the probability of their interaction negligible. With increasing dose and dose rate, however, intertrack interactions contribute increasingly to the process, with the result that the dose–effect curve departs from linearity ("single-hit" kinetics), becomes curvilinear ("multi-hit" kinetics), and approaches a quadratic or power function. With high-LET radiations (such as alpha particles, fast neutrons), the amount of energy deposited by each track as it traverses the cell is large enough so that the contribution from additional tracks makes little difference; hence the dose–effect curve is usually linear from low doses to high doses, and is relatively unaffected by the dose rate.

In attempting to estimate what effects, if any, might occur at the so-called maximum permissible doses and dose rates for radiation workers (roughly 5 rems per year to the whole body) or for the general population (roughly 170 rems per year to the whole body), one must extrapolate from observations at higher levels of exposure, by means of hypotheses which rest on sound use of all cogent data. It is to this question that the following sections of this chapter are primarily addressed.

GENETIC (HERITABLE) EFFECTS

Nature of Genetic Changes

Changes in the hereditary material of the germ cells which are transmissible to descendants of the irradiated individual are generally classified in three major categories: (1) gene mutations, which are alterations in individual genes (so-called point mutations); (2) chromosome aberrations, which result from breakage and rearrangement of chromosomes (the larger aberrations are observable under the microscope, but smaller ones are submicroscopic and may be difficult to distinguish from gene mutations); and (3) changes in chromosome number (aneuploidy).

The structure of the mammalian chromosome and its associated nucleoprotein complex is not known precisely. Hence the molecular effects of radiation on this system cannot be defined fully as yet. Our knowledge of the effects of radiation on DNA, however, has expanded enormously in recent years, amplified by the recognition that effects on DNA are influenced profoundly by repair processes.

Changes in DNA attributed to ionizing radiation include base alteration, base destruction, sugar–phosphate bond cleavage, chain breakage (single strand and double strand), cross-linking of strands (intrastrand and interstrand), and degradation.[5] Although strand breakage has been studied extensively by physicochemical techniques, the molecular changes involved in break formation are not known precisely.[6,7] Double-strand breaks are thought to constitute roughly 7 to 10 percent of all the breaks induced by x-irradiation in mammalian cells and are estimated to require approximately 600 eV per break,[8] as compared with 44 eV per single-strand break.[9] Either type of break may lead indirectly to more complicated molecular changes in the affected DNA if the break is repaired incorrectly. Among the possible results of such "misrepair" are base-pair changes and deletions, such as have been implicated in radiation mutagenesis in Neurospora.[10]

It is amply clear that the mutation process must now be viewed as the end result of a sequence of reactions, the outcome of which may depend as much on the influence of repair mechanisms as on the nature of the primary lesion itself.[4,6,7] At least three types of DNA repair have been noted in bacteria: (1) photoenzymatic repair, (2) excision repair, and (3) postreplication (recombinational) repair.[4,7]

Excision repair, through which pyrimidine dimers induced by ultraviolet light are removed from the affected DNA, is defective in patients suffering from xeroderma pigmentosum, presumably accounting for their photosensitivity.[11] This type of repair also varies markedly among mammalian cell lines.[6] Photoenzymatic repair has not been found in mammals except in marsupials.[4] Because both types of repair involve enzyme systems which are under the influence of genetic, physiologic, metabolic, and environmental factors,[4,7] their role in mutagenesis can be expected to vary markedly among different types of cells, depending on circumstances, and can hence be characterized only in a general way. The assessment of the role of repair is further complicated by our uncertainty concerning the relationship between the DNA in mammalian cells and its associated nucleoprotein complex, which also appears to undergo damage and repair following irradiation.[4,12]

Radiation-induced damage to genes and chromosomes may be expected to manifest itself in subsequent generations as an increase in the frequency of traits and diseases otherwise attributable to naturally occurring mutations and chromosome changes. Among the simpler categories of such genetic damage are the disorders caused by dominant gene mutations, which appear in the first generation. Examples include achondroplasia, polydactyly, and Huntington's chorea. Such conditions, of which there are thought to be several hundred,[13] are estimated collectively to affect roughly 1 percent of the population.

Another category of genetic damage is attributable to recessive mutations, which may not express themselves for many generations. This category includes several hundred diseases,[13] most of which are extremely rare. Among the more common examples are sickle cell anemia, Tay-Sach's disease, cystic fibrosis, and phenylketonuria. Recessive genes located on the X chromosome express themselves as dominants, in contrast to those above, affecting males almost exclusively; hemophilia exemplifies the diseases associated with this group.

Alterations in chromosome number are predominantly lethal to the embryo[14] but may give rise to disturbances in sexual development, systemic disorders such as Down's disease, or other abnormalities.[15]

Chromosome aberrations, which include deletions, translocations, and other less common types of structural alteration, vary in their consequences, depending on the magnitude of the genetic imbalance they produce.[14,15]

Additional categories of genetic detriment include traits and diseases influenced by gene variation in a more complicated way. Although difficult to assess, an elevation in the mutation rate might be expected to increase the frequency of these disorders, with impairment of physical and mental vigor, and reduction in life expectancy.[3]

Dose–Effect Relations for Radiation-Induced Genetic Damage

HUMAN DATA

In contrast to the vast literature on genetic effects of radiation in species other than man, dating from Muller's pioneer work in the 1920s,[16] inherited effects attributable to radiation have yet to be documented conclusively in humans.

Attempts to observe genetic effects of radiation in human populations have been limited thus far to studies of first-generation offspring of irradiated parents, which can be expected to yield data only on chromosomal abnormalities and autosomal dominant and sex-linked mutations. The largest study of this type has been carried out on offspring of atomic-bomb survivors, in Hiroshima and Nagasaki, in whom congenital defects, stillbirths, abortions, infant and child mortality, sex ratio, birth weight, and anthropometric measures were investigated as possible indices of genetic injury.[17,18] Of these indices, only the sex ratio gave any evidence of being altered by radiation, and this effect was inconclusive. In the initial survey,[17] irradiated mothers bore a slightly smaller proportion of sons, and irradiated fathers a slightly larger proportion of sons, than did nonirradiated mothers and fathers, respectively, in keeping with genetic theory; however, these results were of borderline statistical significance and were not borne out by subsequent data on more than 47,000 additional pregnancies.[19] Hence it is not clear whether the change that was observed initially was an artifact.

Similar investigations on other irradiated human populations[20,21] have also given results consistent for the most part with the expectation of a reduction in the proportion of sons born to irradiated mothers, but the data from these studies are even less conclusive than those obtained from the populations of Hiroshima and Nagasaki.[3,20,22]

The negative observations on children of atomic-bomb survivors, although inconclusive, have been interpreted to imply that a radiation dose of at least 50 rems would have been required to double the mutation rate in Hiroshima and Nagasaki.[3,23] Because, moreover, the atomic-bomb radiations were received at an extremely high dose rate, the equivalent doubling dose accumulated through chronic exposure has been estimated to be no less than 3 times larger (150 rems), based on the influence of dose rate in the mouse.[3]

An association between trisomy-21 (Down's disease) and preconceptional diagnostic irradiation of the mother has been observed in several[24–27] but not all[28] studies. On the other hand, the absence of an increased frequency of this condition in offspring of atomic-bomb survivors,[29] whose large numbers lend weight to the observation, has implied that the association with diagnostic irradiation may not depend on the radiation itself but on other factors, such as maternal disease.[3] This interpretation is complicated, however, by more recent data from Japan indicating a dose-dependent increase in sex chromosome trisomy in the progeny of the irradiated population.[3]

Although not directly available for human germ cells, data are available on the incidence of chromosomal changes in human somatic cells, irradiated in vivo as well as in vitro, over a wide range of doses, dose rates, and exposure conditions.[30] An excess of aberrations has been noted in radiation workers, presumably resulting from irradiation at occupational exposure levels.[30-32] Aberrations have also been found to be increased in frequency as a function of the dose in atomic-bomb survivors examined 25 years after irradiation, including those who were exposed in utero during the first trimester of fetal development.[33]

MOUSE DATA

Specific locus (recessive) mutations. Our best information on the induction of mutations in mammals comes from experiments on specific locus mutations in the mouse, which have provided extensive data on recessive mutations at 12 loci affecting external features observable in weanlings.[4,34-36]

From these studies, several conclusions may be drawn:[3,4] (1) the yield of mutations per rad varies with dose, dose rate, dose fractionation, LET, sex, age, and time after irradiation, in a manner that cannot be fully explained on the basis of existing knowledge (Fig. 1-1); (2) in both sexes, the yield is several times lower at low dose rates (<0.1 rad per minute) than at high dose rates (>50 rads per minute) with doses of 100 to 600 rads of low-LET radiation; however, the influence of dose rate, which is tentatively ascribed to repair of premutational injury, is not observed with fast neutron irradiation; (3) at low dose rates, where the mutational effects on a cell are presumed to result from its traversal by a single radiation "track," the yield of mutations in x-irradiated spermatogonia, averaged over all 12 of the loci investigated, is roughly 0.5×10^{-7} mutations per R · gamete (as compared with a spontaneous rate of roughly 8.1×10^{-6} mutations per locus per gamete); however, the corresponding yield induced by fast neutrons under comparable conditions is roughly 20 times higher; (4) in oocytes of adult female mice, the yield of mutations resulting from protracted neutron irradiation is only about 5 percent as high as that in similarly irradiated spermatogonia; however, comparison of the sexes is complicated by the drastic reduction in mutation frequency observed with time after irradiation; i.e., mutations attributable to irradiation have been detected only in offspring conceived within the first 7 weeks after irradiation; in offspring born to females mated at later times, mutagenic effects attributable to irradiation have not been detected, for reasons which remain to be determined.[4] The evidence suggests that oocytes of the female mouse differ from those of other mammals, in terms of maturation schedule and radiosensitivity, with the result that mutation data for female mice cannot be extrapolated to other species without serious qualification.[4]

Because dose rate, dose fractionation, and LET have been observed to influence the yield of specific locus mutations in the manner noted above, it has been suggested that these effects include an appreciable component of small chromosome deletions as well as point mutations; however, this interpretation remains to be verified.[4]

The aforementioned observations on mouse spermatogonia and oocytes are considered to provide the best source of information for estimating the risks of mutations in human offspring,[3,4] since these cells most nearly resemble the human germ cell stages expected to accumulate doses under conditions of low-level irradiation. However, supporting data on radiation-induced mutations come from other studies in animals, plants, insects, microorganisms, and cultured cells.[4]

Dominant mutations. Information is more limited on dominant mutations than on recessive mutations. For dominant visible mutations induced by acute x-irradiation in mouse spermatogonia, the available data imply a yield of roughly 5×10^{-7} per rad per gamete.[4] For dominant mutations affecting the skeletal system, the corresponding rate is roughly 1.1×10^{-5} per gamete per rad, as compared with a spontaneous rate of 2.9×10^{-4} per gamete.[4]

Chromosome abnormalities. Data are available on the yield of radiation-induced translocations in all maturation stages of spermatogenic cells and in late dictyate oocytes of the mouse, based on cytological observations and on genetic analysis of affected offspring for semisterility.[4] As in the case of specific locus mutations, the yield of translocations varies markedly with the dose rate and quality of radiation, chronic gamma irradiation being less than half as effective as acute irradiation and only about one-twentieth as effective as chronic neutron irradiation.[4] Based on the data for semisterility, the yield of translocations from acute x-irradiation has been estimated to be about 3×10^{-5} per gamete per R.[3]

Although translocations represent only about one-third of all the chromosome aberrations observed in newborn babies, they may be expected to represent the bulk of chromosome abnormalities transmitted to the next generation in irradiated male germ cells, based on observations in the mouse implying that reproductive cells carrying other abnormalities are eliminated before they mature.[4] This may be less true of female germ

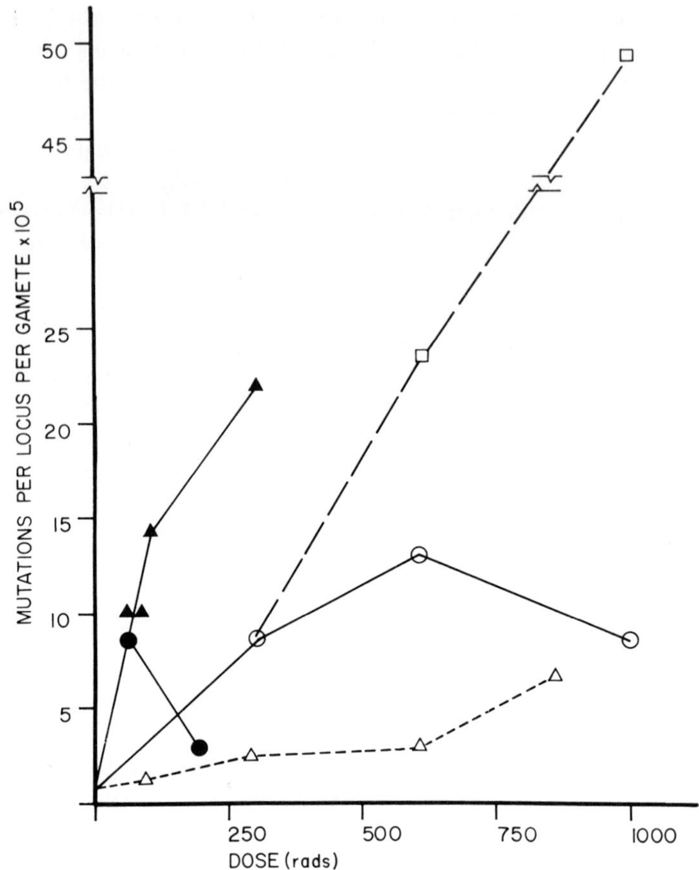

Fig. 1-1. Frequency of specific locus mutations in the mouse, in relation to dose, dose rate, and quality of radiation. (From W. L. Russell et al, cited in a United Nations report.[4] (a) Data for spermatogonia; (b) data for oocytes. Open symbols denote data for x-rays and gamma rays; shaded symbols denote data for fast neutrons: ○ acute (single brief) exposures; △ chronic (daily, protracted) exposures; □ fractionated exposures; ◇ mating more than 7 weeks after irradiation.

cells, however, owing to evidence that offspring missing the X chromosome are produced at a rate of about 5 to 15 per million per rem by appropriate irradiation of inseminated female mice.[4]

Empirical studies of mammalian populations. Direct observation for harmful effects, although seemingly the simplest way to assess offspring for inherited damage, is generally considered to reveal only a part of the total genetic detriment.[3] It is paradoxical, therefore, that this approach has

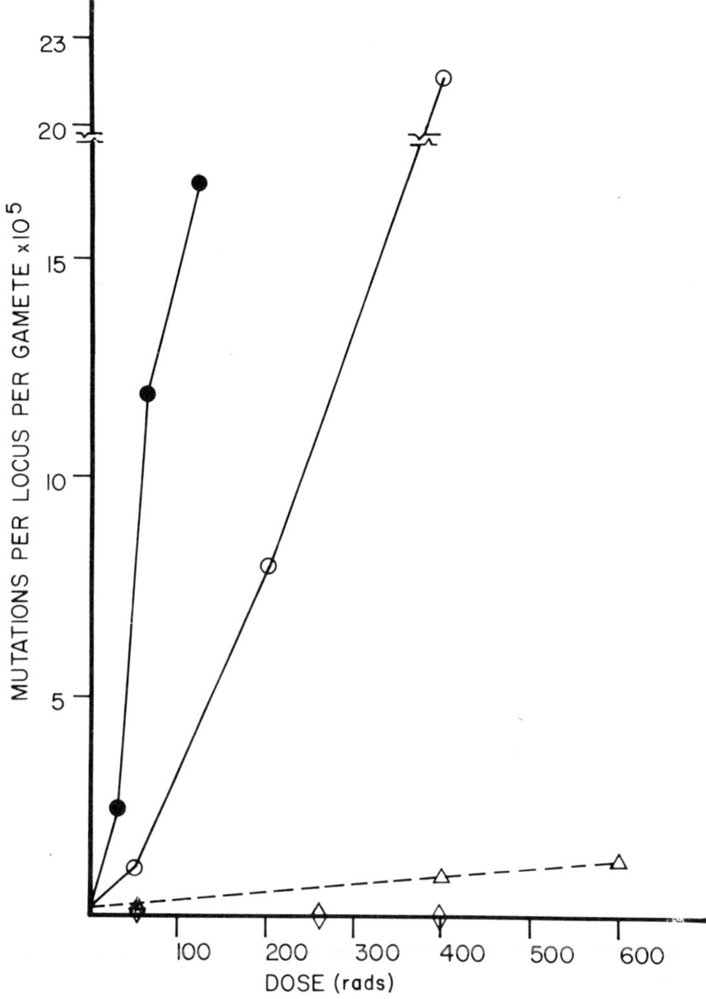

failed to demonstrate the accumulation of genetic injury in populations
of laboratory mammals irradiated serially through successive generations;[37]
however, the negative findings in such animals may be attributable to the
relatively small numbers observed thus far and to their examination by
methods lacking the power to detect small genetic differences in the presence of substantial nongenetic variability.[3,4,37]

Whatever the interpretation of the negative studies mentioned above,
their results, along with other negative findings such as the decreased risk
of mortality in trout embryos derived from lightly irradiated sperm,[38] complicate attempts to estimate the morbidity or mortality attributable to parental irradiation in human populations.

Risk Estimates for Humans

Owing to the absence of direct information on humans, the genetic risks associated with low-level radiation must be estimated largely by extrapolation from animal data. Such estimates have relied heavily on the relevant data from studies in mice, although they have taken into account pertinent information from all other sources. Because, as indicated above, reproductive cells expected to accumulate the greatest dosage on protracted irradiation are spermatogonia and oocytes, it is the mutational response of these cells that is of primary interest.

Based on the foregoing, the risks of genetic effects of low-level radiation in human populations have been estimated in various ways.[3,4] In arriving at such estimates (Table 1-1), 20 to 200 rems has been selected as the range of values bracketing the doubling dose for mutations and chromosome aberrations in man, largely on the basis of the aforementioned

Table 1-1
Estimates of Genetic Detriment per Million Offspring
Attributable to a Gonadal Dose of 5 rems to the
Preceding Generation

Type of genetic detriment	Natural incidence	Effects of 5 rems per generation*	
		First generation	*Equilibrium generations*
Dominant traits and diseases	10,000	5–500	250–5000
Chromosomal and recessive traits and diseases	10,000	<50	<200
Recognized abortions			
Aneuploidy and polyploidy	35,000	55	55
XO	9,000	15	15
Unbalanced rearrangements	11,000	360	460
Congenital chromosomal anomalies			
Unbalanced rearrangements	1,000	60	75
Aneuploidy	4,000	5	5
Other congenital anomalies	15,000		
Anomalies expressed after birth	10,000	5–500	50–5000
Constitutional and degenerative diseases	15,000		
Total (rounded)	120,000	500–1500	900–10,000

* Modified from reports of the National Academy of Sciences[3] and the United Nations[4] based on an assumed doubling dose of 20–200 rems.

data from experiments in the mouse.[3,4] Estimates of the natural frequencies of the traits and diseases listed in Table 1-1 come from various sources.[3,4]

From the estimates tabulated (Table 1-1), it would appear that only a small percentage of naturally occurring diseases of the types listed is attributable to irradiation at doses approaching natural background levels. In addition to the diseases tabulated, however, which include only those with a more or less well-defined genetic component, there are many other unspecified diseases in which the degree of genetic determination is unknown. The mutational component of the latter is presumably smaller than in the diseases tabulated, but it is unlikely to be negligible. It may be assumed, therefore, that any increase in the mutation rate would cause some increase in the overall incidence of disease and thus contribute to the total impairment of mental and physical health in the general population. The magnitude of such an effect cannot be estimated except by crude approximation. Nevertheless, on the assumption that a doubling of the mutation rate would increase the overall level of ill health by one-fifth, it has been estimated that exposure of the population to 5 rems per generation would increase the equilibrium incidence of ill health by 0.5 to 5.0 percent.[3]

The economic costs of such an increase in morbidity have been characterized in terms of a corresponding fraction of the total annual expenditure for medical services in the United States, i.e., 0.5 to 5.0 percent of roughly $400 per capita, or $2 to $20 per person per year.[3]

SOMATIC EFFECTS

Nature of Somatic Effects

Somatic effects differ from genetic effects in that they are manifest in the irradiated individuals themselves, as opposed to their offspring. The various types of somatic effects include some which may be detected soon after irradiation, such as chromosomal and cytological abnormalities, and others which may not appear until weeks, months, or years later.

Certain types of somatic effects, which depend on drastic killing of cells, disorganization of tissue, and disturbance of organ function,[33,34] are not observed at low doses and low dose rates. Other effects, however, such as the induction of chromosomal and cytological abnormalities, result from injury to individual cells and have been observed to vary in frequency as a function of dose down to the lowest doses investigated thus far.[30,33,34] Effects of the latter type, therefore, and their pathologic consequences must be considered in evaluating the biological implications of low-level irradiation.

Included among effects in the latter category, pending further knowledge of their dose–response relations and mechanisms of induction, are cancer, teratologic abnormalities, opacities of the lens of the eye, shortening of the life span from causes other than cancer, impairment of fertility, and effects on the central nervous system. Data on the occurrence of each of these types of effects, as possible consequences of low-level irradiation, are surveyed in the following.

Radiation-Induced Cancer

INTRODUCTION

Only a few years after its discovery, the x-ray was observed to cause skin tumors as an occasional complication of radiodermatitis.[33,35] On wider experience, radiation-induced tumors in other organs were also noted.[33,35] With systematic study, carcinogenic effects of radiation were gradually detected at lower and lower doses, suggesting to some observers the possibility that the risk of certain types of cancer might vary with dose down to natural background radiation levels.[1,3,4,33,36] As a result of these developments, efforts to define the dose–incidence relation and to quantify the risks associated with low-level irradiation have been steadily intensified.[1,3,4,37–39]

Determination of the dose–incidence relationship in humans is complicated by several difficulties: (1) the cancers attributable to radiation are not distinguishable individually from those arising through natural causes and hence are demonstrable only numerically as an excess in irradiated populations; (2) because of the relatively low frequency of cancer of any one type or site, few irradiated populations are large enough to provide quantitative dose–incidence data for any one neoplasm; (3) the average latent period between irradiation and the appearance of cancer is so long (exceeding 15 years from some types of tumors) as to hamper follow-up of the exposed individuals in prospective studies and evaluation of the history of radiation exposure of individuals in retrospective studies; (4) interpretation of dose–incidence data derived from populations exposed to radiation for medical purposes is complicated by the possible influence of underlying disease or of treatments other than radiation on susceptibility to cancer; (5) unexplained variations in the natural incidence of cancer with age, sex, diet, ethnic group, geographic factors, and other variables complicate the interpretation of dose–incidence data obtained from any one population in terms of applicability to another; (6) estimation of the radiation dose that is relevant to the induction of a neoplasm in any given irradiated individual is usually complicated by uncertainties concerning the precise spatial and temporal distribution of the dose in relation to the time and site of origin of the neoplasm.[3,4]

Although complicated by the difficulties just mentioned, an association between radiation exposure and an excess in the frequency of several types of cancer has been documented conclusively. Furthermore, the causal significance of the association is evident from the systematic correlation between dose and incidence, the exclusion of factors other than radiation as alternate causes, and the consonance between the association observed in humans and cogent radiobiological data from experiments in laboratory animals.[3]

LEUKEMIA

Radiation was first implicated in the pathogenesis of leukemia in 1911, when a clustering of cases in radiation workers pointed to occupational exposure as a possible causative factor.[4] More than 200 cases of "radiation-induced" leukemia have since been reported in the literature,[41,42] and the induction of the disease has been studied extensively in laboratory animals of several species.[43]

The most extensive information on the relation between leukemia incidence and radiation dose in human populations comes from epidemiologic studies on atomic-bomb survivors[3,4,44] and British patients given radiotherapy to the spine for ankylosing spondylitis.[3,4,45,46] Supporting evidence has also been obtained from studies on US radiologists, children irradiated therapeutically over the mediastinum in infancy for thymic enlargement or other conditions, women given radiotherapy to the pelvic region for menorrhagia, children exposed to diagnostic irradiation in utero, and other irradiated populations.[3,4,39,47]

The leukemias associated with irradiation include all types except the chronic lymphocytic type. The predominant type varies, depending on age at irradiation. In children, acute lymphatic, or stem cell, leukemias predominate, whereas these forms are rare in adults.[48,49]

The latent period intervening between irradiation and the clinical onset of the disease varies with the hematologic type,[49] and possibly with the radiation dose.[50] In heavily irradiated atomic-bomb survivors, the incidence of acute lymphatic and chronic granulocytic leukemias reached a peak within 5 to 8 years after irradiation and then declined, whereas the incidence of other forms of acute leukemia did not reach maximum until 10 to 15 years after irradiation.[49] In spondylitics, the peak was attained within 4 to 7 years after exposure,[46] as in children exposed to diagnostic radiation in utero.[51] In atomic-bomb survivors and spondylitics the incidence returned toward normal within 20 to 25 years after irradiation, but the excess may not have disappeared entirely by that time.[3] The excess in children exposed prenatally failed to persist beyond the eighth year after birth in one study population[51] but was observed to remain throughout the period of follow-up (i.e., to the 10-year) in another.[52]

Because the incidence of leukemia may vary with age, sex, hematologic type, and time after exposure, it is difficult to interpret the significance of interim dose–incidence data on the overall frequency of leukemias of all types in a population of all ages. Nevertheless, some pooling of incidence data is usually necessary to yield large enough numbers of cases per dose group to enable statistically significant comparisons between dose groups. Such comparisons of pooled leukemia data from atomic-bomb survivors (Table 1-2) reveal a systematic correlation between incidence and dose, for both the acute and chronic forms of the disease. Differences between Hiroshima and Nagasaki are apparent, however, in the incidence and relative proportions of the two forms of leukemia, especially for the 20 to 99 rads dose range. These differences have been tentatively attributed to the difference between the two cities in relative neutron dose, neutrons comprising a significant proportion of the total dose in Hiroshima and virtually none in Nagasaki.[3,44] Based on the likelihood[53] that the relative biological effectiveness (RBE) of the neutrons was substantially higher than that of the gamma rays, the contribution of neutrons to the total effective dose may have appreciably outweighed that of gamma rays in Hiroshima. The dose–incidence curves for the two cities appear dissimilar (Fig. 1-2) unless RBE values in excess of 1.0 are assigned to the neutrons, an RBE of 5.0 being found empirically to give a better approximation than any of the several other values tested[3,44] (Fig. 1-3).

In assessing the curves in Figures 1-2 and 1-3, it must be borne in mind that the number of cases in Nagasaki is too small to give precision to the data, especially at the lower dose levels.[3] Hence, within statistical limits, the points on either curve can be fitted to a straight line, with the slope for the Hiroshima curve corresponding to roughly 1.7 cases per 10^6 per year per rem and that for the Nagasaki curve to roughly 1.0 case per 10^6 per year per rem. The difference in yield between the two cities is due to a greater excess of chronic leukemias in Hiroshima, the excess of acute leukemias being essentially the same in both cities (Table 1-2).[3] An increase in the ratio of chronic to acute forms, most pronounced in Hiroshima, has also been noted in other irradiated populations.[4]

In British patients treated with spinal irradiation for ankylosing spondylitis, a total of 52 cases of leukemia was observed in the 141,496 person-years of observation, as compared with 5.48 cases expected.[3,4,46] Averaged over a follow-up period ranging up to 25 years, the 46.52 excess deaths correspond to 0.88 deaths from leukemia per 10^6 per year per rad mean dose to the marrow.[3,4,46] When the excess is analyzed in relation to age at the onset of radiation therapy, however, it increases steeply (fivefold) with age, the age–incidence curve for the irradiated spondylitics lying above and roughly parallel to that for the nonirradiated populations of England and Wales (Fig. 1-4). The relative excess appears, therefore, to have remained essentially constant, irrespective of age at exposure although the absolute excess increased markedly with age. In contrast, the atomic-

Table 1-2

Incidence of Leukemia in Atomic-Bomb Survivors, 1950–1966*

Range	Dose (rads) *Median values*			Number of subjects	Thousands of person-years	Number of leukemia cases			Leukemia cases/100,000/yr		
	Gamma	Neutron	Total			*Acute*	*Chronic*	*Total*	*Acute*	*Chronic*	*Total*
					Hiroshima						
300+	323	112	427	825	12.1	12	5	17	99.17	41.32	140.5
200–299	185	49	241	606	9.0	2	3	5	22.22	33.33	55.6
100–199	105	27	131	1,652	24.1	8	2	10	33.20	8.30	41.5
50–99	56	13	68	2,611	38.3	3	4	7	7.83	10.44	18.3
20–49	26	5	30	4,555	67.0	6	8	14	8.96	11.94	20.9
5–19	8	2	10	10,541	156.0	4	4	8	2.56	2.56	5.1
Under 5	0	0	0	62,515	915.1	23	4	27	2.51	0.44	3.0
Total	—	—	—	83,305	1222.7	58	30	88	4.74	2.45	7.2
					Nagasaki						
300+	417	7	427	566	8.4	5	1	6	59.52	11.90	71.4
200–299	238	3	240	693	10.4	5	1	6	48.08	9.62	57.7
100–199	145	2	146	1,174	17.7	3	0	3	16.95	0	16.9
50–99	69	0	69	1,173	17.6	0	0	0	0	0	0
20–49	31	0	31	1,354	20.0	0	0	0	0	0	0
5–19	10	0	10	4,501	66.3	1	1	2	1.51	1.51	3.0
Under 5	0	0	0	20,403	297.2	10	2	12	3.36	0.67	4.0
Total	—	—	—	29,864	437.6	24	5	29	5.48	1.14	6.6

* Modified from a National Academy of Sciences report[3] and Ishimaro et al.[44]

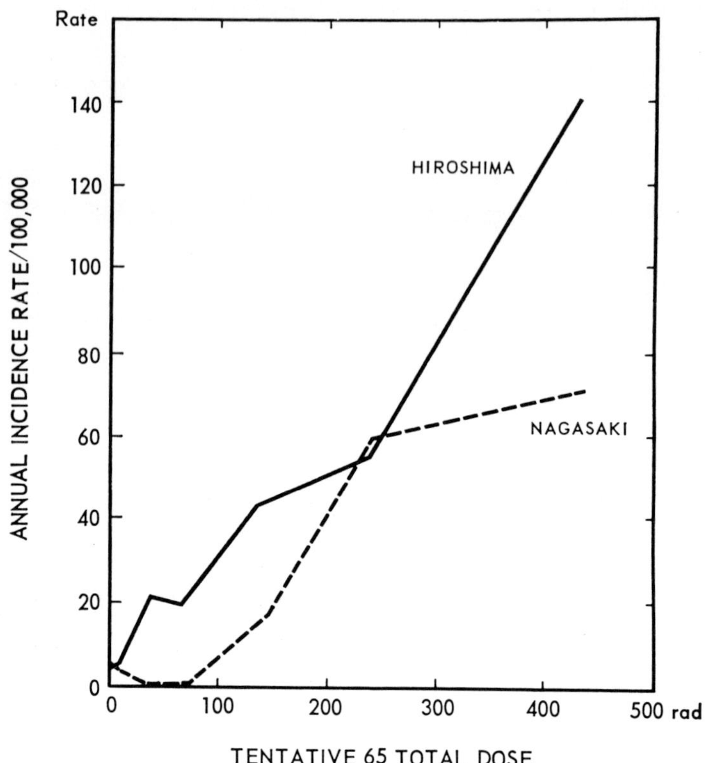

Fig. 1-3.   Incidence of leukemia in atomic-bomb survivors, in relation to estimated dose of radiation in rads (Data from a National Academy of Sciences report[3] and Ishimaru et al.[44])

bomb survivors have shown no significant age-dependent change in either the absolute excess or the relative excess of leukemia, which may be related to the absence in nonirradiated Japanese of the marked age-dependent increase in leukemia which is typical of Western populations.[3,4,48]

In several other irradiated populations, the relation between leukemia incidence and dose is not inconsistent with that observed in atomic-bomb survivors and spondylitics; however, the dose–incidence data for such populations are so imprecise that any similarity may be fortuitous. These populations include US radiologists who entered practice and received their occupational irradiation during the era preceding modern safety standards, children irradiated therapeutically over the mediastinum in infancy for thymic enlargement or other conditions, women sterilized by radiotherapy for treatment and menorrhagia, and children given x-ray therapy to the scalp for tinea capitis.[3,4,47,48]

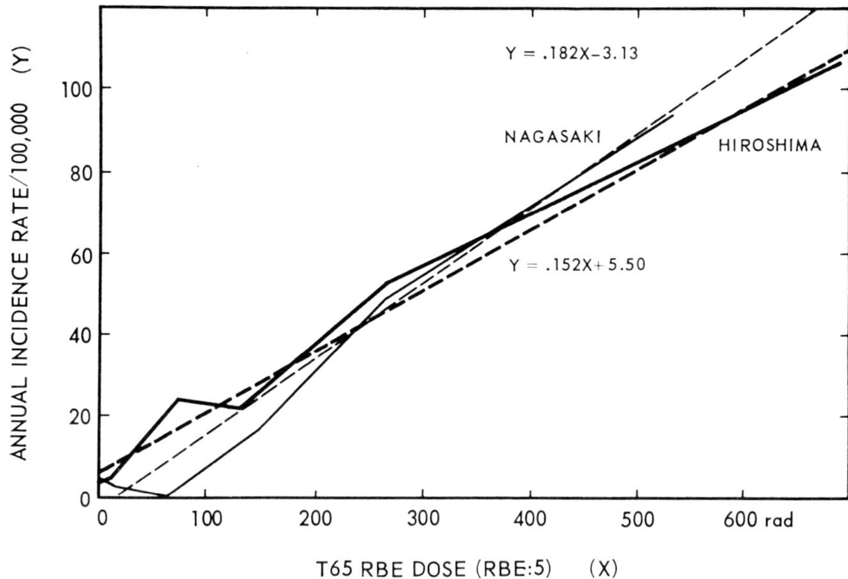

Fig. 1-3.   Incidence of leukemia in atomic-bomb survivors, in relation to estimated dose in rems (RBE of 5 assigned to fast neutrons). (Data from a National Academy of Sciences report[3] and Ishimaru et al.[44])

Other evidence suggesting the induction of leukemia by small amounts of radiation per se comes from the association between leukemia excess and previous radiographic examination. The evidence for such an association although inconclusive as yet in adults,[3,4,39] has been well established in children irradiated prenatally in the radiological examination of their mothers.[3,4,39] A similar increase has also been reported in children. In the largest study to reveal this association, which has involved more than 10,000 cases of juvenile cancer in some 20 million children,[55] and in several large confirmatory investigations, the incidence of leukemia and other cancers has been observed to be higher by about 50 percent in children irradiated before birth than in unirradiated controls.[3,39] The correlation between the magnitude of the excess and the number of abdominal x-ray exposures,[55] and the absence of any discernible cause other than radiation, imply that the association is one of cause and effect; however, the absence of an excess in Japanese children exposed to atomic bomb radiation in utero,[57] and the evidence that factors other than radiation may also affect the risk in irradiated children,[58,59] suggest that radiation might be merely one of a number of responsible etiologic cofactors. Nevertheless, if it is assumed that the observed excess of leukemia is attributable entirely to the dose of radiation received in utero, the excess corresponds to roughly

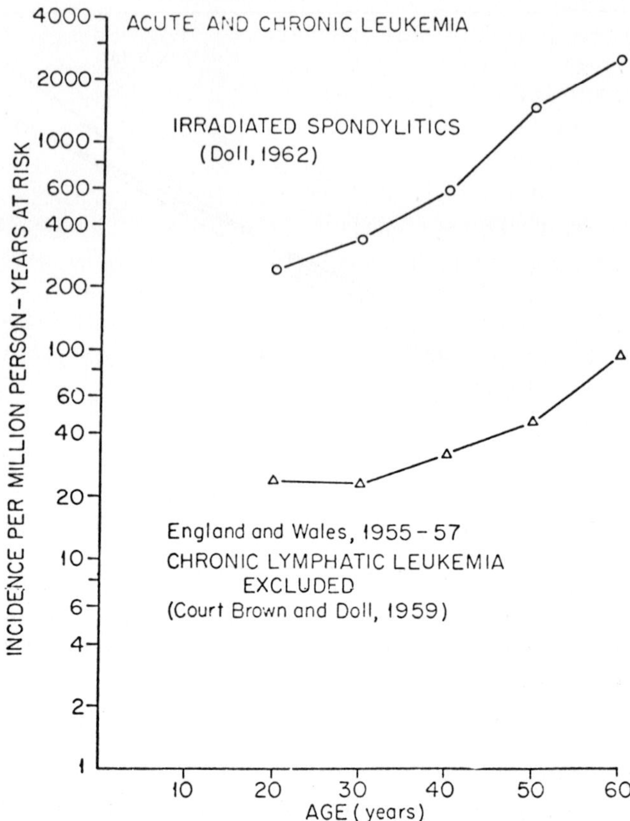

Fig. 1-4.   Incidence of leukemia in British patients treated with spinal radiation for ankylosing spondylitis, in relation to age at onset of irradiation and age-specific incidence in nonirradiated general population of England and Wales, excluding chronic lymphatic leukemia. (Modified from Doll[54] and Upton.[61])

10 to 25 deaths from leukemia per 10^6 per year per rad.[3,4] This rate of induction is an order of magnitude higher than that in atomic-bomb survivors and spondylitics, mentioned above, implying that susceptibility may be correspondingly higher in the fetus.[3,4]

Although irradiation of any fraction of the marrow should be leukemogenic if the incidence of leukemia varies as a linear function of the mean radiation dose to hemopoietic cells, there is evidence that this is not the case in women treated for carcinoma of the cervix by cancericidal doses of radiation delivered to the pelvic region.[3,4] The absence of an excess of leukemia in these patients remains to be explained but may conceivably be due to the possibility that the doses they received were high enough to cause excessive injury to the exposed marrow, since experimental observations imply that the leukemogenic effects of radiation may be overshadowed above a certain dose level by cytotoxicity or other side effects.[43,53,60] Partial-body irradiation has been clearly leukemogenic, on the other hand, in women sterilized by smaller doses of radiation for menorrhagia, in irradiated spondylitics, and in children irradiated therapeutically over the mediastinum in infancy.[3,4]

The influence of dose rate on the leukemogenic effectiveness of a given dose cannot be determined from the available information on humans, but there is ample evidence that x-rays and gamma rays are several times less leukemogenic at low dose rates than at high dose rates in mice.[43,53,61] The excess of leukemia in radiologists, who accumulated their exposure at low dose rates, is not as large per unit dose as that observed in the atomic-bomb survivors and spondylitics, who were exposed at high dose rates, but the difference is not statistically significant.[3] Likewise, although an excess of leukemia has been reported in association with iodine-131 treatment of thyroid carcinoma, phosphorus-32 treatment of polycythemia vera, and thorotrast angiography, interpretation of the excess in terms of dose–incidence relationships is complicated by variables which cannot be adequately evaluated at present.[3,4,62]

On the assumption that the incidence of leukemia is proportional to the dose, at a frequency of 1 case per 10^6 person-years at risk per rem, irrespective of dose and dose rate, it has been estimated that roughly one-tenth of the "spontaneously" occurring cases of leukemia might be attributable to natural background radiation.[36] As yet, however, efforts to relate geographic differences in leukemia incidence to corresponding differences in background radiation have been inconclusive.[39]

The induction of leukemia has been studied extensively in irradiated mice, rats, dogs, swine, guinea pigs, and monkeys.[4,43] The neoplasms include hematologic types similar to those observed in humans, as well as other types peculiar to the species in question. Dose–incidence data over a wide range of doses, dose rates, and LETs are available only in the mouse, in which there are also marked strain variations in the natural incidence of various forms of the disease and in dose–incidence relations. In the mouse, the yield of leukemias following whole-body irradiation is a complex function of dose and dose rate, neutrons being more effective than x-rays or gamma rays and relatively dose-rate independent in effectiveness, x-rays and gamma rays decreasing in effectiveness with decreasing dose and dose rate.[4,43,53]

Studies of the pathogenesis of leukemia in mice have implicated viral agents (which are activated or released by radiation in some unknown way), effects on the integrity of hemopoietic tissues, impairment of immunological competence, and other contributory mechanisms.[4,43] As yet, however, the respective roles of each of these factors remains to be elucidated, as does their potential relevance to the pathogenesis of leukemia in other species, including humans.

THYROID

An association between irradiation of the thyroid gland and the subsequent development of thyroid tumors, first reported by Duffy and Fitzgerald[63] in individuals irradiated during childhood, has since been amply documented, with the further suggestion of such an association in populations irradiated at older ages.[3,4,39] The observed growths include carcinomas, adenomas, and hyperplastic nodules, which have been detected after an average latent period of 10 to 20 years.[3,4,39,64,65,71]

The relation between the incidence of cancer and the dose of radiation to the thyroid gland is not known precisely, but the frequency of nodular growths (which are predominantly benign) has been observed to approach 100 percent in patients whose thyroids received large doses (of the order of 1000 rads or more) of therapeutic radiation in childhood[3,65] and in natives of Rongelap whose thyroids received comparable doses from radioactive fallout (principally from radionuclides of iodine) in childhood.[3,66] In the patients, the excess has approximated 2 to 9 cases per 10^6 per year per rad.[3,4,65,68] In Japanese atomic-bomb survivors, there has also been an excess of thyroid cancer in the dose range 25 to 200 rads, corresponding roughly to 2 to 3 cases per 10^6 per year per rad.[3,4,64]

The excess of thyroid cancer at high dose levels in atomic-bomb survivors who were under 20 years of age at the time of exposure[67] was not so clearly evident in those who were exposed at older ages,[3,64] an age difference which has also been observed in other irradiated populations,[3,70] implying that susceptibility to carcinogenic effects of radiation on the thyroid gland is highest in childhood.[3]

Tumorigenesis following iodine-131 therapy for thyrotoxicosis has not been documented, despite the large numbers of patients so treated,[3,62] possibly because the doses are large enough to leave relatively few epithelial cells in the gland capable of sustained proliferation.[3]

In animals, iodine-131 induces tumors[3,72] about one-tenth as efficiently as x-rays for a given total dose, presumably because of the lower dose rate at which the iodine delivers its radiation.[73] Fast neutrons have been observed to be more effective than x-rays or gamma rays.[61] Tumor formation in animals has been observed to progress through a succession of stages, beginning with hyperplasia, and is subject to promotion or inhibition by hormonal stimulation or other modifying factors.[3]

BREAST

An increased frequency of carcinoma of the breast following irradiation, first reported by MacKenzie in Canadian women subjected to repeated fluoroscopy for pneumothorax therapy of pulmonary tuberculosis (1965), has been confirmed by further observations in such women,[75] in atomic-bomb survivors,[3,4,76] and in women given radiotherapy to the breast for postpartum mastitis.[77] An excess of questionable statistical significance has also been observed in women treated with iodine-131 for thyroid cancer.[62]

The tumors in question have generally developed later than 10 to 15 years after irradiation[3,4] and although the follow-up data are too meager as yet to define the relation between incidence and dose precisely, the findings are consistent with a linear relationship corresponding to roughly 6 to 8 cancers per 10^6 women per year per rem.[3]

Data from the atomic-bomb survivors imply that susceptibility decreases appreciably with increasing age at the time of irradiation.[3]

The induction of breast tumors in animals has been documented repeatedly in several species.[61] Susceptibility varies widely, depending on the influence of genetic background, age, sex, hormonal status, viral agents, and other factors.[3,4,61] In Sprague-Dawley female rats, the majority of which develop breast tumors spontaneously in the second year of life, tumor formation is greatly accelerated by localized irradiation of the mammary gland, the effects being inducible by exposure in vitro as well as in vivo.[3] The dose–incidence relation for x-rays is compatible with linearity down to 25 rads, with relatively little influence of fractionation or protraction on the overall incidence of tumors.[3] The neoplasms comprise chiefly fibroadenomas, with smaller numbers of adenocarcinomas and other growths. The dose–effect curve for fast neutrons rises steeply at far lower doses, resulting in a relative biological effectiveness (RBE) which exceeds 50 at the lowest doses investigated. The dose–effect relation for neutrons at low doses has been interpreted to imply that tumor induction requires radiation-induced alterations in two or more cells as opposed to effects on a single cell alone.[78] These intriguing results are unparalleled in any other carcinogenesis experiments to date.

BONE

An increase in the incidence of skeletal tumors at sites of previous therapeutic irradiation[46,79,80] and in association with high body burdens of radium[81–84] is well documented.[3,4] The tumors include benign as well as malignant types. Osteosarcomas associated with localized radiotherapy, at doses varying from 3000 rads to more than 15,000 rads, have appeared after a latent period averaging 9 years.[79] The benign tumors (chiefly osteochondromas) have been associated primarily with radiotherapy to the mediastinum in infancy, at doses of less than 500 rads, and have appeared after a latent period averaging roughly 11 years.[85-88]

Although the available data indicate clearly that the frequency of skeletal tumors increases with increasing dose to bone, the precise relation between incidence and dose remains to be defined. The most extensive dose–incidence data come from populations with high radium burdens, in which determination of the dose is complicated by several sources of uncertainty: (1) the available measurements relate primarily to the amount of radioactivity that is retained many years after uptake of the radioactive material into the skeleton, with the result that the initial level of radiation and its distribution in space and time are unknown; (2) the radioactivity is characteristically nonuniform in its distribution in space and time within bone, being concentrated in "hotspots," where the dose at the center is so high as to cause extensive killing of potentially transformed and preneoplastic cells, and being translocated gradually with time as a result of the growth and remodeling of bone; (3) the part of the dose responsible for tumor induction cannot be distinguished from that part of the dose received after initiation of the process, and to that extent irrelevant or "wasted"; (4) the relative effectiveness of the alpha particles, as compared with other constituents in the mixture of radiations emitted by radium and its daughter elements, is unknown; and (5) the fraction of the total dose to bone that is delivered to cells at the site or sites of origin of the tumors—for osteosarcomas, presumably the endosteum—cannot be specified precisely.[3,4,62] In view of these sources of uncertainty, any conclusion about the dose–incidence relationship must remain highly tentative at present.

In early painters of luminous dials and in other individuals having high burdens of radium-226, the incidence of osteosarcomas increases as an exponential function of the mean accumulated dose to bone, exceeding 20 percent at doses above 2900 rads.[3,4] On the other hand, in patients treated for tuberculous osteitis or for ankylosing spondylitis with radium-224, which has a half-life of only 3 to 6 days as compared with 1600 years for radium-226, the incidence of tumors increases as an apparently linear function of the dose, exceeding 20 percent at mean accumulated doses above 1345 rads.[3,4] When expressed in relation to the endosteal dose, as opposed to the mean dose throughout bone, the dose–incidence data for both nuclides of radium are brought into closer agreement.[3,4] The excess in these populations corresponds to roughly 0.1 to 0.96 cancer per 10^6 per year per rem mean dose to bone, the higher values being derived from the radium-224 patients.[3,4]

In the radium-224 patients, there is evidence that susceptibility is higher during childhood than during adult life and that the yield of tumors is greater for a given dose when the radiation is accumulated slowly through injections repeated over a period of months or years than when it is received rapidly from a briefer span of injections.[3]

In animals, the induction of bone tumors has been studied extensively in several species, the bulk of the investigations being carried out with bone-seeking internal emitters.[3,4,61,89] When the incidence of osteosarcomas is plotted against the mean accumulated dose to bone, the data for beta emitters consistently yield a sigmoid dose–incidence relationship,[90] whereas those for alpha emitters are usually, but not always, more compatible with linearity.[91]

In mice, a virus has been tentatively implicated in the pathogenesis of certain tumors,[92] but the general significance of viruses in the formation of skeletal tumors remains to be determined.

LUNG

Carcinoma of the lung, long recognized as an occupational disease of pitchblende miners in Saxory and Bohemia,[93] has been observed to occur with increased frequency in uranium miners,[94,95] fluorspar miners,[96] other underground miners exposed occupationally to increased concentrations of radon,[97,98] atomic-bomb survivors,[77,99] and patients treated with x-radiation for ankylosing spondylitis.[46] The neoplasms are predominantly epidermoid, small cell, and undifferentiated carcinomas, occurring in the hilar region some 15 to 20 years after the onset of exposure.[3,4,98–100]

Evaluation of the dose–incidence relation in miners is complicated by dosimetric difficulties, since the dose to the bronchial epithelium can be estimated only approximately from fragmentary data on the concentration of radon measured sporadically at varying locations in the air of the mines.[3] Exposure for one "working level" month, for example, has been estimated to deliver a dose to the bronchial epithelium varying from less than 0.1 rad to more than 20 rads.[101] Evaluation of the dose–incidence relation in atomic-bomb survivors and spondylitics is hampered by other uncertainties, including the paucity of cases observed to date.[3,4] From the limited information available, the excess incidence of bronchial cancer in the populations mentioned above has been estimated to approximate 1 case per 10^6 per year per rem;[3] however, the possible influence of cigarette smoking cannot be excluded as a significant contributing factor, in view of data suggesting that the effects of smoking and radiation are multiplicative rather than additive in affected miners.[102]

In laboratory animals, pulmonary neoplasms of a variety of types have been induced by irradiation, depending on the circumstances of exposure and the species irradiated.[3,4,61,103,104] In general, the doses required to increase the incidence of bronchial carcinomas are higher than those required to increase the incidence of adenomas by a comparable amount. For both benign and malignant tumors, high-LET radiations have been found to be more effective than low-LET radiations, and to give dose–effect curves which are more nearly consistent with linearity than are the curves for low-LET radiation.[103]

GASTROINTESTINAL TRACT

An excess of tumors of the gastrointestinal tract has been observed in patients treated with spinal irradiation for ankylosing spondylitis, 80 tumors being observed in the stomach, pancreas, pharynx, and colon, as opposed to the 40 cases expected (Table 1-3). In 277 patients treated with pelvic irradiation for menorrhagia, deaths from tumors of the rectum and large intestine have also occurred in excess of expectation, 7 deaths being observed, as opposed to the 1.5 expected during 12 to 25 years of follow-up.[105] An excess of salivary gland tumors, benign as well as malignant, has been noted in patients exposed to therapeutic irradiation of the neck region in childhood[1,88,106] and in atomic-bomb survivors of all age groups.[107] The overall incidence of gastrointestinal cancers in atomic-bomb survivors, however, has shown no significant excess to date,[1,3,4] possibly because of the high natural frequency of gastric tumors in Japanese.[108]

Although the data are too fragmentary to define the shape of the dose–incidence relation, the overall excess of tumors of the gastrointestinal tract noted after therapeutic irradiation, as mentioned above, has been estimated to approximate 1 fatal case per 10^6 per year per rem.[3]

Neoplasms of the organs of the gastrointestinal tract have been induced by irradiation in animals,[4,61] but dose–incidence data for such tumors are relatively meager. In general, such neoplasms are induced in lower frequency for a given dose than are neoplasms of the other types and sites discussed in the foregoing.

SKIN

Carcinoma of the skin, developing in an area of radiodermatitis on the hand of a radiation worker more than 70 years ago,[109] was the first neoplasm attributed to radiation.[35] It was followed by scores of similar tumors in other pioneer radiation workers and radiologists during the decades preceding modern safety standards.[35] The tumors include epidermoid carcinomas, basal cell carcinomas, and fibrosarcomas, arising after latent periods generally ranging from 10 to 30 years.[110] In most instances, tumor formation has been preceded by long-standing radiodermatitis, but some neoplasms have arisen in skin that appeared clinically "normal."[111]

The available data do not enable estimation of the numerical relationship between the incidence of skin tumors and the dose; however, the evidence implies that the susceptibility of the skin to radiation carcinogenesis may not be as high as that of the other tissues mentioned above.[1,3]

Table 1-3

Cancer of Heavily Irradiated Sites in Ankylosing Spondylitics*

Subgroup in which the difference between the observed and expected cancer incidence was statistically significant ($P < 0.025$ on a one-tailed test)	Number of cases		Excess over expected	
	Observed	*Expected*	*Number of cases*	*Rate per thousand persons*
Leukemia	60	7	53.3	4.7
Aplastic anemia	16	1	15.4	
Cancer of bronchus	96	54	41.8	2.9
Other cancers (mostly carcinomatosis, primary unknown)	24	7	17.2	1.2
Cancer of stomach	38	24	14.4	1.0
Malignant disease of lymphatic and hematopoietic tissues other than leukemia†	10	3	6.6	
Cancer of pancreas	12	6	6.3	
Cancer of pharynx	5	1	4.0	0.3–0.5
Bone cancer	5	1	3.9§	
Subgroup in which the difference between the observed and expected cancer incidence was not statistically significant				
Cancer of ovary	4	2	1.8	(0.8)
larynx	2	2	0.2	
esophagus	3	3	−0.4	
skin	0	1	−1.4	
Hodgkin's disease	1	2	−1.5	0.02 or less
Cancer which may be clinically associated with ankylosing spondylitis				
Cancer of colon	25	15	5.0††	0.4

* From a report of the International Commission on Radiological Protection[1] and Court-Brown and Doll.[46]

† Lymphosarcoma, reticulosarcoma, lymphoma unspecified (8 cases altogether), and myelomatosis (2 cases) as compared with 2.9 cases expected.

†† An excess of 10.2 was recorded by Court-Brown and Doll,[46] who reckoned that at least one-half of the excess might be attributed to the associations of cancer of the colon with ulcerative colitis and of ulcerative colitis with anklyosing spondylitis.

§ The reliability of the diagnosis of primary bone tumors on a death certificate is not high. The excess of confirmed deaths due to bone sarcoma was 2.4.

Cutaneous tumors have been induced by irradiation in several species of experimental animals.[3,4,61] In a series of experiments with rats, the yield of tumors was observed to be correlated closely with the incidence of irreparably damaged hair follicles, rising steeply above a dose of 1000 rems, passing through a maximum at 2000 to 4000 rems, and decreasing sharply at higher doses.[112] In mice, on the other hand, the yield has been found to increase as the square of the dose with superficial beta irradiation.[113] In general, the skin has appeared to be less susceptible to radiation carcinogenesis in experimental animals than have most of the other tissues mentioned above.

OTHER CANCERS

Neoplasms of types other than those discussed in the foregoing are reported to have been induced by irradiation, but the pertinent evidence is less quantitative than that for the neoplasms already discussed. The other types include lymphomas in atomic-bomb survivors[114–116] and irradiated spondylitics,[46] multiple myelomas in atomic-bomb survivors[114] and US radiologists,[117] tumors of the pharynx in patients given therapeutic external irradiation for thyrotoxicosis or other lesions in the neck,[118] cancer of the uterus in atomic-bomb survivors,[1] carcinomas or paranasal and mastoid sinuses in individuals with high radium burdens,[82,84] cholangiomas and hemagioendothelomas of the liver in individuals injected intravascularly with thorium dioxide (thorotrast),[119] tumors of the central nervous system and other sites in children exposed to diagnostic irradiation in utero,[1,3,4,39,51,52,55] and miscellaneous neoplasms at sites of intensive localized therapeutic irradiation.[1,3,4,35,39,106]

Although the diversity of observed neoplasms indicates that different tissues of the body are susceptible to radiation carcinogenesis, the relative susceptibility of different organs and tissues cannot yet be specified precisely. The long latent period required for development of radiation-induced tumors, as compared with the relatively short follow-up of most irradiated populations investigated to date, makes it likely that further study will significantly extend the existing data.[1,3,4,46] At present, the combined excess of mortality from all cancers other than leukemia and cancers of the thyroid, breast, bone, lung, and gastrointestinal tract, taken collectively, is estimated to approximate 1 death per 10^6 per year per rem,[3] implying that neoplasms of other types and sites are induced in relatively small numbers (or after a relatively long latency) as compared with those discussed above.

From the findings to date, the human data are consistent with observations in experimental animals,[4,61] indicating that the carcinogenic effects of radiation do not affect all organs equally and are not fully manifest until virtually all members of a population at risk have been followed until death, particularly after irradiation at low dose levels.

ESTIMATION OF THE CANCER RISKS ASSOCIATED WITH LOW-LEVEL RADIATION

In the absence of more complete information than is now available, the risks of cancer induction by irradiation at low doses and low dose rates can be estimated only by extrapolation from effects observed at higher doses and higher dose rates, based on tentative assumptions about the dose–incidence relationship, the mechanisms of carcinogenesis, and the susceptibility of the population at risk. There are ample reasons for expecting that the dose–incidence relationship will not be linear over all doses, dose rates, and variations in LET.[3,4,61,78,111] Nevertheless, practical expediency has dictated use of the linear, nonthreshold dose–incidence hypothesis as a basis for estimating upper limits of risk in radiation protection.[1,3] The estimates derived by this approach, as reported by the National Academy of Sciences, National Research Council Advisory Committee on the Biological Effects of Ionizing Radiation,[3] are summarized in Table 1-4. Insofar as these estimates, which are based largely on effects observed at high doses and high dose rates, fail to allow for the likelihood that x-rays, gamma rays, and other low-LET radiations will be several times less carcinogenic per unit dose at low doses and low dose rates, they may be expected to exaggerate the risks of low-level irradiation, and thus to provide conservative estimates of the upper limits of risk. Also because of limitations in the data and other possible sources of error, the estimates can be taken to represent no more than crude approximations.

It will be evident on inspection of the table that higher estimates are yielded by the relative risk model than by the absolute risk model. According to the former, the excess mortality attributable to radiation is assumed to be a constant percentage of the natural cancer mortality rate, while according to the latter the excess is assumed to be a constant number of cancer deaths per unit dose. It is not possible from existing data to reject either model, although the evidence available at present is more consistent with the absolute risk model,[1] except in the case of leukemia.[3] In either case, the total number of cancer deaths attributable to background radiation exposure is estimated to be only a small percentage of those occurring naturally (i.e., 0.6–2.9 percent).

Several factors argue against the assumption of a simple, linear dose–incidence relation for low-LET radiation, independent of dose rate, such as formed the basis for extrapolation in deriving the estimates shown in Table 1-4. The most compelling argument is the well-known difference in relative biological effectiveness (RBE) between low-LET radiations (such as x-rays and gamma rays) and high-LET radiations (such as alpha

Table 1-4

Upper Limit Estimate of Cancer Mortality in the US Population Attributable to Continual Exposure at a Rate of 0.1 rem per year (Roughly Equivalent to Natural Background)*

Age at irradiation	Type of cancer	Duration of latent period (years)	Duration of period of increased risk (years)	Absolute risk model		Relative risk model	
				No. deaths per 10⁶ per year per rem	Total excess deaths in population	Percentage increase in deaths per year	Total excess deaths in population
In utero	Leukemia	0	10	25	75		
	All other cancers	0	10	25	75	50	56
						50	56
0–9 years	Leukemia	2	25	2.0	164	5.0	93
	All other cancers	15	(a) 30	1.0	73	2.0	715
			(b) Life	1.0	122	2.0	5869
10+ years	Leukemia	2	25	1.0	277	2.0	589
	All other cancers	15	(a) 30	5.0	1062	0.2	1665
			(b) Life	5.0	1288	0.2	2415
All ages combined	Leukemia				516		738
	All other cancers		(a)		1210		2436
			(b)		1485		8340
All ages combined			(a)		1726 (= 0.6%)†		3174 (= 1.0%)†
	Total		(b)		2001 (= 0.6%)†		9078 (= 2.9%)†

* From a National Academy of Sciences report.[3]

† Values in parentheses denote percentage of natural cancer deaths per year in US population, based on vital statistics for 1967.

particles and fast neutrons). In most experimental radiobiological systems, including all cogent dose–incidence studies of radiation-induced neoplasms in laboratory animals, high-LET radiations have been observed to have a high RBE, which increases with decreasing dose and dose rate. The change in RBE observed under these conditions is due primarily to decrease in the effectiveness of the low-LET radiation with decreasing dose and dose rate, the effectiveness of the high-LET radiation remaining relatively constant.[3,43,53,61] This relationship is consistent with a linear response for the high-LET radiations and a curvilinear, or sigmoid, response for low-LET radiations, such as is suggested by the dose–incidence curves for leukemia in Hiroshima and Nagasaki, respectively (Fig. 1-2). Other arguments against the assumption that the dose–incidence relation for low-LET radiation would be linear and independent of dose rate are discussed elsewhere.[3,4,82,120]

On the other hand, it may be expected on physical grounds that the dose–incidence relation will be linear in the low-dose region, where there is a negligible probability of a cell being traversed by more than one radiation track, provided that effects of radiation on single cells can increase the likelihood of neoplasia.[1,121] Evidence for the clonal theory of cancer argues in favor of this interpretation, but the possibility remains that carcinogenesis may require more complicated interactions between altered cells, at least in certain stages of the process or in certain instances.[78] In any case, the region of dose and dose rate where the dose–incidence curve might be expected to obey single track kinetics is considerably lower than the region in which the bulk of known effects have been observed. Hence, there are grounds for expecting that use of a linear extrapolation from the high-dose region will overestimate the risks at low doses and low dose rates.

MORTALITY FROM EFFECTS OTHER THAN CANCER

Observations in experimental animals have been interpreted to indicate that radiation at relatively high dose levels may shorten the life span through late effects other than cancer, the severity of such life shortening increasing with the dose.[1,3,122–126] Based on such findings, it has been suggested that irradiation might reduce the life expectancy in human beings by 1 to 5 days per rem.[122,123]

Comparable information for human populations is largely unavailable. Elderly US radiologists have disclosed an excess in age-adjusted mortality which cannot be attributed entirely to cancer, but the excess has not been evident in those entering practice after 1939, during the time when modern safety standards have been in general use.[3,127,128] No definite excess in mortality from causes other than cancer has been attributable to radiation in atomic-bomb survivors[76] or other irradiated populations.[3] Hence mortality at any time during life from causes other than cancer is no longer considered likely to be one of the risks associated with low-level irradiation.[1,3]

CATARACT

The observation of radiation cataracts in 10 cyclotron workers in 1949[129] was followed quickly by reports of similar cases in other cyclotron workers,[130] reactor accident victims,[131] and atomic-bomb survivors.[132-134] The occurrence of cataracts in these subjects, who were exposed to radiations containing fast neutrons, was interpreted to be consistent with experimental data indicating a high relative biological effectiveness of fast neutrons for cataract formation in laboratory animals.[135,136]

The findings in the subjects just discussed contrast with the absence of radiation cataracts in radiotherapy patients exposed to x-rays and other low-LET radiations at doses below 200 to 600 rems.[137-141] In such patients, the dose–effect data indicate, moreover, that (1) fractionation or protraction of irradiation increases the threshold for cataract induction by a factor of 3 or more; (2) the time required for appearance of cataracts varies in relation to the dose and dose rate, ranging from less than 1 year to more than 10 years; (3) the lens opacities may progress in severity, remain stationary, or regress, the probability of progression increasing with the dose; and (4) all opacities detectable by ophthalmological examination as "radiation cataracts" are not necessarily severe enough to cause significant impairment of vision.

In view of the sigmoid nature of the dose–response relation for cataract induction by low-LET radiation, a similar response has been inferred to exist for high-LET radiation, with an effective threshold at approximately 75 to 100 rads.[1,136] The human lens is thus considered to be appreciably less radiosensitive than the mouse lens, in which less than 1 rad of fast neutrons can induce microscopically detectable opacities.[142] This conclusion is consistent with evidence that the lens is unusually sensitive in the mouse, as compared with larger mammals.[1] In light of all available human and animal data, the induction of cataracts is not expected to result from low-level irradiation in human populations.[1]

IMPAIRMENT OF FERTILITY

Spermatogonia and oocytes have long been recognized as being among the most radiosensitive cells in the human body. Drastic depression of the sperm count can be induced by acute exposure to a dose as low as 15 rems,[143,144] and temporary sterility can be induced in either sex by 200 to 300 rems delivered in a single brief exposure.[144,145] The doses required for permanent sterility, however, are substantially higher, depending on age, and may exceed the mean lethal dose if administered to the whole body in a single exposure.[144,145] It is not astonishing, therefore, that atomic-bomb survivors have manifested no lasting impairment of fertility attributable to irradiation.[146]

Data on the effects of protracted irradiation on human fertility are fragmentary. Fractionation and protraction within certain limits have been observed to increase the injury from a given dose of x-radiation to the spermatogenic epithelium;[144] however, systematic follow-up studies on chronically irradiated dogs have revealed no change in sperm count at or below a dose rate of 0.6 rem per week.[147] Protraction of exposure has generally been observed to reduce the killing of oocytes.[145]

Based on the above-mentioned findings, effects on human fertility are not expected at dose rates compatible with existing radiation protection standards.[1]

Effects on Growth and Development (Teratogenesis)

The high radiosensitivity of embryonal, fetal, and juvenile animals has long been recognized. Disturbances in growth and development have been produced in experimental animals by doses as low as 25 rems delivered during critical stages in organogenesis. Similarly, atomic-bomb survivors who were irradiated under 16 weeks of fetal age have shown an increased incidence of micocephaly at doses down to 25 rads.

The complexity of the effects, in which cell killing undoubtably plays a significant role, complicates estimation of dose–response relationships in the low-dose range, effects differing in kind, severity, and stage during development when they may be most easily induced. Susceptibility to any one effect is characteristically confined to a sharply circumscribed "critical" period that may not coincide with the "critical" period for another. At low dose rates, the amount of radiation received during the stage of sensitivity to any given effect is relatively small. In experimental animals, effects have not been detected at dose rates under 1 rem per day.[3]

The existing dose–response data are interpreted to suggest that effects on growth and development will not be detectable at present maximum permissible dose levels.[1,3]

Effects on the Central Nervous System

Although small doses are known to elicit transitory physiological responses in the central nervous system, retina, and olfactory apparatus, lasting effects on the structure, function, or performance of the nervous system have not been documented at doses below 10 to 20 rems, except in the developing embryo.[3,30] For this reason, harmful effects on these organs are not expected at dose levels compatible with present radiation protection standards.[3]

Effects on the Immune Response

It is well established that large doses of radiation (of the order of 100 rems) can impair the immune response, and that such an effect may have far-reaching implications for the affected individual. Such effects have not been detected, however, at doses below 20 rems.[4]

Cytological Abnormalities

An increase in the frequency of bilobed lymphocytes and other cytological abnormalities has been observed in humans exposed to diagnostic x-radiation of dose levels of the order of 1 rad.[148] The biological significance of such effects remains to be determined, as does that of the chromosomal aberrations which have been detectable at comparable dose levels in the circulating lymphocytes of exposed subjects.[30] Because such effects may conceivably represent a type of cellular injury that can occasionally be amplified to clinical significance, in the form of cancer, autoimmune disease, or other disorders, they deserve to be investigated further.

SUMMARY

Although the biological effects of ionizing radiation are probably better known than those of any other physical or chemical agent in the environment, our information about such effects has come from observations at doses and dose rates which are orders of magnitude higher than natural background environmental radiation levels. Whether, therefore, biological effects occur in response to such low levels can be estimated only by extrapolation, based on assumptions about the dose–effect relationship and the mechanisms of the effects in question.

Present knowledge suggests the possibility that several types of biological effects may result from low-level irradiation. The induction of heritable genetic changes in germ cells and carcinogenic changes in somatic cells are considered to be the most important from the standpoint of their potential threat to health. On the basis of existing data, it is possible to make only tentative upper limit estimates of the risks of these effects at low doses.

The estimates imply that the frequency of such effects attributable to exposure at natural background radiation levels would constitute only a small fraction of their natural incidence.

REFERENCES

1. International Commission on Radiological Protection. Publication 14: Radiosensitivity and Spatial Distribution of Dose. Reports prepared by two Task Groups of Committee 1 of the International Commission on Radiological Protection, New York, Pergamon Press, 1969
2. National Council on Radiation Protection and Measurements: Basic Radiation Protection Criteria, NCRP Report No 39, Jan 15 1971, 135 pp
3. The Effects on Populations of Exposure to Low Levels of Ionizing Radiation. Report of the Advisory Committee on the Biological Effects of Ionizing Radiations, National Academy of Sciences, National Research Council, Washington DC, 1972
4. Ionizing Radiation: Levels and Effects. A Report of the United Nations Scientific Committee on the Effects of Atomic Radiation to the General Assembly. Official Records of the General Assembly, Twenty-seventh Session, Suppl No 25 (A/8725). New York, United Nations, 1972
5. Kanazir DT: Radiation-induced alterations in the structure of deoxyribonucleic acid and their biological consequences, in Progress in Nucleic Acid Research and Molecular Biology, vol 9. New York, Academic Press, 1969, pp 117–222
6. Painter RE: Repair of DNA in mammalian cells, in Ebert M, Howard A (eds): Current Topics in Radiation Research Quarterly, vol 7, Amsterdam, North Holland, 1970, pp 45–70
7. Fox BW, Lajtha LG: Radiation damage and repair. Br Med Bull 29:16–22, 1973
8. Corry PM, Cole A: Radiation-induced double-strand scission of the DNA of mammalian metaphase chromosomes. Radiat Res 36:528–543, 1968
9. Lehman AR, Ormerod MG: The replication of DNA in murine lymphoma cells (L5178Y). 1. Rate of replication. Biochim Biophys Acta 204:128–143, 1970
10. Malling HV, De Serres EJ: Identification of the spectrums of x-ray-induced intragenic alterations at the molecular level in Neurospora crassa. Jap J Genet 44, Suppl 2:61, 1969
11. Cleaver JE: Xeroderma pigmentosum: A human disease in which an initial stage of DNA repair is defective. Proc Natl Acad Sci USA 63:428–435, 1969
12. Elkind MM, Kamper C: Biophys J 10:237, 1970, cited in Elkind MM: Damage and repair processes relative to neutron (and charged particle) irradiation, in Ebert M, Howard A (eds): Current Topics in Radiation Research Quarterly, vol 7. Amsterdam, North Holland, 1970, pp 1–44
13. McKusic VA: Mendelian Inheritance in Man. Baltimore, The Johns Hopkins Press, 1971
14. Carr DH: Chromosomes and abortion, in Harris H, Hirschorn K (eds): Advances in Human Genetics, New York, Plenum Press, vol 2. 1971, pp 201–257

15. Court-Brown WM, Smith PG: Human population cytogenetics. Br Med Bull 25:74–80, 1969
16. Muller HJ: The production of mutations by x-rays. Proc Natl Acad Sci USA 14:714–726, 1928
17. Neel JV, Schull WJ: The effect of exposure to the atomic bombs on pregnancy termination in Hiroshima and Nagasaki. Natl Acad Sci Publ 461, 1956
18. Kato H, Schull WJ, Neel JV: Survival in children of parents exposed to the atomic bomb, a cohort study. Amer J Human Genetics 18:339–373, 1966
19. Schull WJ, Neel JV, Hashizume A: Some further observations on the sex ratio among infants born to survivors of the atomic bombings of Hiroshima and Nagasaki. Am J Hum Genet 18:328–338, 1966
20. Schull WJ: Hereditary effects. Nucleonics 21(3):54–57, 1963
21. Meyer MB, Merz T, Diamond EL: Investigation of the effects of prenatal x-ray exposure of human oogonia and oocytes as measured by later reproductive performance. Am J Epidemiol 89:619–635, 1969
22. Purdom CE: Genetic Effects of Radiations. New York, Academic Press, 1963
23. Neel JV: Atomic bombs, inbreeding, and Japanese genes: The Russell lecture for 1966. Univ Mich Med Center J 32:107–116, 1966
24. Uchida IA, Curtis EJ: A possible association between maternal radiation and mongolism. Lancet ii:848–850, 1961
25. Sigler AT, Lilienfeld AM, Cohen HB, Westlake JE: Radiation exposure in parents of children with mongolism (Down's Syndrome). Bull Johns Hopkins Hosp 117:374–399, 1965
26. Uchida IA, Holunga R, Lawler C: Maternal radiation and chromosomal aberrations. Lancet ii:1045–1049, 1968
27. Albermann E, Polani TE, Fraser Roberts JA, Spicer CC, Elliott M, Armstrong E: Parental exposure to x-irradiation and Down's Syndrome. Ann Hum Genet 36:195–208, 1972
28. Carter CO, Evans KA, Stewart AM: Maternal radiation and Down's Syndrome (mongolism). Lancet ii:1042, 1961
29. Schull WJ, Neel JV: Maternal radiation and mongolism. Lancet i:537, 1962
30. Report of the United Nations Scientific Committee on the Effects of Atomic Radiation, Official Records of the General Assembly, Twenty-fourth Session, Suppl No 13 (A/7613). New York, United Nations, 1969
31. Court-Brown WM, Buckton KE, McLean AJ: Quantitative studies of chromosome aberrations in man following acute and chronic exposure to x-rays and gamma rays. Lancet 1:1239–41, 1965
32. Norman A, Sasaki, MS, Ottoman RE, Veomett, RC: Chromosome aberrations in radiation workers. Radiat Res 23:282–289, 1964
33. Bloom AD: Induced chromosomal aberrations in man. Adv Hum Genet 3:99–172, 1972
34. Rubin P, Casarett GW: Clinical Radiation Pathology, vol 1. Philadelphia, WB Saunders, 1968, pp 1–61
35. Furth J, Lorenz E: Carcinogenesis by ionizing radiations, in Hollaender A (ed): Radiation Biology, vol 1. New York, McGraw-Hill, 1954, pp 1145–1201
36. Lewis EB: Leukemia and ionizing radiation. Science 125:965–972, 1957
37. Brues AM: Critique of the linear theory of carcinogenesis. Science 128:693–699, 1958
38. Brues AM: Somatic effects, in Brues AM (ed): Low Level Irradiation. Washington DC, Am Assoc Adv Sci, 1959, pp 73–78

39. Report of the United Nations Scientific Committee on the Effects of Atomic Radiation. General Assembly, Nineteenth Session. Official Records, Suppl No 14 (A/5814). New York, United Nations, 1964

40. Von Jagie N, Scwarz G., Von Sienbenrock L: Blutbefunde bei Rontgenologen. Berl Klin Wochscr 48:1220–1222, 1911

41. Cronkite EP, Moloney W, Bond VP: Radiation leukemogenesis, an analysis of the problem. Am J Med 5:673–682, 1960

42. Heyssel R, Brill AB: The risk of leukemia in man following radiation exposure, in Meneely GR (ed): Radioactivity in man. Springfield, Illinois, Charles C Thomas, 1961, pp 266–281

43. Upton AC, Cosgrove GE Jr: Radiation-induced leukemia, in Rich MA (ed): Experimental Leukemia. New York, Appleton-Century Crofts, 1968, pp 131–158

44. Ishimaru T, Hoshimo T, Ichimaru M, Okada A, Tomiyasu T, Tsuchimoto T, Pamamoto T: Leukemia in atomic bomb survivors of Hiroshima and Nagasaki, 1 October 1950–30 September 1966. Radiat Res 45:216–233, 1971

45. Court-Brown WM, Doll R: Leukemia and aplastic anemia in patients irradiated for ankylosing spondylitis. Medical Research Council Report Series No 295. London, HMSO, 1957

46. Court-Brown WM, Doll R: Mortality from cancer and other causes after radiotherapy for ankylosing spondylitis. Br Med J ii:1327–1332, 1965

47. Lillienfeld AM: Epidemiological studies of the leukemogenic effects of radiation. Yale J Biol Med 39:143–146, 1966

48. Brill AB, Tomonaga M, Heyssel RM: Leukemia in man following exposure to ionizing radiation: a summary of the findings in Hiroshima and Nagasaki, and a comparison with other human experience. Am Inst Med 56:590–609, 1962

49. Bizzozero OJ Jr, Johnson KG, Ciocco A, Kawaski S, Toyoda S: Radiation-related leukaemia in Hiroshima and Nagasaki 1946–1964. II. Observations on type-specific leukaemia, survivorship, and clinical behavior. Ann Int Med 66:522–530, 1967

50. Bizzozero OJ Jr, Johnson KG, Ciocco A: Radiation-related leukaemia in Hiroshima and Nagasaki 1946–64. I. New Engl J Med 274:1095–1101, 1966

51. MacMahon B: Prenatal x-ray exposure and childhood cancer. J Natl Cancer Inst 28:1173–1191, 1962

52. Stewart A, Webb J, Hewitt D: A survey of childhood malignancies, Br Med J i: 1495–1508, 1958

53. Upton AC, Randolph ML, Conklin JW: Late effects of fast neutrons and gamma-rays in mice as influenced by the dose rate of irradiation: induction of neoplasia. Radiat Res 41:467–491, 1970

54. Doll R: The age factor in the susceptibility of man and animals to radiation. Br J Radiol 35:31–36, 1962

55. Stewart A, Kneale GW: Radiation dose effects in relation to obstetric x-rays and childhood cancers. Lancet i: 1185–1188, 1970

56. Graham S, Levin ML, Schuman LM, Gibson R, Dowd JE, Hempelmann LH, Lilienfeld AM: Preconception, intrauterine and postnatal irradiation as related to leukaemia. Natl Cancer Inst Monogr No 19:347–371, 1966

57. Jablon S, Kato H: Childhood cancer in relation to prenatal exposure to atomic-bomb radiation. Lancet ii:1000–1003, 1970

58. Gibson RW, Bross ID, Graham S, Lillienfeld AM, Schuman LM, Levin ML, Dowd JE: Leukemia in children exposed to multiple risk factors. N Engl J Med 279:906–909, 1968

59. Bross ID, Natarajan N: Leukemia from low-level radiation: identification of susceptible children. N Engl J Med 287:109–110, 1972

60. Gray LH: Radiation biology and cancer, in Cellular Radiation Biology, 18th M.D. Anderson Hospital and Tumor Institute Symposium on Fundamental Cancer Research. Baltimore, Williams & Wilkins, 1965, pp 7–25

61. Upton AC: Comparative observations on radiation carcinogenesis in man and animals, in Carcinogenesis: A Broad Critique. Proceedings of the 20th Annual Symposium on Fundamental Cancer Research. Baltimore, Williams & Wilkins, 1967, pp 631–635

62. Pochin EE: Frequency of induction of malignancies in man by ionizing radiation, in Zuppinger A, Hug O (eds): Encyclopedia of Medical Radiology. Berlin, Springer-Verlag, 1972, pp 341–355

63. Duffy BJ Jr, Fitzgerald PJ: Thyroid cancer in childhood and adolescence: a report on 28 cases. Cancer 3:1018–1032, 1950

64. Wood JW, Tamagaki H, Nerishi S, Jato T, Sheldon WF, Archer PG, Hamilton HB, Johnson KG: Thyroid carcinoma in atomic bomb survivors, Hiroshima and Nagasaki. Am J Epidemiol 89:4–14, 1969

65. Hempelman LH: Risk of thyroid neoplasms after irradiation in childhood. Science 160:159–163, 1968

66. Conard RA, Dobyns BM, Sutow WW: Thyroid neoplasia as late effects of exposure to radioactive iodine in fallout. JAMA 214:316–324, 1972

67. Jablon S, Belsky JL, Tsachikawa K, Steer A: Cancer in Japanese exposed as children to atomic bombs. Lancet i:927–932, 1971

68. Beach SA, Dolphin GW: A study of the relationship of x-ray dose delivered to the thyroids of children and subsequent development of malignant tumors. Phys Med Biol 6:583–598, 1962

69. Green M, Wilson GM: Thyrotoxicosis treated by surgery or iodine-131, with special reference to development of hypothyroidism. Br Med J i:1005–1010, 1964

70. DeLawter DS, Winship T: Follow-up study of adults treated with roentgen rays for thyroid disease. Cancer 16:1028–1031, 1963

71. Sampson RJ, Key CR, Buncher CR, Iyima S: Thyroid carcinoma in Hiroshima and Nagasaki, JAMA 209:65–70, 1969

72. Lindsay S, Chaikoff IL: The effects of irradiation on the thyroid gland with particular reference to the induction of thyroid neoplasms. Cancer Res 24:1099–1107, 1964

73. Doniach I: Effects including carcinogenesis of I-131 and x-rays on the thyroid of experimental animals. Health Phys 9:1357–1362, 1963

74. Mackenzie I: Breast cancer following multiple fluoroscopies. Br J Cancer 19:1–8, 1965

75. Myrden JA, Hiltz JE: Breast cancer following multiple fluoroscopies during artificial pneumothorax treatment of pulmonary tuberculosis. Can Med Assoc J 100:1032–1034, 1969

76. Jablon S, Kato H: Studies of the mortality of a-bomb survivors. 5. Radiation dose and mortality, 1950–1970. Radiat Res 50:649–698, 1972

77. Mettler FA, Hempelmann LH, Dutton AM, Pifer JW, Toyooka ET, Ames WR: Breast neoplasms in women treated with x-rays for acute postpartum mastitis, a pilot study. J Natl Cancer Inst 43:803–811, 1969

78. Rossi HH, Kellerer AM: Radiation carcinogenesis at low doses. Science 175:200–202, 1972

79. Bloch C: Postirradiation osteogenic sarcoma. Report of a case and review of literature. Am J Roentgenol 87:1157–1162, 1962

80. Pifer JW, Toyooka ET, Murray RW, Ames RW, Hempelmann LH: Neoplasms in children treated with x-rays for thymic enlargement. 1. Neoplasms and mortality. J Natl Cancer Inst 31:1333–1356, 1963

81. Marinelli LD: Radioactivity and the human skeleton. Am J Roentgenol 80:729–739, 1958

82. Evans RD, Keane AT, Shanahan MM: Radiogenic effects in man of long-term alpha-irradiation, in Stover BJ, Jee SS (eds): Radiobiology of Plutonium. Salt Lake City, JW Press, 1972, pp 431–468

83. Spiess H, Mays CW: Bone cancers induced by 224 Ra (Th X) in children and adults. Health Phys 19:713–720, 1970

84. Finkel AJ, Miller CE, Hasterlik RJ: Radium-induced malignant tumors in children and adults, in Mays CW, Jee WSS, Lloyd RD, Stover BJ, Daugherty JH, Taylor GN (eds): Delayed Effects of Bone-seeking Radionuclides. Salt Lake City, University of Utah Press, 1969, pp 195–225

85. Toyooka ET, Pifer JW, Crump BL, Dutton AM, Hempelmann LH: Neoplasms in children treated with x-rays for thymic enlargement. II. Tumor incidence as a function of radiation factors. J Natl Cancer Inst 31:1357–1377, 1963

86. Toyooka ET, Pifer JW, Hempelmann LH: Neoplasms in children treated with x-rays for thymic enlargement. III. Clinical description of cases. J Natl Cancer Inst 31:1379–1405, 1963

87. Hempelmann LH, Pifer JW, Burke GJ, Terry R, Ames WR: Neoplasms in persons treated with x-rays in infancy for thymic enlargement. A report of the third follow-up survey. J Natl Cancer Inst 38:317–341, 1967

88. Pifer JW, Hempelmann LH, Dodge HJ: Neoplasms in the Ann Arbor series of thymus-irradiated children; a second survey. Am J Roentgenol Radium Ther Nucl Med 103:13–18, 1968

89. Mays CW, Jee WSS, Lloyd RD (eds): Delayed Effects of Bone-Seeking Radionuclides. Salt Lake City, University of Utah Press, 1969

90. Mays CW, Lloyd RD: Bone sarcoma risk from ^{90}Sr, in Goldman M, Bustad LK (eds): Biomedical Implications of Radiostrontium Exposure. Oak Ridge, Tennessee, USAEC, Office of Information Services, 1972, pp 352–370

91. Mays CW, Lloyd RD: Bone sarcome incidence vs. alpha particle dose, in Jee WSS, Stover BJ (eds): The Radiobiology of Plutonium. Salt Lake City, JW Press, 1972, pp 409–430

92. Finkel MP, Biskis BO: Osteosarcomas induced in mice by FBJ virus and 90-strontium, in Mays CW, Jee SS, Lloyd RD, Stover BJ, Dougherty JH, Taylor GN (eds): Delayed Effects of Bone-Seeking Radionuclides. Salt Lake City, University of Utah Press, 1969, pp 417–435

93. Weller CV: Causal Factors in Cancer of the Lung. Springfield, Illinois, Charles C Thomas, 1956, pp 43–47

94. Wagoner JK, Archer VE, Lundin FE Jr, Holaday DA, Lloyd JW: Radiation as the cause of lung cancer among uranium miners. New Engl J Med 273:181–188, 1965

95. Lundin FE Jr, Wagoner JK, Archer VE: Radon daughter exposure and respiratory cancer, quantitative and temporal aspects. Report from the epidemiological study of United States uranium miners. National Institute for Occupational Safety and Health, National Institute for Environmental Health Sciences, Joint Monograph No 1, 1971, US Dept Health, Education, and Welfare, National Tech Info Service, US Dept of Commerce, Springfield, Va 22151

96. deVilliers AJ, Windish JP: Lung cancer in a fluorspar mining community. I. Radiation, dust, and mortality experience. Br J Med 21:94–109, 1964

97. Boyd JT, Doll R, Faulds JS, Lieper J: Cancer of the lung in iron ore (haematite) miners. Br J Ind Med 27:97–105, 1970

98. Wagoner JK, Miller RW, Lundin FE, Fraumeni JF Jr, Haij ME: Unusual cancer mortality among a group of underground metal miners. New Engl J Med 269:284, 1963

99. Wanebo CK, Johnson KG, Sato K, Thorslund TW: Lung cancer following atomic radiation. Am Rev Respir Dis 98:778–787, 1968

100. Saccomanno G, Archer VE, Auerbach O, Kuschner M, Saunders RP, Klein MG: Histologic types of lung cancer among uranium miners. Cancer 27(3):515–523, 1971

101. Hague AKMM, Collinson AJL: Radiation dose to the respiratory system due to radon and its daughter products. Health Phys 13:431–443, 1967

102. Lundin FE Jr, Lloyd JW, Smith EM, Arther VE, Holaday DA: Mortality of uranium miners in relation to exposure, hard-rock mining and cigarette smoking—1950 through September 1967. Health Phys 16:571–578, 1969

103. Sanders CL, Thompson RC, Bair WJ: Lung cancer; dose response studies with radionuclides, in Inhalation Carcinogenesis. Oak Ridge, Tennessee, USAEC Symposium Series No 18, 1970, pp 285–302

104. Laskin S, Kuschner M, Drew RT: Studies in pulmonary carcinogenesis, in Hanna MG, Nettesheim P, Gilbert JR (eds): Inhalation Carcinogenesis. Oak Ridge, Tennessee, USAEC, Division Technical Information, 1970, pp 321–351

105. Brinkley D, Haybittle JL: The late effects of artificial menopause by x-radiation. Br J Radiol 42:519–521, 1969

106. Hazen RW, Pifer JW, Toyooka ET, Livingood J, Hempelmann, LH: Neoplasms following irradiation of the head. Cancer Res 26:305–311, 1966

107. Belsky JL, Takeichi N, Yamamoto T, Cihak RW, Hirose F, Ezaki H, Inoue S, Blot W: Salivary gland neoplasms following atomic irradiation. ABCC TR, 1972, pp 23–72

108. Yamamoto T, Kato H, Ishida K, Tahara E, McGregor DH: Gastric carcinoma in a fixed population: Hiroshima and Nagasaki. ABCC TR, 1970, pp 6–70

109. Frieben A: Demonstration eines Cancroids des rechten Handruckens, das sich nach langdaurnder Einwirkung von Rontgenstrahlen entwickelt hatte. Fortschr Geb Roentgenstr 6:106, 1902

110. Traenkle HL: X-Ray-induced skin cancer in man, in Urbach F (ed): The First International Conference on the Biology of Cutaneous Cancer (National Cancer Institute Monograph 10). Washington DC, 1963, pp 423–432

111. Mole RH: Late effects of radiation: carcinogenesis, Br Med Bull 29:78–83, 1973

112. Burnes FJ, Albert RE, Heimbach RD: RBE for skin tumors and hair follicle damage in the rat following irradiation with alpha particles and electrons. Radiat Res 36:225–241, 1968

113. Hulse EV, Mole RH: Skin tumor incidence in CBA mice given fractionated exposures to low-energy beta particles. Br J Cancer 23:452–463, 1969

114. Anderson RE, Ishida K: Malignant lymphoma in survivors of the atomic bomb in Hiroshima, Am Inst Med 61:853–862, 1964

115. Angevine DM, Jablon S: Late radiation effects of neoplasia and other diseases in Japan. Ann NY Acad Sci 114:823–831, 1964

116. Shimizu K: Epidemiological study on malignant lymphoma among A-bomb survivors in Hiroshima. Hiroshima J Med Sci 15:201–211, 1966

117. Lewis EB: Leukaemia, multiple myeloma, and aplastic anemia in American radiologists. Science 142:1492–1494, 1963

118. Goolden AWG: Radiation cancer. A review with special reference to radiation tumours in the pharynx, larynx, and thyroid. Br J Radiol 30:626–640, 1957

119. International Atomic Energy Authority Technical Report 106. The dosimetry and toxicity of thorotrast. Int. Atomic Energy Authority, Vienna, 1968

120. Mole RH: Radiation effects in man: current views and prospects. Health Phys 20:485–490, 1971

121. Borek C, Hall EJ: Transformation of mammalian cells in vitro by low doses of x-rays. Nature 243:450–453, 1973

122. Failla G, McClement P: The shortening of life by chronic whole-body irradiation. J Roentgenol Radium Ther Nucl Med 78:946–954, 1957

123. Jones HB: The Nature of Radioactive Fallout and Its Effects. Washington DC, US Government Printing Office, 1957

124. Van Cleave, CD: Late somatic effects of ionizing radiation. Oak Ridge, Tennessee, USAEC Division of Technical Information Extension, 1968, pp 23–77

125. Upton AC, Randolph ML, Conklin JW: Late effects of fast neutrons and gamma rays in mice as influenced by the dose rate of irradiation life shortening. Radiat Res 32:493–509, 1967

126. Grahn D: Biological effects of protracted low dose radiation exposure of man and animals, in Fry RM, Griem ML, Rust JH (eds): Late Effects of Radiation. London, Taylor and Francis Ltd, 1970, pp 101–136

127. Seltser R, Sartwell PE: The influence of occupational exposure to radiation on the mortality of American radiologists and other medical specialists. Am J Epidemiol 81:2–22, 1965

128. Warren S: The basis for the limit on whole-body exposure—experience of radiologists. Health Phys 12:737–741, 1966

129. Abelson PH, Kruger PG: Cyclotron-induced radiation cataracts. Science 110:665–7, 1949

130. Dollfus MA: Cataracts par radiations issues du cyclotron. Bull Soc Ophthalmol Fr 5:459–466, 1950

131. Hempelmann LH, Lisco H, Hoffman, JG: The acute radiation syndrome: a study of nine cases and a review of the problem. Ann Int Med 36:279–510, 1952

132. Cogan DG, Martin SF, Kimura SJ, Ikui H: Ophthalmological survey of atomic bomb survivors in Japan 1949. Trans Am Ophthalmol Soc 48:62–87, 1950

133. Fillmore PG: The medical examination of Hiroshima patients with radiation cataracts. Science 116:322–323, 1952

134. Sinskey RM: The status of lenticular opacities caused by atomic radiation. Am J Ophthalmol 39:285–293, 1955

135. Woods AC: Cyclotron cataracts. Am J Ophthalmol 47, Part II:20–28, 1959

136. Ham WT Jr: Fast neutron radiation hazards, in Marion JB and Fowler JL (eds): Fast Neutron Physics. London, Interscience, 1960, Chap. IV–H, pp 841–927

137. Cogan DG, Dreisler KK: Minimal amount of x-ray exposure causing lens opacities in the human eye. Arch Ophthalmol 50:30–34, 1953

138. Merriam GR, Focht EF: A clinical study of radiation cataracts and the relationship to dose. Am J Roentgenol 77:759–785, 1957

139. Qvist CF, Zachau-Christiansen B: Radiation cataract following fractionated radium therapy in childhood. Acta Radiol 51:207–216, 1959

140. Britten MJA, Halnan KE, Meredith WJ: Radiation cataract: New evidence on radiation dosage to the lens. Br J Radiol 39:612–17, 1966

141. Natter G, Walstam R, Wikholm L: Radiation-induced cataracts after radium therapy in children. Acta Radiol Suppl 254:87–92, 1966
142. Bateman JL, Rossi HH, Kellerer AM, Robinson CV, Bond VP: Dose-dependence of fast neutron RBE for lens opacification in mice. Radiat Res 51:381–390, 1972
143. Heller CG: cited in Langham WH (ed): Radiobiological Factors in Manned Space Flight. National Academy of Science, National Research Council Publication 1487, Washington DC, 1967, pp 127–129
144. Rubin P, Casarett GW: Clinical Radiation Pathology, vol 1. Philadelphia, WB Saunders, 1968, pp 374–422
145. Baker TG: Radiosensitivity of mammalian oocytes with particular reference to the human female. Am J Obstet Gynecol 110:746–761, 1971
146. Blot WJ, Sawada H: Fertility among female survivors of the atomic bombs of Hiroshima and Nagasaki. Am J Hum Genet 24:613–622, 1972
147. Casarett GW, Eddy HA: Fractionation of dose in radiation-induced male sterility, in Brown DG, Cragle RG, Noonan RR (eds): Dose Rate in Mammalian Radiation Biology. CONF 680410. Oak Ridge, Tennessee, USAEC Division of Technical Information, 1968, pp 14.1–14.6
148. Upton AC: Effects of radiation on man. Am Rev Nucl Sci 18:495–528, 1968

Thomas F. Budinger

2

Quantitative Nuclear Medicine Imaging: Application of Computers to the Gamma Camera and Whole-Body Scanner

INTRODUCTION

A major goal of radionuclide imaging is the three-dimensional spatial and temporal quantitative description of isotope distribution. In contrast to conventional roentgenography, the majority of nuclear medicine procedures involve the in vivo delineation of biochemical activity, cell membrane transport, or organ fluid dynamics in space and time. In order to gain reliable quantitative information, the scintillation probe scanners and cameras have been interfaced to digital computers and electrooptical devices with increasing frequency over the past 10 years. Advances in digital engineering and computer science have enabled the nuclear medicine researcher and clinician to acquire and manipulate two-dimensional image data in a fashion that was only a hope or dream 5 to 10 years ago when pioneering papers emphasized this adjunct to nuclear medicine.[19,22,36,54,82,97,98,106,115,126,132,148,158,184,192,201]

Some of the recent major papers and innovations on digital quantitation have come from universities and nuclear medicine laboratories in Belgium, Czechoslovakia, England, France, Germany, and the United States.[5,9,25,33,35,36,40,89,99,119,128,138,142,151,166,171,183,207,208,210,213] Over the past 4 years it has become increasingly apparent to researchers and clinicians that the hardware and electronic devices interfaced to the scintillation camera were not able to perform even the simplest techniques of selected area cardiac function without 30 to 50 percent data loss. In many instances cumbersome manipulations would distract and discourage most busy clinicians and technicians. Now these problems have for the most part been overcome, and it is possible to acquire, manipulate, and display images that give quantitative functional dynamic information of value to the diagnosis and care of patients. The goals of this chapter are to review progress in techniques of quantitating the organ concentration of radionuclides in static and rapid sequential quantitative studies. The plan of this chapter is first to review the properties of computer systems. Then we investigate the properties of a single projection. Next, benefits of conjugate views are described as applied to whole-body sequential quantitative scanning, after which a detailed exposition of three-dimensional reconstruction from multiple gamma-camera views is attempted. Finally, progress in quantitative cardioangiography is reviewed in order to present most of the mathematical and practical techniques applicable to quantitation of organ function by nuclear medicine imaging techniques.

PROPERTIES OF COMPUTER SYSTEMS FOR NUCLEAR MEDICINE QUANTITATION

Requirements for Data Acquisition from Gamma Cameras

In addition to the image distortion associated with scattering in the body and the collimator, and intrinsic resolution of the detector, other problems of spatial nonuniformity and count rate nonlinearity seriously affect the quantitative capability of a nuclear medicine imaging system. The sources of distortion are basically of two types: the count loss due to dead time of the imaging device including the dead time of the analog to digital converter (ADC); and secondly, spatial distortion due to variation in sensitivity across the detector and inadequate spatial sampling by the analog to digital conversion process.

DATA LOSS DUE TO CAMERA AND
COMPUTER DEAD TIME

In commercially available scintillation cameras the dead time of the scintillation process, photomultiplier, and electronic circuits results in a pulse pair resolution greater than 2 μsec. Most of the commercial scintillation cameras have dead times greater than 4 μsec. A comparison of four commercial cameras is shown in Figure 2-1, where it can be seen that even for a relatively small dead time such as 10 μsec, the data loss at relatively low counting rates of 20,000 counts/sec is significant. This is due to the Poisson distribution of the physical process wherein a significant number of events fall within time intervals less than the pulse pair resolution of the camera. The average operating dead time for the Pho/Gamma

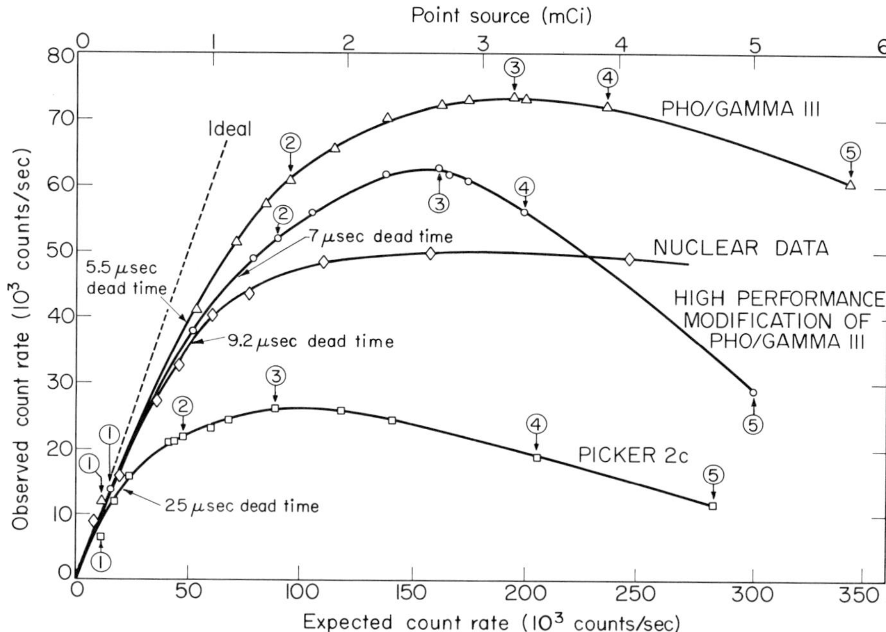

Fig. 2-1. Measurements of performance at high counting rate for four different cameras. All cameras maintain resolution up to and sometimes beyond the point of saturation, with the exception of the Pho/Gamma-III. The Ohio Nuclear camera (not shown) has performance superior to the others.

camera (Searle Radiographics) and Radicamera (Nuclear Data) is approximately 10 μsec. During the routine 10-mCi ^{99}Tc-pertechnetate or -albumin cardiac study, the data rate of the photopeak events is 40,000 counts/sec during 2 to 3 sec of the study. With a dead time of 10 μsec the loss of data is 27 percent, and for 20 μsec, 62 percent. One can show that the maximum counting rate as a source isotope increases without limit is the reciprocal of the dead time, which for the 40-μsec system is 25 kc/sec. This presumes that the camera is of the nonparalyzing type. For the paralyzing situation, the maximum rate is $1/(2.7\tau)$. Slow cameras not only limit statistics but give uptake–washout or flow curves that are distorted and must be corrected before they can be used for quantitative work. This is particularly important in cardiac flow studies.[45,99,112] If in addition to the camera dead time there is a computer ADC dead time significantly greater than that of the camera, the data are further distorted. Dead time can be measured conveniently by the classical methods of dual source substitution or addition of known amounts of source (Fig. 2-1);[46] however, data correction is not a desirable procedure for two reasons. First, it has been well established that the dead time for the Anger scintillation camera varies with count rate[2,46] as can be seen by applying the usual equation for dead-time measurement to the data depicted in Figure 2-1:

$$\tau = \frac{1}{R_0} - \frac{1}{R_t}.$$

(1)

Here R_0 and R_t are the observed and true counting rates, respectively. The second problem is that correction of the observed counts to the true counts in some interval using the equation

$$R_t = \frac{R_0}{1 - R_0 \tau}$$

(2)

is subject to the error corresponding to the statistics of the original observation and the errors inherent in the count rate and the dead-time determination. It turns out that the standard deviation of the corrected count N_c for the time interval T on a system with a dead time τ will be

$$\sigma(N_c) = \sqrt{N_c} \left[1 + \frac{2N_c^3 \, \mathrm{var}(\tau)}{T^2} \right]^{1/2}.$$

(3)

Thus the error is greater than merely $\sqrt{N_c}/N_c$, but as shown by Heiss and co-workers,[99] this error is less than the error that might be expected from the observed statistics.

A recent development has been the incorporation of high-speed ADC's in the high-speed small computer system, which will give a pulse pair resolution of 3 μsec, with a capability of data accumulation at 82,000 counts/sec in list mode and 300,000 counts/sec in histogram mode. The ADCs have been designed by the Hewlett-Packard Company and are incorporated in their system HP-5407.[45] The clock time of the dual ADCs is 200 mHz, and the system will match all scintillation cameras presently commercially available. Not all researchers and clinicians have this system available, and thus each digital system should have the dead-time determination as a function of count rate and the time–activity or uptake–washout curves should be corrected for the data loss. The seriousness of the problem can be seen by examination of Figure 2-2 which shows the effect of data dropout where the uptake–washout curve is simulated for 0, 20, and 40 μsec dead times. The analog to digital conversion speed can be effectively increased by the addition of a few levels of analog derandomization buffers. Very fast ADC's using the successive approximation design have the fundamental defect of possible spatial distortion, and thus caution must be exercised in choosing a very fast ADC to avoid spatial sampling errors, particularly when high spatial resolution is required. The criterion for the

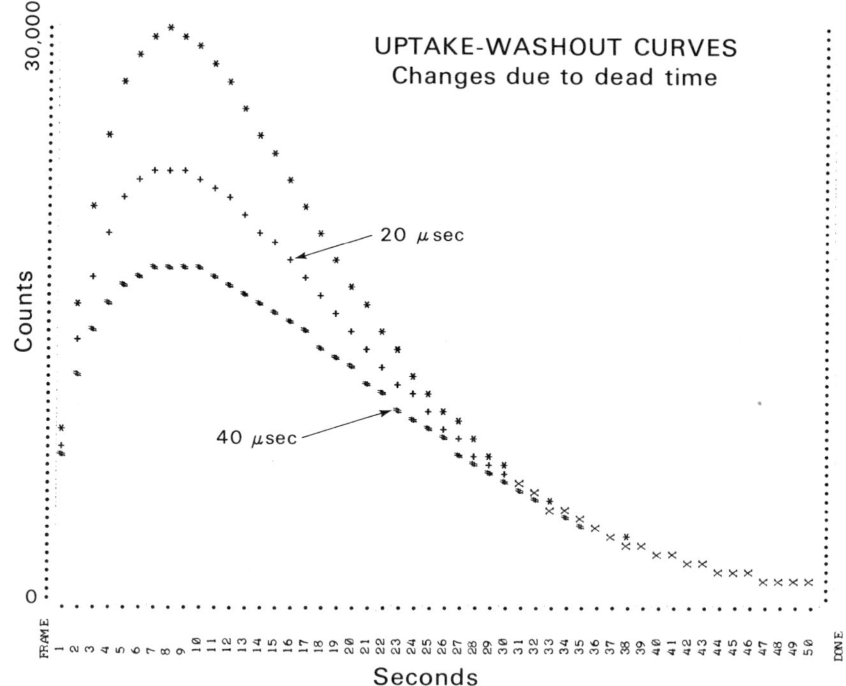

Fig. 2-2. Comparison of uptake–washout curves for a study recorded with dead times of 0, 20, and 40 μsec.

successive approximation ADC's sampling accuracy or digitizing accuracy is given by the differential linearity which should be less than 1 percent for nuclear medicine studies.

SPATIAL AND TEMPORAL SAMPLING FREQUENCY

The framing speed is the speed at which a two-dimensional image is acquired and stored as a discrete entity. Image data can be collected either in list mode or frame mode (histogram mode). In list mode the data are collected as individual counts and stored as computer words indicating the x, y position, and sometimes also energy of each event. It is possible to collect a list of counts during a flow study and then reconstitute the data into frames representing whatever time interval the investigator desires to examine. In the Hewlett-Packard HP-5407 system the time marks are put in every 10 msec; thus it is easy to frame data in 50-msec intervals, which is particularly appropriate for studying the flow of isotopes through the intercardiac chambers in premature infants with heart rates of 180. Since the digitization is limited only by the computer word size, for a 16-bit word it is possible to obtain data with an effective resolution of 256×256 without burdening the computer memory. However, in list mode the data storage capacity is seriously taxed after accumulating approximately 1 million computer words or scintillation events. Thus with presently available small computer data store systems it is not feasible to accumulate high-speed list mode indefinitely without reconstituting the data for more efficient storage.

In contrast, the histogram mode provides the ability for convenient reconstitution of data and storage in terms of frames or images; however, in this mode of accumulation both the resolution and the framing speed are seriously limited. Most commercial systems have a framing rate of 7 to 10 frames per second, which Lange and co-workers[134] find adequate for their cardiac studies; however, we find 15 to 20 per second is needed. The basic frame data require 16K core for 128×128, and 4K for 64×64; thus it is necessary to have at least an 8K memory in a small computer system to acquire and store 64×64 frames. The argument for setting up a system with a resolution of 64×64 or 32×32 is that it is convenient for a particular 12- or 16-bit word computer. As has been shown by Brill and Erickson[34] from changes in the modulation transfer function, one needs more than 64×64 elements across a 25.4-cm crystal. They showed that the modulation transfer function from a 128-point sampling across the crystal is very similar to that from a 256-point sampling, while that of a 64-point sampling is degraded by 10 to 15 percent in the range 0.2 to 0.7 cycles/cm. The 32-point sampling is degraded by as much as 40 percent, as shown in Figure 2-3, lower left. One can present another argument for the data array size. If a 25.4-cm crystal can resolve a sinusoidal wave of 0.8-cm wavelength, we expect $25.4/0.8 = 31.7$ wavelengths or cycles. The uniform sampling theorem in the spatial domain asserts that if a real space function $f(x)$ contains no frequency components greater than $s_{\max}$ cycles per unit distance, then $f(x)$ can be completely determined by its value at uniform intervals less than $(2s_{\max})^{-1}$. Thus for a 0.8-cm resolution we need 63 sample points and for a 0.5-cm resolution we need 102 sample points. The resolution pattern is not a simple sine wave, and higher order components constitute the bar pattern frequency spectrum. A resolution greater than 100×100 is required for faithful reproduction of camera images, as shown in Figure 2-3; thus a system limited to 64×64 resolution will lose anatomical information present in the camera. However, this does not mean to imply a loss in quantitative information, as it has been found that a 64×64 resolution is adequate for delineation of cardiac chambers, kidneys, and other regions of the body being studied. This is particularly true for deep-lying organs as the smearing due to scatter limits the obtainable resolution of the scintillation camera; thus a sampling of 64×64 under 10-cm scattering conditions will faithfully represent the data.

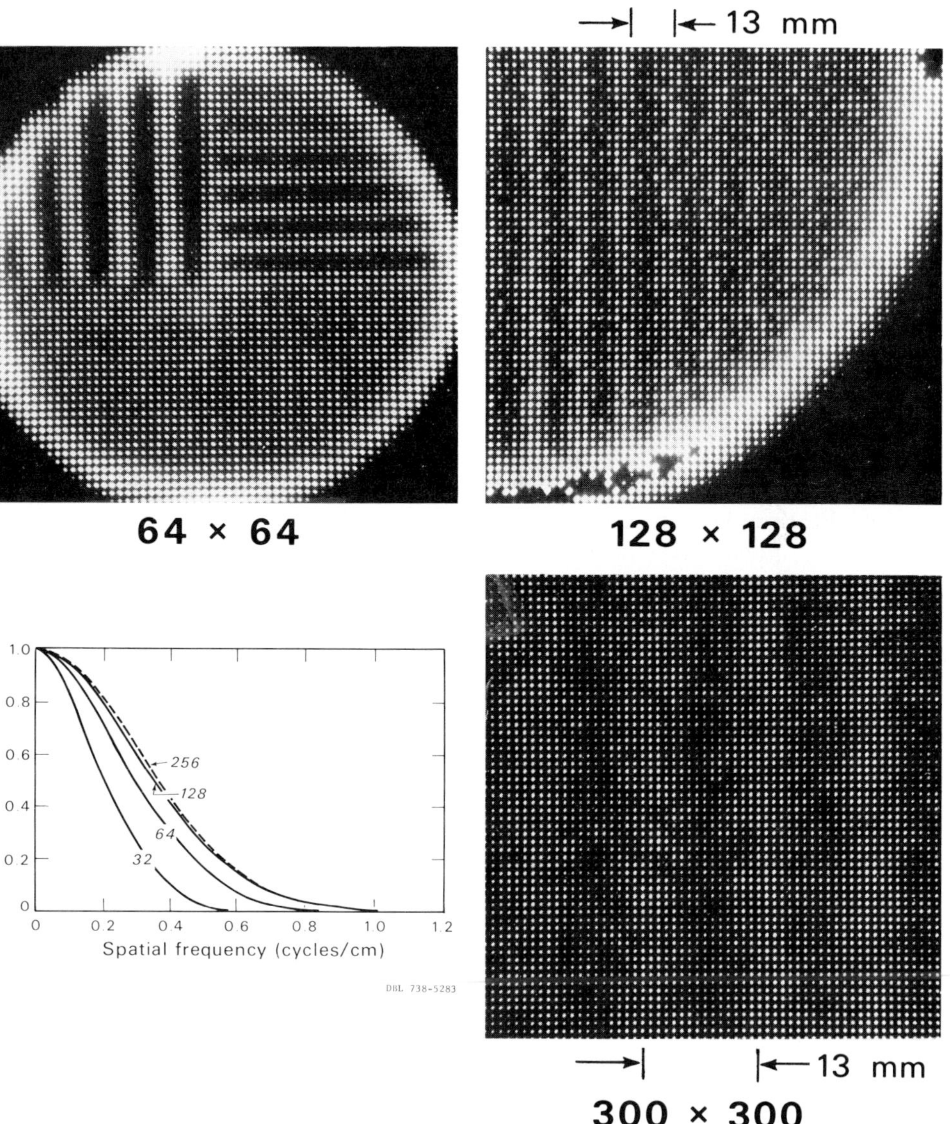

Fig. 2-3.   Illustration of the inadequacy of 64 × 64 resolution digitization. The upper right shows the 128 × 128 resolution for the right lower quadrant of the upper left scintigraph (bars 6.5 mm wide separated by 6.5 mm). The effective resolution of 300 × 300 was obtained by zooming the ADCs to look at part of the crystal. Lower left shows a change in the impulse response measured by Brill and Erickson[34] for line sources digitized at various spatial frequencies.

Data Accumulation and Manipulation Systems

The pioneering efforts of many researchers in the field of digital computers in nuclear medicine have been based on inventiveness in using multichannel analyzers and small computers such as the PDP-8, PDP-12, PDP-15, HP-2116, HP-2100, NOVA, and other minicomputers. From the early work of the Intertechinque Corporation and Nuclear Data Corporation, other commercial computer systems have evolved which acquire, store, and manipulate data in a fashion that is convenient for many research and clinical applications. Most systems can be operated by a technician, and provide the ability to perform the quantitative nuclear medicine procedures discussed in this chapter. A review of some of these systems and discussions of various attributes can be found in articles by Wagner and Natarajan,[208] Budinger,[45] and Silber and Sorenson.[190] The system we are using is shown schematically in Figure 2-4. The major systems now commercially available are offered by Baird-Atomic, Digital Equipment, General Electric, Hewlett-Packard, Medical Data Systems, Nuclear Data, Ohio Nuclear, Picker, Raytheon, and Searle Radiographics (Nuclear Chicago). A major European system is manufactured by the French company Intertechnique.

QUANTITATIVE INFORMATION FROM A SINGLE VIEW

The analysis of the relation between organ isotope concentration and detected projections of the isotope distribution falls naturally into two topics. The first category involves the relationship of the three-dimensional distribution of the emissivity or isotope concentration to the detected two-dimensional projection. This category includes considerations of scattered photons, collimator penetration, camera sensitivity, and inherent spatial resolution of the imaging device. The second topic concerns what types of quantitative information can be gleaned from a single camera view.

Relation between the Object and the Image

Absorption, scattering, the impulse response or spread function of the detector, and information contributed by underlying and overlying tissues result in a smearing of the ideal projection of the organ of interest. In addition, further distortion can occur if there are spatial and temporal nonlinearities of the detector or recording system, as discussed in the preceding section. The scintigraphic process leading to an image can be considered to be the result of a convolution of the detector response with the radionuclide distribution of the object. Thus for a three-dimensional self-

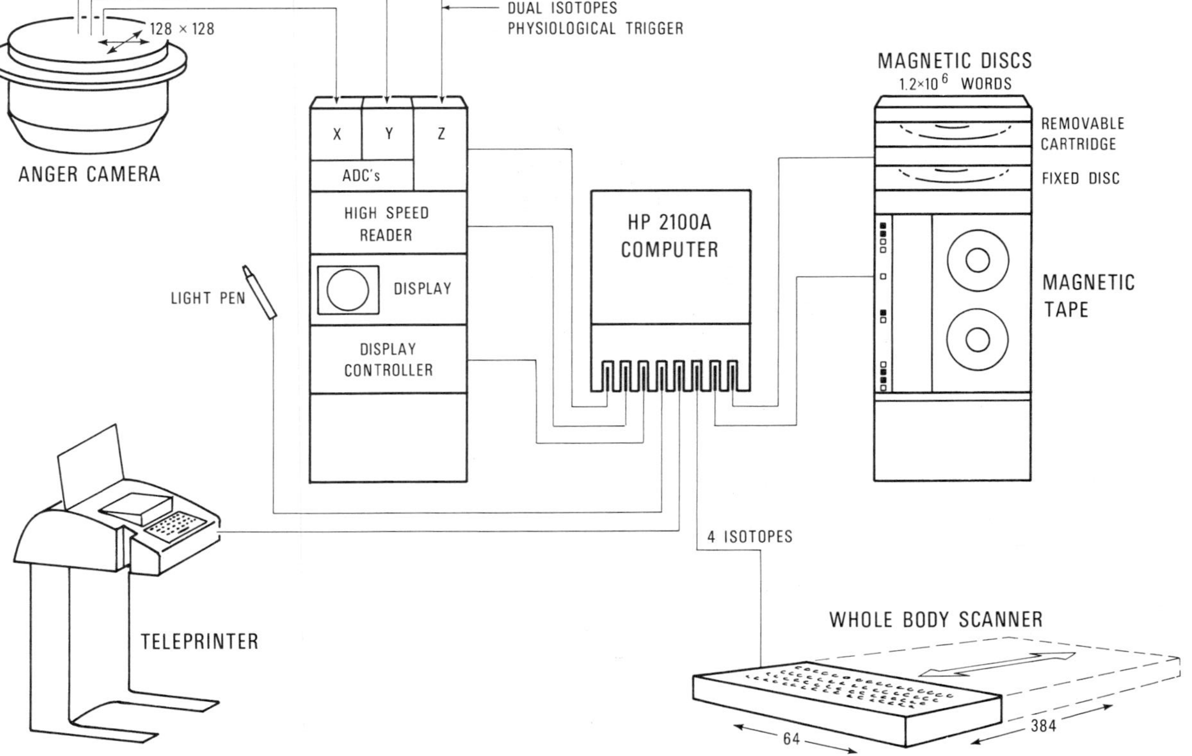

Fig. 2-4. Schematic of the digital system configuration at Donner Laboratory. A second Anger camera is now part of this system. The hardware and most of the software, with the exception of the whole-body scanner, are now commercially available as the Hewlett-Packard HP-5407 system.

radiant distribution of radionuclide atoms, each point in the image is the summation of the contributions of some part of each small object volume modified by the point spread function or impulse response function of the imaging system. The impulse response is invariant over the plane of the detector, but is not invariant with distance from the camera.

This is equivalent to saying that a given impulse response applies only to a particular focal distance. In some situations the "depth of focus" is great and one need find only one impulse response function; thus the image is given in cylindrical coordinates as

$$I(r) = \int \rho(r', z) h(r - r') \, dr' \tag{4}$$

where $\rho(r,z)$ is the isotope distribution and $h(r)$ is the impulse response. Unfortunately the nuclear medicine image is the superposition of the convolutions of many impulse response functions for many distances between the detector and planes in the organ; thus

$$I(r) = \int_{\text{organ}} dz \int \rho(r', z) h(r - r', z) \, dr' + N(r). \tag{5}$$

The last term was added to emphasize the presence of noise. The Fourier convolution theorem suggests a technique whereby the ideal image might be restored if the impulse response is known. Thus the term $\rho(r, z)$ can be deconvoluted from Eq. (4) by

$$\rho(r, z) = \mathcal{F}^{-1}\{\mathcal{F}(\rho(r,z))\} = \mathcal{F}^{-1}\left\{\frac{\mathcal{F}(I)}{\mathcal{F}(h)}\right\}. \tag{6}*$$

However, the presence of both additive and multiplicative noise and the dependence of the transfer function on depth of the organ leave us with a far more difficult task—namely, deconvolution of $\rho(r, z)$ from Eq. (5). Some attempts have been made to improve images using linear filters and Wiener filters,[43,90a,107,118,143,156] and scintigrams with improved visual impact can be seen in the careful work of these authors, who also recognize the fundamental limitations of linear systems theory as applied to nuclear medicine images. It has not been established whether there is any clinical value in this type of processing or, for that matter, other somewhat equivalent smoothing techniques.[129] There is a distinct clinical qualitative advantage of image enhancement through thresholding and contrast enhancement because proper treatment of the image can lead to a visual impact that will

* The symbol $\mathcal{F}$ denotes the Fourier transform operation on some function:

$$\mathcal{F}(f(x)) = \int f(x) \exp\left(-i2\pi x \cdot s\right) dx.$$

make the diagnosis easier to communicate to the nonspecialist, as shown in Figure 2-5, which demonstrates simple smoothing, contrast enhancement, and thresholding as first explored by Bender and Blau[18] and others.[52,95]

The impulse response of a camera system includes the distortions due to scattered radiation in the patient. The pulse amplitude spectra due to scattered and unscattered photons overlap; thus only through special analysis techniques can the true unscattered image information be separated from the observed image.[14,15] The problem of scattered radiation is important to the subject of quantitation from the standpoint of the spatial resolution of quantitative validity and statistical significance of the data. The importance of scattered events in reducing the resolution is shown in Figure 2-6.[15] As the energy discrimination improves, the size of a defect or lesion that can be detected decreases; however, the sensitivity of the camera or statistics of the data decrease, as illustrated by Rollo and Schultz[181] in Figure 2-7. The resolution of the gamma camera at 10 cm distance from the parallel-hole collimator is such that we should expect to quantitate absolute quantities in organs with 1.5 cm resolution.

One can take advantage of an imaging system that has an impulse response, which is a sensitive function of focal distance, by reconstructing the image appropriate to a particular plane. An example of this is laminography or longitudinal tomography discussed in Chapter 5. By taking advantage of the fact of Eq. (5), one can determine the distribution of sources from one view of the gamma camera by minimizing the difference between the digitized image and a set of constructed images each of which is calculated from some guessed-at source distribution. The image of any unit cube in the object space is calculated from the line source response functions measured at different depths in a scattering medium.[81]

The potential for reconstructing planes parallel to the camera from a single view can also be seen for the reconstruction of isotope distribution from a Fresnel hologram.[11,12,180]

It can be shown[48] that the image is related to the Fourier transform of the Fresnel hologram after an appropriate quadratic phase shift. This relationship is

$$I(x, y) = \mathcal{F}\left\{ H(s_x, s_y) \exp\left[\frac{i\pi(s_x^2 + s_y^2)}{r_1^2} \right] \right\} \tag{7}$$

where $H(s_x, s_y)$ is the two-dimensional scintigram of the Fresnel coded image, and r_1 is the radius of the inner ring of the Fresnel zone plate projected on the detector. This is related to the focal distance of the object, f, and the distance between the zone plate and the detector, s, as

$$r_1 = r_0(1 + s/f) \tag{8}$$

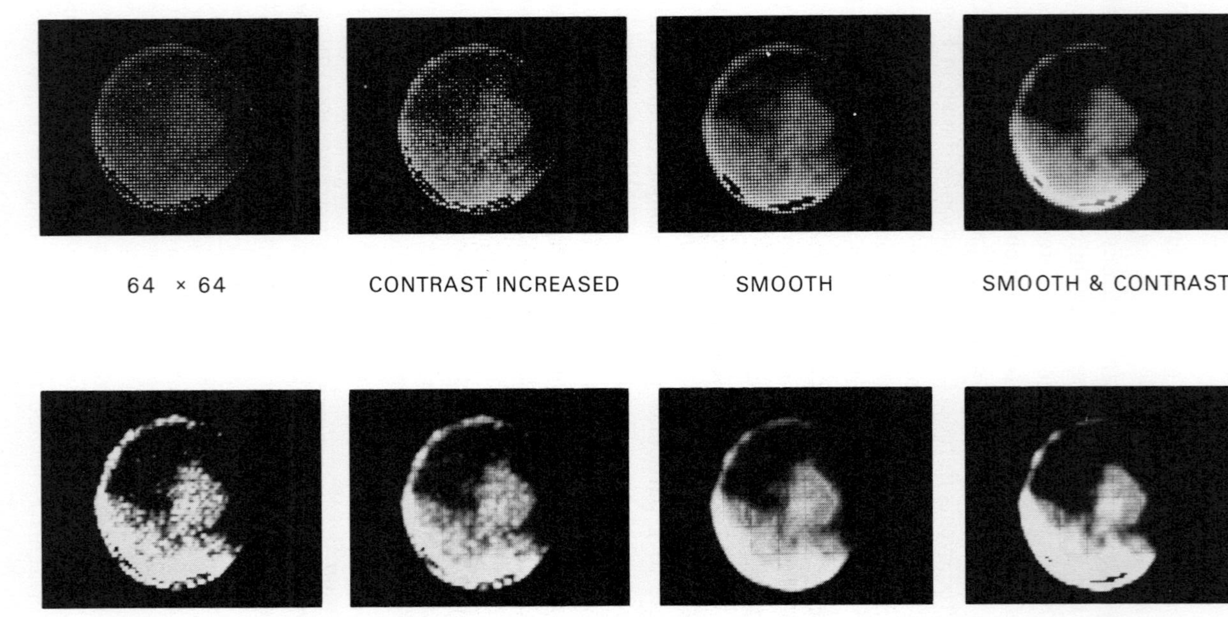

Fig. 2-5. Demonstration of the use of thresholding and contrast enhancement in the presentation of scintigraphs. Upper left is the linear image; lower images show the combination of defocusing, contrast enhancement, and subtraction of background by thresholding using the cathode ray brightness and contrast controls.

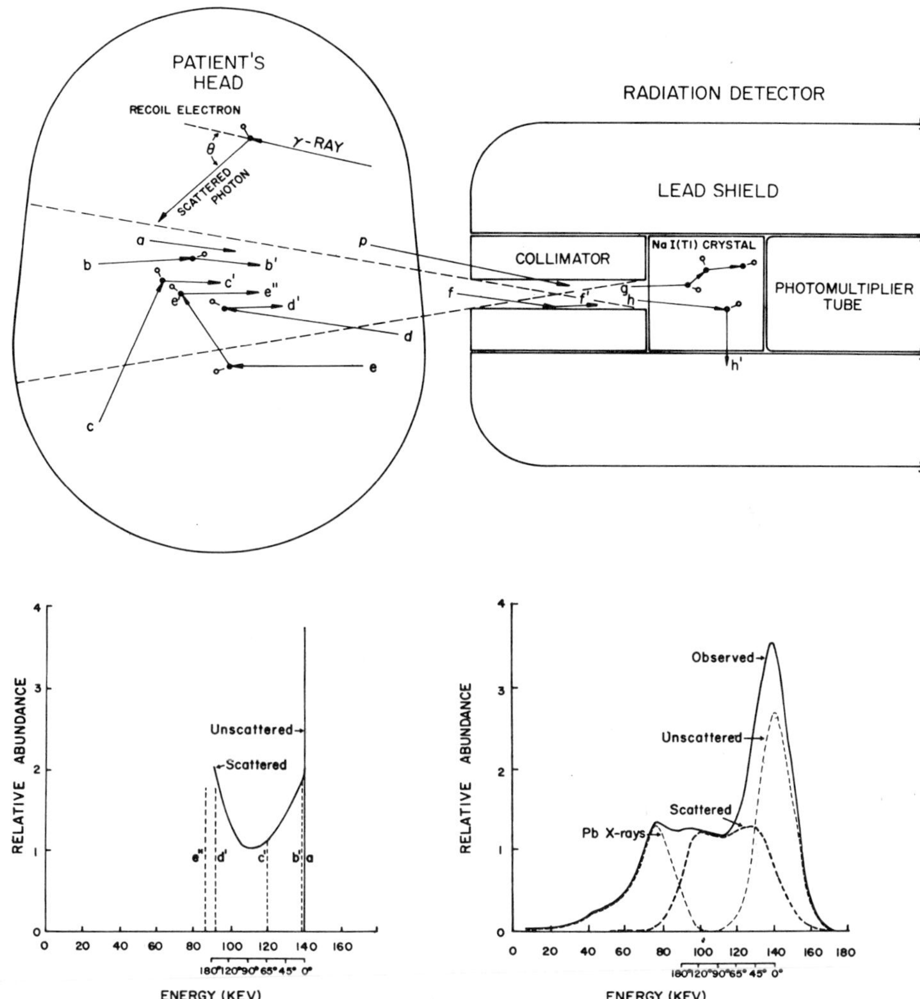

Fig. 2-6. Demonstration of the multiple scattering processes (upper) that result in a serious overlap between the true photopeak events and scattered events detected by the imaging device. Lower left shows the relative abundance of scattered photons for various scattering angles, and demonstrates that photons scattered by as much as 65° might be detected in a window with a baseline of 120 keV for technetium. (From Beck et al.[15])

where r_0 is the actual radius of the zone plate. The digital reconstruction can be done in two ways. The acquired data are placed in a 64×64 frame and the phase shift of Eq. (7) is effected, after which the complex Fourier transform is made on the phase-shifted amplitudes. This is done automatically for different object planes by incrementing r_1 by 1 for each operation. The result is 32 transformed images that represent 32 planes through the

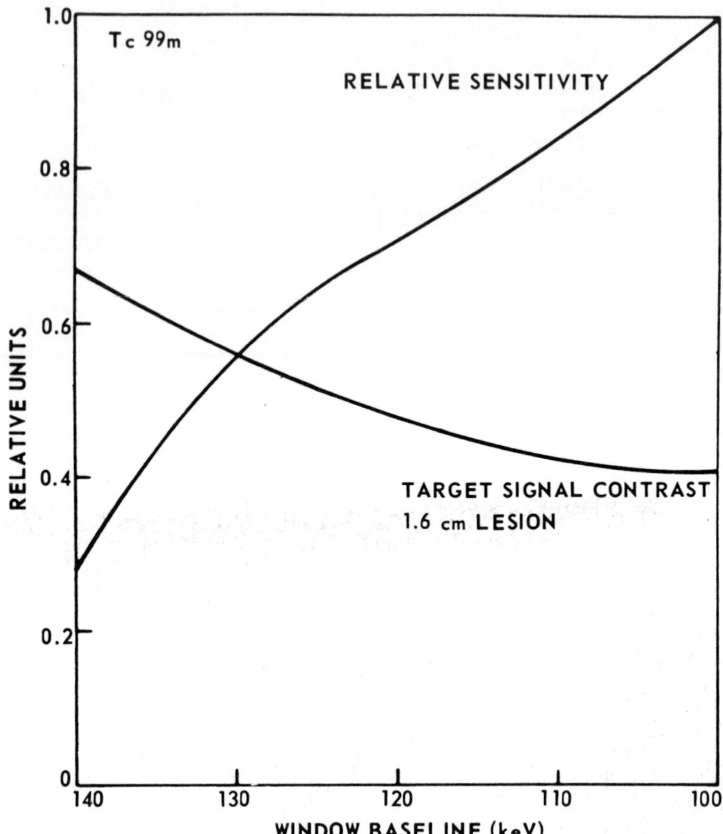

Fig. 2-7.   Demonstration of the cost in sensitivity or statistics occasioned by narrowing the acceptance window for detection of events. (With permission.[181])

object. This operation can be done in a small computer with 12K core such that each plane is reconstructed in 1 min. The alternate technique involves writing the acquired digital frame onto tape and performing the reconstruction on a larger machine where the Fourier transforms are done on arrays up to 1024×1024. These arrays are needed for the high spatial resolution of multiwire chambers. These techniques facilitate a comparison of the pinhole coding to Fresnel zone plate coding for understanding the efficacy of Fresnel zone plate imaging in nuclear medicine.

An example of the reconstruction of two sources at a distance 50 cm from the camera is shown in Figure 2-8. Similar techniques can be applied to multiple pinhole views or other gamma camera lens systems. The presence of noise and artifacts in both the optical and digital reconstruction techniques limit practical quantitative potentials of this approach.

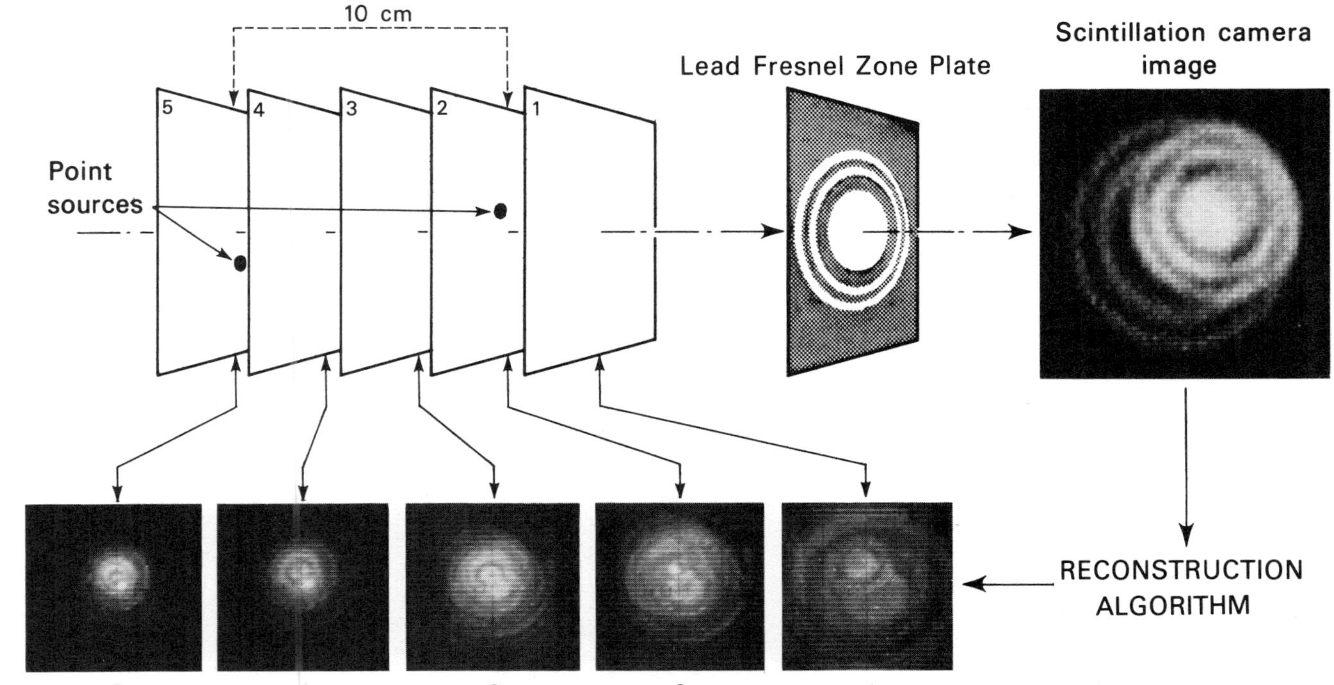

Fig. 2-8.   A demonstration of the ability to perform digital reconstruction of the Fresnel-coded scintigraph using the Anger scintillation camera. A large background has been subtracted from the reconstruction image to present this figure. The data were digitized and transformed at 64 × 64.

Only one camera view is required for conventional techniques of tomography (see Chapter 5). The digital computer can be used to perform nonquantitative three-dimensional imaging such as reconstruction of planes from the Fresnel hologram or simulation of the distribution of activity in the three-dimensional object by taking advantage of the known impulse response dependence on distance from the collimator. Digital tomography is possible using a rectilinear scanner with focusing collimator.[8] Using the scintillation camera with a pinhole collimator, digital reconstruction of object planes in the tomographic sense has been successfully implemented by Dr. Lucien Mathieu (Lyon, France) in collaboration with the author However, when the target-to-nontarget ratio is small, when precise anatomical location is important, and when organ concentration versus background concentration is desired, the problem of quantitation or reconstructing a three-dimensional distribution of isotope requires multiple views.

Relation between the Object and Its Projection

The difference between the detected activity and actual concentration distribution in a portion of the body is dependent on the volume of the organ or cavity, the isotope concentration, the volume of contiguous tissues, and the target-to-nontarget ratios. In Figure 2-9 the actual concentration distribution through a portion of the body containing an organ or tumor of interest is compared to the projection of this distribution as detected by an ideal scintillation camera. If the detector response is ideal, the information in one picture element of the camera is the projection of activity through a portion of the body, which is merely the line integral along a ray normal to the camera (Fig. 2-10):

$$P(r) = \int_k A \, dl + \int_k B \, dl \tag{9}$$

or for digital implementation:

$$P_{k(\theta)} = \sum_{i,j \in k(\theta)} A(i, j) + \sum_{i,j \in k(\theta)} B(i, j) \tag{10}$$

where A is the target tissue and B is the nontarget or interfering background. There is no simple way of recovering $\{A(i, j)\}$ from $P_{k(\theta)}$ using one camera view. In the section on three-dimensional reconstruction from projections we explore the practical solution of this problem by using multiple views and three-dimensional reconstruction techniques.

Thus with all these problems, what quantitative information can be deduced from a single view? There are three categories of quantitative manipulations from one camera or detector plane of view: objective analysis

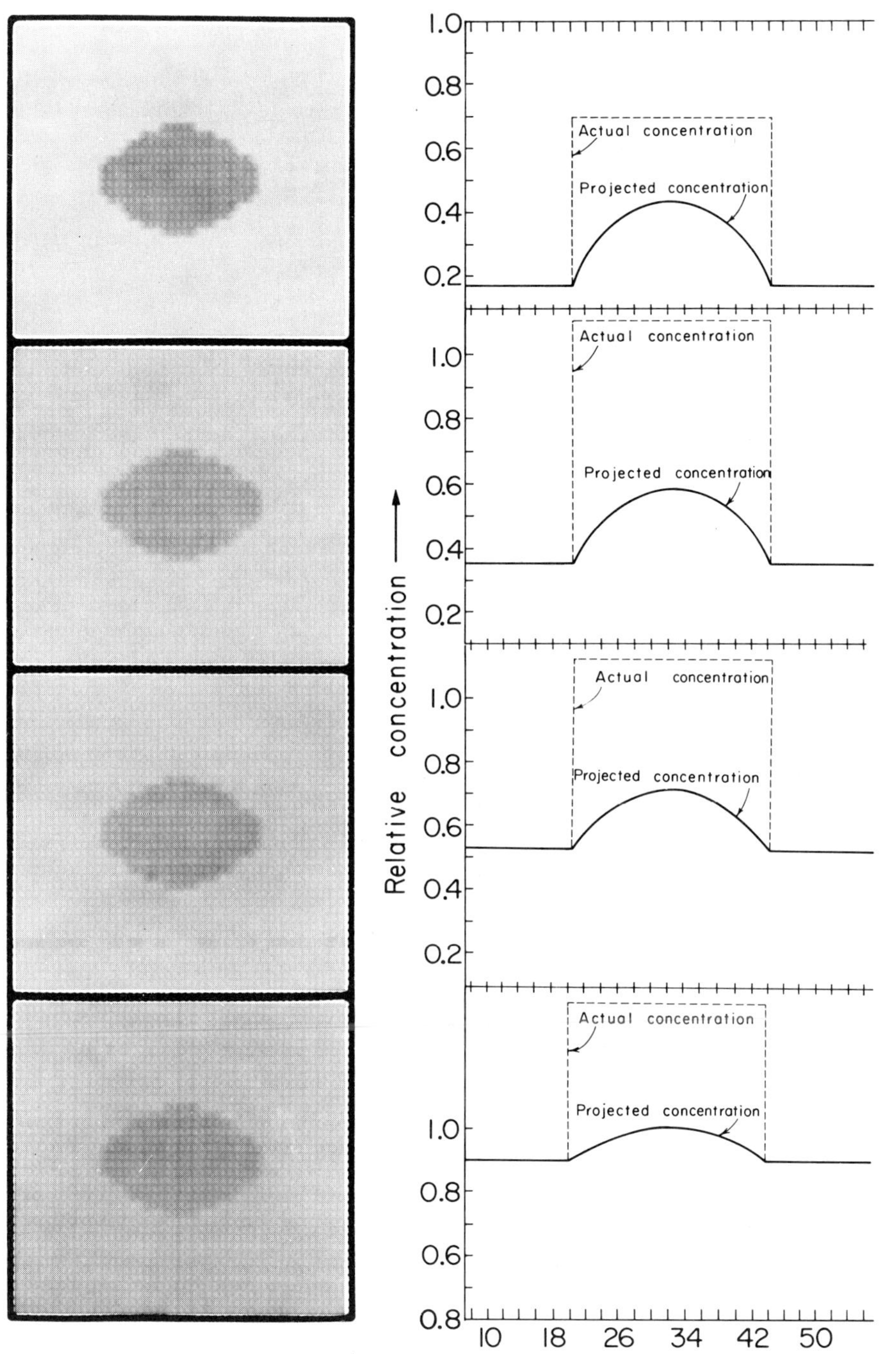

Fig. 2-9. Projected profiles (right) demonstrate the difficulty in ascertaining the actual concentration of isotope in a target, as the target-to-nontarget ratio changes from 8:1 (upper) to 8:6 (lower).

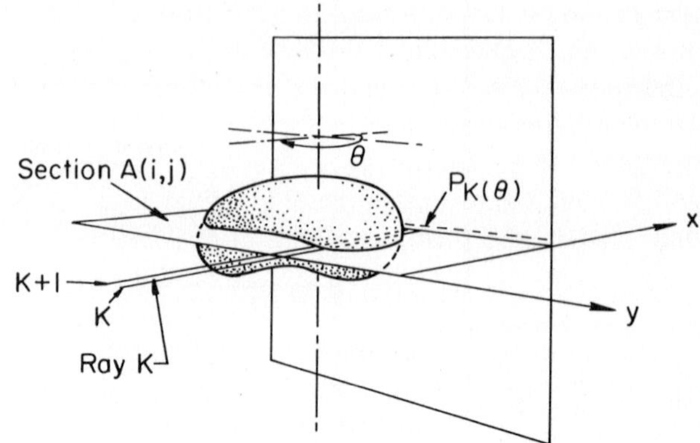

Fig. 2-10.   The projection onto a plane of a two-dimensional slice from a three-dimensional object. The value at each point in the plane $P_{k(\theta)}$ is the line integral along ray k.

of images; presentation of functional or parametric images; and extraction of kinetic information from time–activity curves.

Objective Evaluation of Static Images

The ability to perform objective image analysis and defect versus artifact diagnoses involves quantitative data acquisition, numerical manipulation, and numerical or quantitative displays. The objective of many early uses of numerical or computerized images has been the determination of the statistical significance of an apparent "hole" or "hot spot" on the image.[22,137,201] In fact, the need for quantitative information was a prime motivating influence on the construction of devices that would digitize camera or rectilinear scanner data and print out pictures of numbers or some other means of displaying counts (gray level) using color or isopleths of equal counts (contours).[2] Examples of computer-processed quantitative images are shown in Figure 2-11. Relative quantitation for ascertaining optimum scanning times and quantitative measurements of uptake of bone scanning agents also have a continuing role in nuclear medicine.[90]

If we assume that a lesion can be detected if the counts in the lesion N_t differ from the detected events N_c from the contiguous tissues by 3 standard deviations, then for the Poisson case we require

$$\frac{N_t - N_c}{\sqrt{N_t + N_c}} > 3. \tag{11}$$

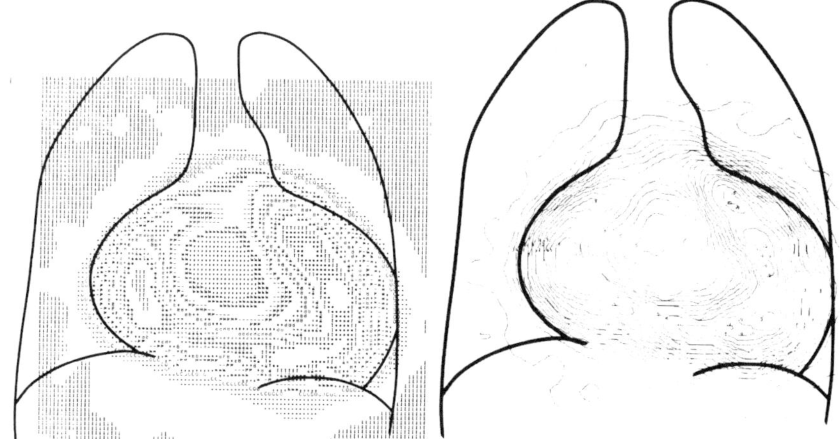

Fig. 2-11. Computer-processed images of scintigraphic data from a study of the distribution of radioiodinated human serum albumin after interpericardial injection in a patient with myxedema. The digitized plot from a high-speed printer is at left, and an isointensity contour plot from an x, y plotter shows quantitatively 20 levels of activity on the right. (With permission.[202])

Using this criterion Benua and co-workers[22] have objectively evaluated static scintigrams for the detection of defects.

Contrast enhancement is easily effected by adjustment of brightness and contrast control on the display CRT (cathode rag tube). This is equivalent to raising the counts in such picture elements to some power (usually ~ 2). This is frequently of value to consider when comparing a flat or linear response scintigraph to one with enhanced contrast (Fig. 2-5). This is not a quantitative technique in the spirit of this chapter, but if enhancement is necessary for communicating diagnostic impressions, then it is of value to have numerical control over the enhancement process.

The Functional or Parametric Image

CLEARANCE RATE IMAGE

The availability of instrumentation for the quantitative acquisition of scintillation events has led to techniques of extracting two-dimensional distributions of functional parameters such as the clearance rate λ, resulting in images depicting relative flow, perfusion, and ventilation, particularly in studies of the lung.[16,49a,108,113,151,159] The clearance image shows the magnitude of the rate constant λ_{ij} for each picture element. One measure of the specific topographic function of any organ is the rate of clearance of some substance, and this rate can be a measure of perfusion or metabolism. As a first approximation flow is derived by multiplying the fractional clearance rate by the amount initially present for a simple washout situation,

$$F = A_{t=0}\lambda. \tag{12}$$

Thus flow can be determined by letting $A_{t=0}$ be the equilibrium count rate of xenon before exhalation. For a somewhat more complicated system, such as the two-compartment model for iodohippurate mixing and excretion, flow in separate regions of the kidney can be depicted as a two-dimensional image where the intensity is proportional to the flow parameter magnitude

$$F = \frac{I\lambda_1\lambda_2}{A\lambda_2 + B\lambda_1}. \tag{13}$$

Here I equals the injected dose, and A and B are the intercepts for the fast component and the slow component of the kidney washout, respectively.[28]

The washout images applied to heart, lungs, and kidneys require calculation of λ_{ij} in many regions of the sequential images. This parameter can be approximated by assuming single exponential kinetics. The determination is made using successive frames collected during a study such as exhalation of xenon gas from the lung. One method is to calculate λ_{ij} for pixel ij by assuming the observed counts $A(t)$ are given by $A_0e^{-\lambda t}$ and fitting $\ln A(t) = \ln A_0 - \lambda t$. Unfortunately this solution employs an improper weighting resulting from treatment of $\ln A(t) = \ln A_0 - \lambda t$ as the linear function $Y = Bx$. In effect we have minimized $\Sigma[\ln A_0 - \lambda t - \ln \bar{A}(t)]^2$.
This gives

$$\lambda_{ij} = \frac{\Sigma t \, \Sigma \ln A(t) - N \, \Sigma t \ln A(t)}{N \, \Sigma t^2 - [\Sigma t]^2} \tag{14}$$

A valid approach that minimizes $\Sigma[A_0e^{-\lambda t} - \bar{A}(t)]^2$ and assumes a weighting by the square root of the observed count value $A(t)$ leads to a solution

$$\lambda = \frac{\Sigma A(t) \, t \, \Sigma[A(t) \times \ln A(t)] - \Sigma tA(t) \ln A(t) \, \Sigma A(t)}{\Sigma A(t) \, \Sigma[t^2 A(t)] - [\Sigma tA(t)]^2}. \tag{15}$$

An alternate technique for computing λ is based on the maximum likelihood principle, and is probably more valid than the foregoing because it applies to the Poisson statistics of the imaging situation. In this case λ is estimated by the ratio of the zeroth moment to the first moment[5]

$$\lambda = \frac{\Sigma A(t)}{\Sigma tA(t)}. \tag{16}$$

The clinical utility of the washout functional image has been explored by Burdine and co-workers[49a] and others cited above. Little work has been done with the kidney primarily because the statistics are very poor for calculating $\{\lambda_{ij}\}$. This will change when ^{123}I-hippuran is readily available (cf. Chapter 3).

TRANSIT-TIME IMAGE

Another useful parameter is the mean transit time, which can be used to create an image of regional flow or perfusion of brain, heart, lungs, kidneys, and liver. The mean transit time, well known for over 70 years,[198] is given as

$$\bar{t} = V/F \tag{17}$$

where F is the flow rate through the system and V is the volume of distribution of the isotope. The simple equation (17), known as the central volume principle, presents problems because the interpretation of the quantities V and F is seldom straightforward. The operational definition of the mean transit time depends on the specific type of experiment performed.[179,218,219] Thus for most external detection situations such as cerebral blood flow (Fig. 2-12) the applicable equation is

$$\bar{t} = \int_0^\infty \frac{A(t)\,dt}{A_0} \tag{18}$$

where A_0 is the total amount of material going through the system under study. Unfortunately it is not possible to perform the integration of Eq. (18) unless a nondiffusible agent is used and there is a means of extrapolating the time–activity curve to zero (Fig. 2-13) in order to overcome the distortion due to recirculation. The usual technique of completing the integration of Eq. (18) is to extrapolate from the point of recirculation to infinity using a single exponential. Thus the area under the recirculation portion B (Fig. 2-13) is given by

$$B = \int_0^\infty A_r(t)e^{-\lambda t}\,dt = A_r(t)/\lambda = A_r \times \text{mean transit time} \tag{19}$$

where $A_r(t)$ is the activity at the point of recirculation and λ is the rate constant determined from earlier portions of the curve. This is a successful technique for the determination of cardiac output (discussed below in the subsection on cardiac output and stroke volume), but of doubtful value in brain, myocardium, and kidney studies because the clearance from these regions does not follow a single exponential. The random walk of tracer through these systems[102] can probably be fit better by the gamma variate function, as noted by Thompson and co-workers[202a] and Starmer and

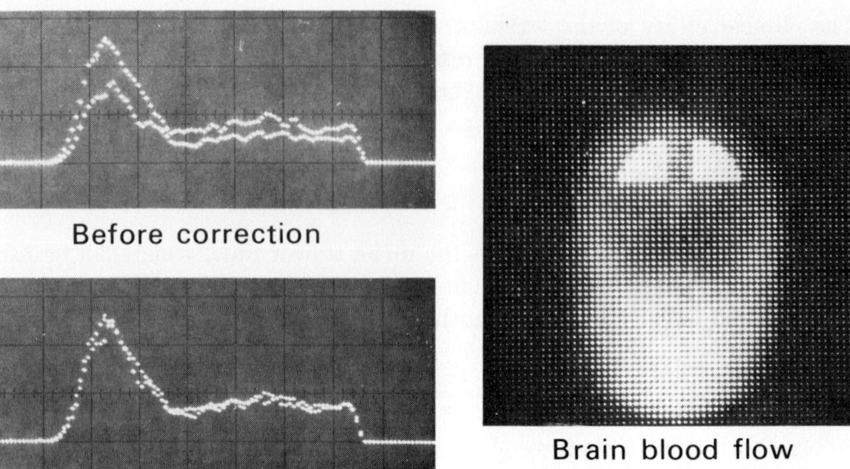

Fig. 2-12. Brain blood flow study after antecubital injection of 15 mCi of technetium-albumin demonstrates the ability to obtain quantitative uptake–washout curves. To obtain $\int A(t)\ dt$, the washout must be extrapolated to the baseline or background. The peak number of counts per 50 picture elements is 300 to 400. The figure also illustrates an artifactual discrepancy between the left and right sides occasioned by a nonuniform sensitivity of scintillation camera.

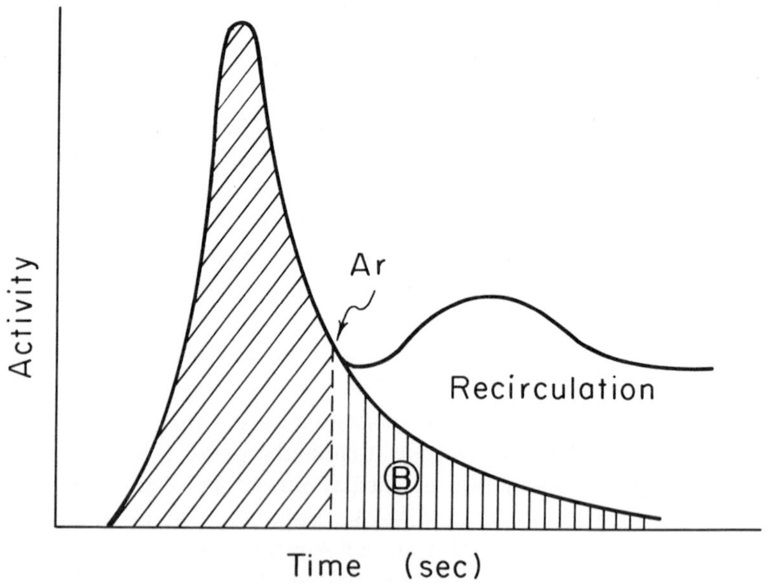

Fig. 2-13. Uptake–washout curves for blood flow studies are quantitated after extrapolation of the washout curve.

Clark.[197] This function allows extrapolation through the terminal portion of the washout curves to be automated more readily than the usual single exponential approach. The function is

$$A(t_i) = k(t_i - t_a)^\alpha \exp\left[-(t_i - t_a)/\beta\right] \tag{20}$$

where k, α, and β are arbitrary parameters and t_a is appearance time. Another general density function[42] which will fit these data well is

$$A(t) = 2\alpha(t - t_a)A(0) \exp\left[-\alpha(t - t_a)^2\right]. \tag{21}$$

A convenient means for exploring these methods of extending and smoothing time–activity curves for subsequent extraction of parameters and even formal deconvolution has just become available in many nuclear medicine laboratories. Halko and co-workers[92] present images of transit-time parameters for kidney studies.

RATE OF UPTAKE IMAGE

Functional images representing regional myocardial perfusion have been presented by Smith and co-workers.[193] The method is an important development from the early work of Love and Burch.[145] The technique is as follows. An intravenous infusion of radionuclide such as ^{42}K, ^{43}K, ^{81}Rb, ^{129}Cs is started and regulated such that a constant blood concentration is present. Using a rectilinear scanner or gamma camera, sequential quantitative images are obtained and for each pixel $A(i, j)$ the rate of uptake is determined by a straight line fit to the activity points. This gives a parameter m for the rate of uptake.

The line $y = mA + b$, fit to the data points of each pixel on successive frames, is extrapolated to give an ordinate intercept that is related to the time of appearance. Using this technique, Smith and co-workers[193] have demonstrated a correlation between perfusion defects, collateral circulation, and nonperfusion situations in dogs and more recently in man. We used this technique with ^{129}Cs in man in 1972, but found no difference between uptake and static images; however, our subjects were found to be normal, and thus no difference should have been expected. Functional images from selective coronary arteriography have recently been described and this technique has been found to be a clinically useful adjunct to contrast coronary arteriography.[191]

GATED IMAGE

Another type of functional image is one in which various states of the organ activity are compared, such as is shown in Figure 2-14. This image was derived from retrospective gating using the following technique. After i.v. injection of ^{99m}Tc-pertechnetate the time–activity curve was ascer-

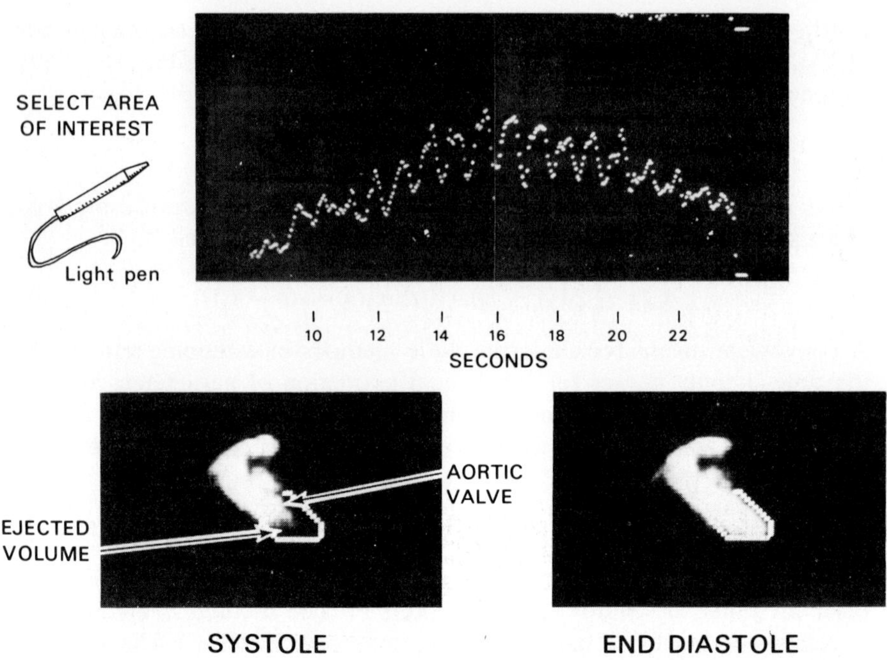

Fig. 2-14.   Demonstration of images reflecting different physiological states (see text for details).

tained by selecting an area of interest over the left ventricle, and obtaining information at 50-msec intervals (upper Fig. 2-14). The first derivative of this time–activity curve was taken, after which the zeros of this function were grouped according to whether the information represented a maximum (end-diastole) or minimum (end-systole). This automatic procedure allows one to delineate the aortic valve and gives an image of end-diastole with adequate statistics for volume calculation as outlined in the section on quantitative cardiac radioangiography. Another method[199,215,216] involves electronic gating of the camera and is also discussed in the section just mentioned.

SUBTRACTED IMAGE AND DUAL ISOTOPE IMAGE

The subtracted image, or ratio image, has been shown to have clinical value in dual isotope studies such as pancreas extraction from ^{75}Se-methionine and ^{99m}Tc-sulfur colloid (Fig. 2-15) or dual isotope studies of the liver and thyroid using technetium and gallium or selenomethionine (e.g., see Blanquet et al,[27] Hundeshagen et al,[102] Desgrez et al,[69] and Hamamoto

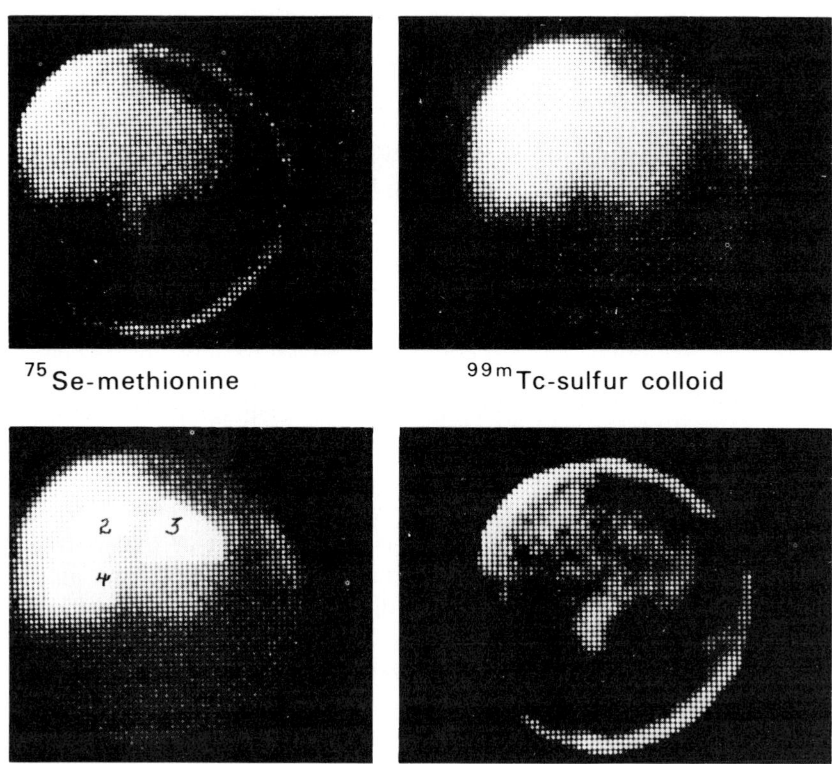

Fig. 2-15. A demonstration of pancreas delineation by subtracting the information obtained from technetium-sulfur colloid study from the two-dimensional data from selenium-75 methionine after normalization. In regions 2, 3, and 4 the variations for the ratio of uptake of sulfur colloid to the ^{75}Se methionine are 10 percent.

et al[93]). Color is a useful technique whereby multiple functions can be delineated in one image, as has been done by the simple insertion of filters between the cathode ray tube of a computer display and Polaroid 180 film.[46,163]

MOTION IMAGING AND MOTION EXTRACTION

The problem of high-resolution isotope distribution imaging in the myocardium and ventricle is complicated by organ motion. For understanding the central circulation dynamics we seek an analysis of motion; however, for static imaging of a moving organ we seek a means of extracting motion. This is particularly the case when imaging the myocardium; thus recent approaches to motion extraction or compensation such as the digital filter approach[186a] or other techniques[160a] are of great importance in the quantitative evaluation of image defects. For example, the paucity of alkali metal (potassium-43, rubidium-81, or cesium-129) in the heart apex, which we have noted in numerous studies, is in the main due to the fact that the apex has a high motion amplitude during the 4 min (^{81}Rb) to 15 min (^{129}Cs) imaging interval. Motion can be removed by gating the camera, or a better technique is to gather information with respect to respiration motion, and heartbeat during the study so that retrospectively the image can be reconstituted using only that information in a specified interval relative to the physiologic marker.

Another technique of analyzing motion, which we have been exploring at Donner Laboratory, involves the calculation of the two-dimensional distribution of Fourier coefficients for the temporal frequency. This approach requires the collection of 32, 64, or 128 sequential frames of spatial activity. The counts for a specific pixel on each conventional frame are extracted to form a time domain function, which is then Fourier transformed (one dimensional) to give the temporal frequency spectrum of that particular spatial point in the patient. This operation is done 4096 times and the result displayed as frames of the spatial distribution of Fourier coefficients. For a cardiac flow study in a patient with a heart rate of 70 sec^{-1}, the frame representing 70 sec^{-1} will show the left ventricle activity. On transmission studies of the heart silhouette, the frame of 70 min^{-1} will show the edge of the beating heart and the frame of 12 min^{-1} will show the movement of the lungs if the respiration rate is 12 min^{-1}.

Time—Activity Curves from Selected Areas

Quantitative nuclear medicine imaging includes the ability to extract from sequential images, curves of concentration or activity versus time. Thus the rapid sequence of isotope flow through the circulatory system can be recorded simultaneously as a series of input–output dilution or metabolic extraction processes from specific regions such as each kidney, bladder, aorta, and background. In brain flow studies distinct uptake–washout curves for the left and right anterior (Fig. 2-12), middle, and posterior cerebral artery distributions can be delineated. The central cardiac circulation has received increasing attention in the past few years; thus aspects of quantitative radioangiography are covered in a separate section later in this chapter. The preceding section discussed the presentation of parameters such as rate constants, transit times, and motion using each picture element or a small cluster of picture elements as the selected area for the description of the flow or metabolic activity using an image to present the data. In many situations where there is not adequate statistical information from the small region of a picture element, there is sufficient information from the entire organ, or a distinct region of an organ such as the cortex of the kidney. By suitable background-subtraction techniques one can overcome some of the problems illustrated in Figure 2-9. By the extraction of data from selected regions using digital techniques and light pen or other means of flagging areas of interest, it is possible to improve upon the techniques of quantitative function study such as thyroid uptake, renography (Fig. 2-16), brain blood flow (Fig. 2-12), and cardiac hemodynamics.

CLEARANCE TECHNIQUES

Glomerular filtration rates and renal effective blood flow have been determined by well-founded methods which rely on measurement of the plasma concentration of some glomerular agent (^{125}I-iodothalamate or ^{99m}Tc-DTPA) or a tubular agent (^{123}I-hippurate), and the amount of activity which appears in the urine. The method of Blaufox, Potchen, and Merrill[28] involves assumption of two compartments and calculation of flow according to Eq. (13). This method is used if urine collections cannot be reliably made. Four or more plasma samples taken over 3 to 4 hr are counted and two exponential components extracted from the plot of these values on semilogarithmic paper. Clearance is calculated from the intercept B of the curve with relatively long half-life T_2 and the intercept A of the curve with the shorter half-life T_1. Equation (13) written in terms of half-lives is

$$C = \frac{\ln 2 \cdot I}{AT_2 + BT_1} \tag{22}$$

where I is the total dose administered. When urine collections are reliable, clearance can be calculated from measuring the amount of isotope in urine and 3 plasma samples taken during an interval between 2 and 4 hr after injection. The formula is

$$C = \frac{\ln 2 \cdot U}{T_2(P_1 - P_2)} \tag{23}$$

where U is the number of counts in the urine collected between times when plasma samples P_1 and P_2 were collected. The half-time of the plasma clearance curve is T_2. Note that the area under the single exponential clearance curve is given as P_1/λ or $T_2P_1/\ln 2$; thus it must be equally valid to calculate renal clearance from the quotient of the activity in the urine, and the area under the plasma clearance curve for the period of collection between times t_1 and t_2 given by

$$\int_{t_1}^{t_2} P(t)\, dt = (P_1 - P_2)/\lambda. \tag{24}$$

Whereas these methods give good clinical evaluations and correlate well with creatinine clearance,[10] they involve multiple venipuncture and urine

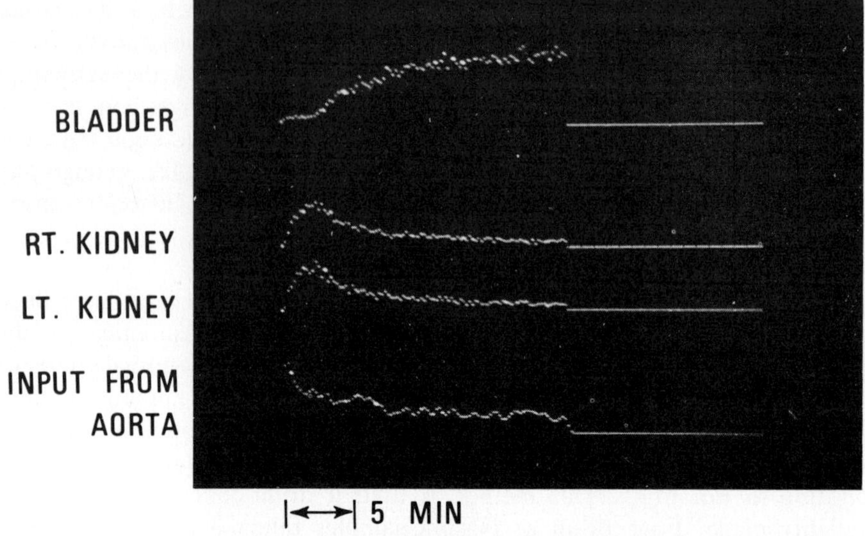

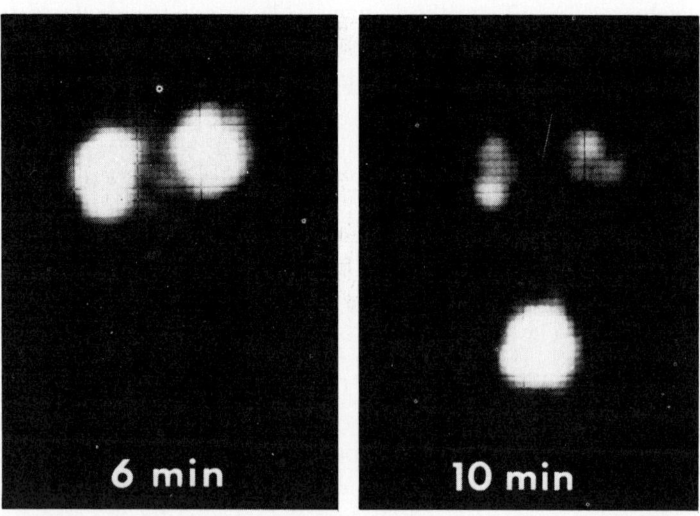

Fig. 2-16. Demonstration of a renal study with iodohippurate wherein areas of interest over the bladder, kidneys, and aorta were extracted after selection of irregular regions of interest. Lower images demonstrate qualitatively the excretion of hippuran from kidneys (upper) into the bladder (right lower). Normal study.

collections. Dual isotope studies using external monitoring by camera rather than blood sampling for input into the equations given above have not been promising, primarily because the "distribution volume" and rate constants seen by the camera include extravascular space.[170] The technique of blood-background subtraction of Britton and Brown[35] has been implemented using selected areas with the camera–computer system, and is now undergoing clinical trials.[65,73,212]

An alternate approach to the analysis of renal function from time–activity curves uses an estimation theory approach that seeks the best estimate of clearance parameters by successive guesses at the parameters for the various compartments.[70,111] A comparison of what the time–activity curves will be under these guesses is made to the observed curves, after which the deviations between the calculated time–activity curves and the observed curves are noted and new parameter estimates are made until the calculated curves agree with the observed curves within some criterion of goodness-of-fit.

In studies of De Grazia and co-workers[64] a multiparameter fit is made to ascertain renal tubular function using hippurate and the results of this program, which utilizes time functions from the kidney, bladder, and precordium, give very good comparisons to the far more costly and morbid retrograde catheterization studies. Our work at Donner Laboratory using a 27-parameter program with a five-compartment model corroborates their approach to this complicated problem of ascertaining tubular function by noninvasive external monitoring using area of interest capability of computer–camera quantitative systems.

FLOW FROM GAS WASHOUT

One of the most extensive analytical uses of the time–activity curves from both cameras and probe detectors has been the determination of flow in myocardial, cerebral, and peripheral muscle tissues.[4,139,182] The principle is as follows. Let the rate of change in amount of radioactive gas such as xenon-133 or krypton-85 be expressed in terms of flow (Fick principle):

$$\frac{dA(t)}{dt} = F(A_a(t) - A_v(t)) \tag{25}$$

where F is flow and A_a and A_v are the arterial and venous activities, respectively. After passage of the injected bolus in, say, the coronary artery, $A_a = 0$ and the venous concentration can be expressed as

$$A_v(t) = \frac{A(t)}{V \cdot f} \tag{26}$$

where A is the organ activity, V is the myocardium volume and f is the partition coefficient[116] between myocardium and blood (about 0.7). Thus Eqs. (25) and (26) give

$$\frac{dA(t)}{dt} = -\frac{A(t) \cdot F}{V \cdot f} \tag{27}$$

which has as its solution

$$A(t) = A_0 e^{-kt} \tag{28}$$

where $k = F/(V \cdot f)$ is the slope of the disappearance curve. The myocardium volume can be expressed as mass over specific gravity, thus flow can be expressed on the basis of 100 gm myocardium by the simple relation

$$F = \frac{100 \cdot f \cdot k}{\text{sp gr}} \; (\text{cc}/100 \text{ gm}). \tag{29}$$

In situations where an injection can be made in the coronary or carotid artery this technique is a valuable clinical measure of relative flow.[182,209] Peripheral muscles can be injected and occlusive disease evaluated effectively by this method.[135]

APPLICATION OF TRANSFER FUNCTION THEORY

Both the Fourier transform and the Laplace transform have important applications to the time–activity curves representing the response of a compartment or organ to some input of radionuclide ion or radiopharmaceutical. Whereas the deconvolution of the ideal image from the detected image using linear systems theory is subject to serious errors due to the variation of the impulse response with distance from the detector, the kinetics of isotope distribution does follow linear systems theory to the point of recirculation or feedback. Recently an adequate theory of handling deconvolution in the presence of multiplicative noise has become available and Fourier transform programs have been implemented on small machines for convenient application of these "black box" techniques.

In principle the extraction of the impulse response is done by calculating the inverse Fourier transform of the ratio of the Fourier transform of the output to the Fourier transform of the input. In theory the response of the system, be it systemic circulation or lung perfusion, is invariant with respect to the input function. Thus, if we have a known input function and a known output, we can determine the transfer function, and therefore the distribution of transit times of the system. This is a practical application of the linear systems theory and can be accomplished if the statistics are good, which is the case for many situations of intercavitary heart hemodynamics. The system response $h(t)$ is the inverse transform of the ratio of the Fourier transform of the output time function (B) to the input time function (A):

$$h(t) = \mathfrak{F}^{-1}\left[\frac{\mathfrak{F}(B)}{\mathfrak{F}(A)}\right] \tag{30}$$

and the mean transit time is simply

$$\bar{t} = \int th(t)\, dt. \tag{31}$$

This is a nice approach to the calculation of mean transit time if there is some measure of the input function and the data are noise free.[38,39,43,51] There are two approaches which take into account noise. We seek a solution which minimizes the mean squared value of the noise.[43] In this case the system response is determined from the cross-power spectrum of the output and the input S_{AB} and the power spectrum of the input

$$h(t) = \frac{S_{AB}}{S_{AA}} = \frac{\mathfrak{F}\{R_{AB}\}}{\mathfrak{F}\{R_{AA}\}} \tag{32}$$

where R_{AB} and R_{AA} are the cross correlation of input and output and the autocorrelation of the input functions, respectively. Solution for the impulse response using Eq. (32) takes about 10 sec using the fast Fourier transform. Another approach has been elaborated by Hunt[104] which also involves calculation of the impulse response in the presence of noisy data using Fourier transform techniques. Neither of these approaches has been applied in other than exploratory fashion for the analysis of the time–activity curves in nuclear medicine, but have great potential combined with techniques of fitting and extending time–activity curves beyond points of recirculation, such as discussed for the gamma variate[197,202a] in the section on the transit time image.

Application of the Laplace transform to determination of heart chamber volumes has been successful in the hands of Ishii and MacIntyre.[109] They use the law of conservation of mass, and model the central circulatory system as a series of vascular compartments interconnected in a cascade fashion with or without time delay. The system is assumed to be stationary and linear with no feedback (valvular regurgitation) and the concentration of isotope $A_i(t)$ in the ith compartment is homogeneous. The total amount of isotope in the ith compartment at time t is thus the difference between the input flowing into that compartment up to time t and the output that leaves the compartment until time t. Thus

$$V_i A_i(t) = F\left[\int_0^t A_{i-1}(t)\, dt - \int_0^t A_i(t)\, dt\right] \tag{33}$$

where V_i is the volume of distribution in the ith vascular compartment. Delay can be introduced easily if there is no dispersion of the tracer between compartments $i - 1$ and i:

$$V_i A_i(t) = F \left[\int_0^t A_{i-1}(t - \tau_i) \, dt - \int_0^t A_i(t) \, dt \right]. \tag{34}$$

Note that in both Eqs. (33) and (34) the identity of mass equals the mass (i.e., vol $\times$ mass/vol = vol/time $\times$ mass/vol $\times$ time). The differential equation corresponding to Eq. (34) is

$$\frac{V_i}{F} \frac{dA_i(t)}{dt} = T_i \frac{dA_i(t)}{dt} = A_{i-1}(t - \tau_i) - A_i(t) \tag{35}$$

where τ_i is the time constant of a first-order lag system. The Laplace transform of Eq. (35) yields

$$\alpha_i(s) = \alpha_{i-1}(s) \left[\frac{\exp \, (-\tau_i s)}{(T_i s + 1)} \right] \tag{36}$$

where the *transfer function* in brackets is the operator on the input $\alpha_{i-1}(s)$ to give the output $\alpha_i(s)$. Ishii and MacIntyre[109] adjust the lag parameter τ_i and then T_i in an analog computer until the measured output $\alpha_i^m(s)$ is fit by the operation on the known input $\alpha_{i-1}(s)$. The input to the superior vena cava is assumed to be a square wave. The lag τ is used only for pulmonary lag, i.e., from the right ventricle to the left atrium. Once τ_i is known, then from the cardiac output (CO) the volume can be calculated from $V_i = \text{CO} \times T_i$ (cf. the section on quantitative cardiac radioangiography).

A more general theory for analysis of a catenary tracer-kinetic system has been presented by Shephard[188] who analyzed the frequency function for transit times in terms of coefficients of a power series of the Laplace transform of the frequency function.

QUANTITATION USING TWO CONJUGATE VIEWS

Quantitative Whole-Body Scanning

Quantitative measures of the changes in the spatial and temporal distribution of isotopes and radiopharmaceuticals through the whole body are vital to the analysis of the metabolic fate of injected or ingested substances as well as to the precise calculations of radiation dose. The problems of precise regional quantitation have been analyzed since 1937 when Robley

Evans successfully estimated the amount of radioactivity in radium dial painters. The following variables are involved:

1. Patient thickness.[74,195]
2. Source thickness and homogeneity.[82,195]
3. Photon attenuation coefficient.
4. Geometry effect.
5. Source position.

For rectilinear scanners and whole-body scanners the geometry effect can be neglected if appropriate collimation is used. The crystal array of 64 detectors in the Mark II whole-body scanner[7] is not collimated by an exact parallel-hole straight bore array; rather each collimator has a focus approximately 11 ft away. If the quantitation is done on an organ region basis rather than an element-by-element basis using both supine and prone scans (conjugate scanning), then the geometry effect should be negligible for most situations. The slight geometry effect was found to be insignificant and has not been included in this analysis.

The Geometric Mean

The rationale for conjugate scanning and estimation of activity from the square root of the product of supine and prone scans versus the sum or average can be seen by comparing the mathematical description of the two situations.

The detected activity from the supine and prone scans can be represented as

$$A^s = A_0 \exp(-\mu x_1), \qquad A^p = A_0 \exp(-\mu x_2) \tag{37}$$

where A^s and A^p are the detected activity from the supine and prone scans and x_1 and x_2 are the respective distances through the patient from the source A_0. The average value is

$$A_{av} = A_0[\exp(-\mu x_1) + \exp(-\mu x_2)]/2 \tag{38}$$

whereas the geometric mean is

$$A_{geo} = \sqrt{A^s A^p} = \sqrt{A_0 A_0} \exp[-\mu/2(x_1 + x_2)]. \tag{39}$$

Since $x_1 + x_2 = T$, the patient thickness, the reconstitution of true activity from observed conjugate scans is a simple matter of inverting Eq. (39). Thus

$$A_0 = C\sqrt{A^s A^p} \exp(+\mu T/2) \tag{40}$$

and is easily effected because μ is known and T can be measured physically or by a transmission attenuation experiment, and C is a calibration factor. Activity calculated from Eq. (38) will be in error by ± 10 percent, whereas Eq. (40) will give less than 3 percent error for tissues 20 to 30 cm thick.

This analysis is incomplete as it assumes a point source or a homogeneous small source. The analysis applicable to any size source or multiple sources through the body region being evaluated is somewhat more complicated, but the implementation of this analysis is as simple as Eq. (40) with a correction coefficient modifying the calibration factor above. This new correction factor is

$$C' = \frac{Ce^{\mu T/2}\,f\mu T/2}{\sinh(f\mu T/2)}. \tag{41}$$

Correction for Source Thickness and Attenuation

Source thickness was taken into account by Genna[82] and source homogeneity was included in the analysis by Sorenson.[195] The analysis applicable to the Donner whole-body scanner starts by assuming that we can measure the body mass thickness at each point T_{ij} in a 64×384 array by scanning the patient under a source of ^{241}Am, ^{99m}Tc, or ^{57}Co. The measured attenuation of photons by the presence of the body gives a good measure of effective body mass thickness:

$$T_{ij} = +\ln(N_{\rm b}/N_{\rm a})\mu^{-1} \tag{42}$$

where $N_{\rm b}$ and $N_{\rm a}$ are the counts before and after the patient is positioned, respectively. A practical and presently acceptable method is to measure the body thickness at 20 points using an outside caliber. The derivation of the absolute concentration is as follows. During a supine scan the isotope emission counts $dA^{\rm s}$ contributed by a small thickness increment dx of the body is related to the activity from that portion of the body as $A_{\rm o}\,dA/T_{ij}f$, where f (>0) is the linear fraction of the body thickness wherein the isotope is distributed. It is also related to the attenuation coefficient and the depth of the increment in the body; thus

$$dA_{ij} = A_{ij}^{0}/fT_{ij}(e^{-\mu x}\,dx)(1/C) \tag{43}$$

where C is a sensitivity and calibration factor. We integrate this over the body thickness to obtain

$$A_{ij}^{\rm s} = \frac{A_{ij}^{0}e^{-\mu m}\,\sinh(f\mu T_{ij}/2)}{f\mu T_{ij}/2}\left(\frac{1}{C}\right) \tag{44}$$

where m is the mean source depth which will cancel when the prone scan is included. [Note: $\sinh z = \frac{1}{2}(e^z - e^{-z})$.] A similar expression is obtained for the prone scan:

$$A_{ij}^{p} = \frac{A_{ij}^{0}\ e^{[-\mu(T-m)]}\ \sinh(f\mu T_{ij}/2)}{f\mu T_{ij}/2}\left(\frac{1}{C}\right).$$

(45)

The activity A_{ij}^{0} is determined from the geometric mean $(A^sA^p)^{1/2}$ as

$$A_{ij}^{0} = \frac{(A_{ij}^{p}A_{ij}^{s})^{1/2}e^{\mu T/2}f\mu T_{ij}/2}{\sinh(f\mu T_{ij}/2)}\ C.$$

(46)

An estimate of $f = \frac{2}{3}$ has been shown by Sorenson[195] to be adequate, and our analysis corroborates his work. The importance of body thickness on the accuracy is reflected in the relationship of the change in correction factor C'/C as body thickness increases (Fig. 2-17). For a given thickness this correction factor will change according to the fraction of body thickness f over which the isotope is considered to be distributed; however, this is shown to be of little importance (Fig. 2-17).

The contribution from attenuation through the body is not accurately given by a constant attentuation coefficient μ; however, for photons above ~ 100 keV we do not expect this to lead to significant errors.

Results of Whole-Body Quantitation

Initial results using Eq. (46) showed we can calculate the amount of activity in a body region with 3 percent precision and ± 10 percent accuracy for ^{99}Tc.

Representative results from calibration trials are shown in Table 2-1 for both ^{99m}Tc and ^{131}I. Sources of different concentrations in different volumes attenuated by various thicknesses of scattering media were used with the whole-body scanner.

The classic work on the quantitative determination of iron kinetics and hemoglobin synthesis in human subjects by Pollycove and Mortimer[169] was limited by the inability to delineate areas of interest (spleen, liver, and bone marrow) though their analysis was quite complete. The advances in equipment and analysis of this section allow the clinician to perform those kinetic analyses conveniently by selecting regions of interest such as spleen, bone marrow, heart, and so on, by light pen. Practical results with patients are in progress for the sequential whole-body quantitation of ^{111}InCl, ^{99m}Tc-pertechnetate, ^{131}I-iodocholesterol, ^{43}K, ^{51}Cr, ^{24}Na, ^{22}Na,

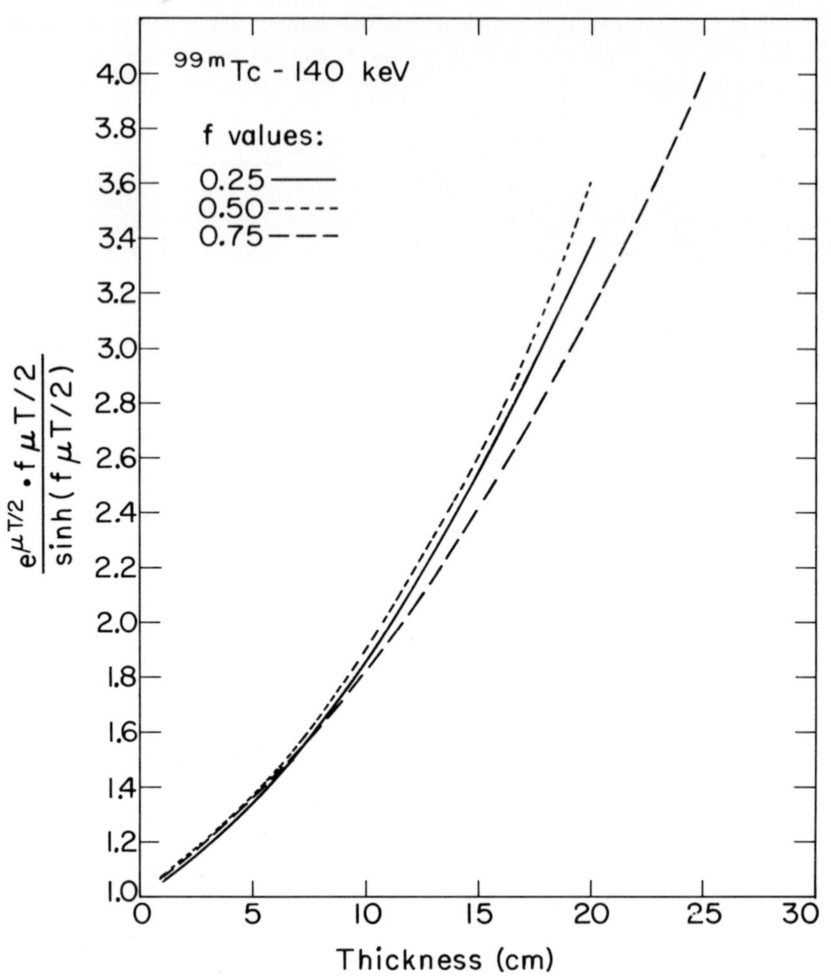

Fig. 2-17. Correction factor applied to the results of the geometric mean of supine and prone scans described as a function of thickness of the patient. The factor is not very sensitive to the fraction of the thickness wherein the isotope is distributed.

[37]Br, [52]Fe, ^{75}Se-selenomethionine, [81]Rb, and other radionuclides and radio-pharmaceuticals. An example of sequential studies extending to nine half-lives for [81]Rb is shown as Figure 2-18 and the sequential distribution of ^{131}I-iodocholesterol over a period of 7 days is shown as Figure 2-19. The quantitative regional distribution for ^{131}I-iodocholesterol is described by Table 2-2 where the fraction of the injected dose for each important body region has been calculated.

Table 2-1
Accuracy of Calculated Activity Using Eq. (1)

Thickness (cm)	True activity	Calculated activity*	Percent error
^{99M}Tc *(Efficiency factor: 3.2 $\times$ 10^{-3})*			
2.0	16.0	15.3	-4.4
7.0	16.0	16.1	$+0.6$
7.0	52.8	54.8	$+3.78$
10.0	52.8	52.8	0.0
12.5	52.8	51.5	-2.46
^{131}I *(Efficiency factor: 7.4 $\times$ 10^{-3})*			
10.3	28	27.5	-1.78
10.3	114	110	-3.5
12.4	28	26.6	-5.0
12.4	114	119	$+4.38$
13.0	36	33.3	-7.5
13.0	81	75.8	-6.41
14.4	28	26.4	-5.7
14.4	114	118	$+3.5$

* Calculated from efficiency factor $\times$ C_t (Fig. 2-2) $\times$ geometric mean.

Organ Function by Whole-Body Clearance Rate

In addition to the direct quantitation discussed above, the whole-body scanner provides a unique opportunity to determine organ clearance of substances which are removed from the blood by only one organ. It is assumed that the rate of excretion or disappearance of a substance is proportional to the concentration of that substance in the plasma:

$$\frac{dA_t(t)}{dt} = \lambda A_p(t) \tag{47}$$

where $-dA_t/dt$ is the rate of whole-body disappearance and $A_p(t)$ is the amount in the plasma. To relate Eq. (47) to clearance rate, we note that $A_p = C_p \times V_p$, where C_p and V_p are, respectively, plasma concentration and plasma volume. Thus the volume clearance rate C_v is

$$C_v(t) = -\left(\frac{dA_t(t)}{dt}\right)\bigg/ C_p(t) \text{ ml/sec.} \tag{48}$$

Thus we can determine the instantaneous extraction rate of a particular organ by measuring the rate of change of the substance in the body and the plasma concentration. The derivative $dA_t(t)/dt$ is an excretion rate

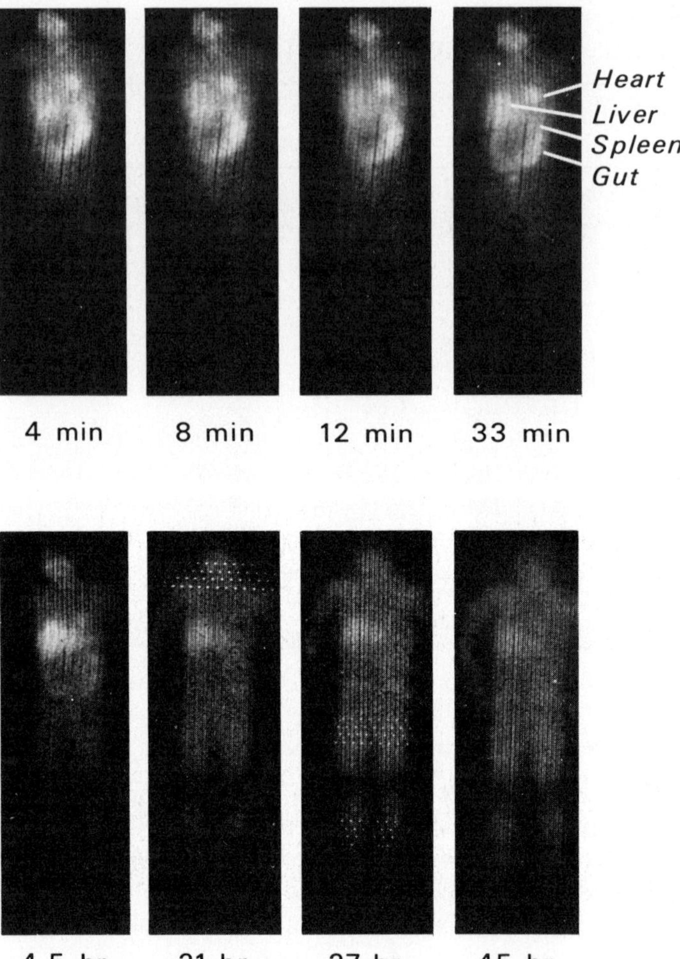

Fig. 2-18. Results of a sequential imaging after 3 mCi injection of rubidium-81 (contaminated with 20 percent rubidium-82m) using the Mark II whole-body scanner. The shift from central circulation to liver and peripheral tissues can now be quantitated with an accuracy of about 10 percent.

from the entire body. Usually the clearance function being evaluated, such as glomerular filtration rate or liver extraction, is estimated by the accumulation into the organ of interest, and not extraction out of the rest of the body. The conventional clearance rate method is limited by the degree to which the extracted material returns to the plasma or moves out of the organ, such as into the tubules in the case of kidneys, and into the biliary tree in the case of the liver. The apparent organ extraction, $+dA_0(t)/dt$, is proportional not only to the clearance but also to the rate of removal

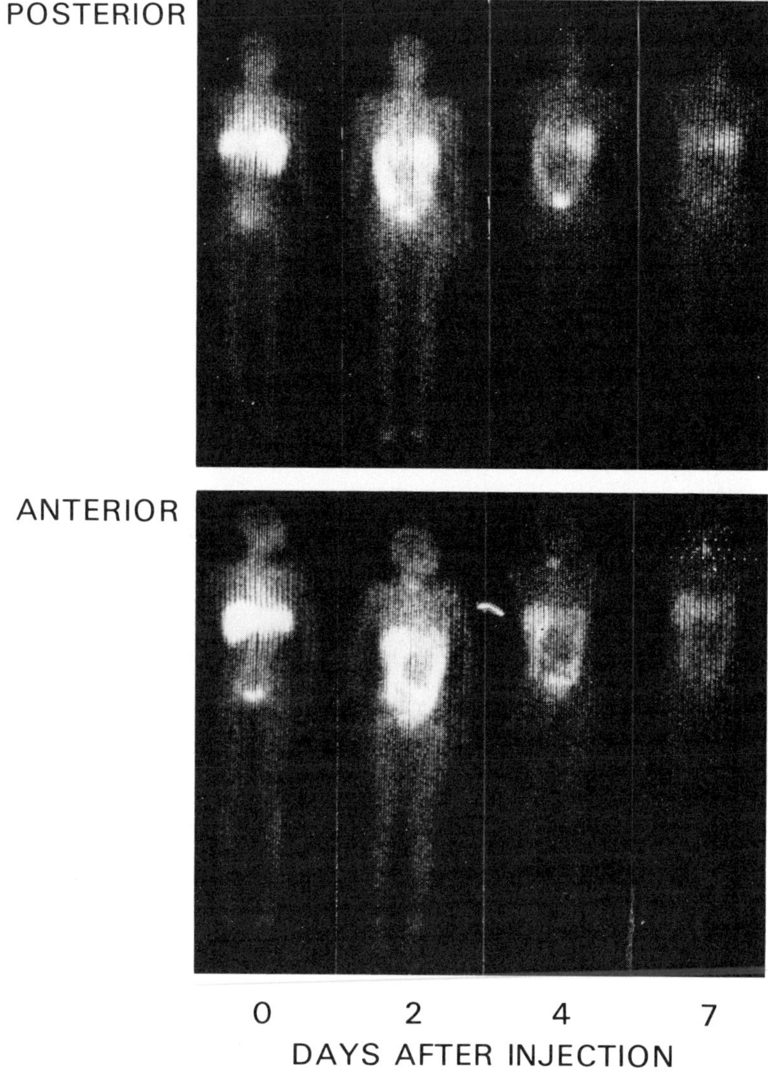

Fig. 2-19. Anterior and posterior whole-body scans show the sequential distribution of a radiopharmaceutical and allow one to extract quantitative data on the fractional distribution of the dose with respect to regions in the body and time (see Table 2-2).

Table 2-2
Percentages of Initial Activity in Body Regions

					Day					
Area/Time	0	1 (19 hr)	2 (47 hr)	4	6	8	11	13	18	22
Skull	0.2	0.22	0.14	0.07	0.05	0.04	0.04	0.02	0.02	—
Brain	1.6	0.87	0.64	0.29	0.17	0.13	0.12	0.12	0.14	—
Face	3.4	2.2	1.3	0.72	0.42	0.34	0.32	0.30	0.22	—
Thyroid	0.9	0.7	0.55	0.36	0.35	0.34	0.28	0.31	0.33	0.43
Chest	16.2	8.2	5.6	3.0	2.2	1.4	1.8	1.32	0.93	0.89
Liver	24.4	12.5	7.1	4.1	2.4	1.4	1.2	1.08	0.74	0.71
Spleen	3.3	2.5	1.7	0.74	0.54	0.32	0.27	0.23	—	—
Gut	24.4	26.5	17.7	8.2	6.3	4.7	4.1	3.50	2.59	—
Bladder	1.7	2.8	2.0	0.69	0.68	0.35	0.27	0.36	0.16	—
Arms	7.8	4.5	2.9	1.7	1.3	1.2	1.0	0.66	0.61	—
Legs	15.9	11.5	6.0	4.0	3.0	2.7	1.9	2.2	1.77	—
Gallbladder	—	2.2	1.2	0.93	0.49	0.31	0.24	0.20	0.12	—

from the organ of interest. Thus, if the relative change in whole-body counts is known, and from this we exclude the contribution from the organ of interest and compartment to which the cleared substance is excreted, we have a simple measure of function insofar as the assumption of Eq. (47) is correct. The whole-body scanner quantitation system allows one to implement these ideas readily because the change in counts over the whole body, exclusive of the organ of interest, can be determined by subtracting the organ contribution using a light pen for removing regional counts. This is an improvement over shielded whole-body counter methods.[160,203]

Organ Exchange Rate Quantitation Using the Whole-Body Scanner

The specific activity of any organ exchanging isotope with the blood pool is related to the uptake by all the other organs and the specific uptake or exchange rate of the organ of interest which we designate as K. If there is one exponential rate of plasma clearance λ, then

$$\lambda = -\frac{dA(t)/dt}{A(t)}. \tag{49}$$

If K is the constant exchange rate between a specific organ and the plasma, then

$$dS/dt = -K(S - A) \tag{50}$$

where S is the organ activity and A is the blood activity. Solving for the specific activity S gives

$$S = \frac{KA_0}{K - \lambda} (e^{-\lambda t} - e^{-KT}). \tag{51}$$

For the realistic situation of multiple compartments exchanging with the blood pool, the plasma curve becomes

$$A(t) = A_1 \exp(-\lambda_1 t) + A_2 \exp(-\lambda_2 t) + \cdots + A_n \exp(-\lambda_n t)$$

and the solution is

$$S = \frac{KA_1}{K - \lambda_1} [\exp(-\lambda_1 t) - e^{-Kt}] + \frac{KA_2}{K - \lambda_2} [\exp(-\lambda_2 t) - e^{-Kt}]$$

$$+ \cdots + \frac{KA_n}{K - \lambda_n} [\exp(-\lambda_n t) - e^{-Kt}]. \tag{52}$$

The exchange rate for a specific organ K_i can thus be determined by the sequential quantitative whole-body scans by solving Eq. (52) numerically. This parameter extraction project has not reached clinical trials as yet.

THREE-DIMENSIONAL RECONSTRUCTION FROM PROJECTIONS

Introduction

An advanced goal in nuclear medicine imaging is the quantitative evaluation of the three-dimensional distribution of radionuclide in the body. There are two general categories of imaging techniques applicable to this tractable problem: tomoscanning, which is an imaging technique similar to x-ray laminography or tomography (cf. Chapter 5); and digital reconstruction of three-dimensional information from two-dimensional projections. The latter category has been variously termed transverse section imaging or scanning, computerized transverse axial tomography, or three-dimensional reconstruction by Fourier or arithmetic methods. This section is an overview of the known techniques for digital computer reconstruction of radionuclide distribution. Results using the gamma camera are given for phantom and patient studies. Sufficient detail is given here for the practical implementation of reconstruction techniques on small computers available to the nuclear medicine clinician and researcher. This and the preceding section are the major contributions of this chapter and constitute new work.[49]

The methods of reconstructing a density distribution from multiple views of an object can be divided into thirteen distinct categories, all of which can be shown to be equivalent under special conditions of transformation. The methods are as follows

1. Direct matrix techniques, generalized inverse and pseudo-inverse[49]
2. Summation, linear superposition, back projection, moiré, or simple transverse section scanning[125,127,205]
3. Algebraic reconstruction technique[88,101]
4. Algebraic reconstruction technique modified for noise
5. Simultaneous iterative reconstruction technique[83]
6. Orthogonal tangent correction[131]
7. Iterative least squares technique[87,49]
8. Summation of compensated projections[49]

9. Summation of filtered back projections, convolution technique[32,49,85,165,174]
10. Geometric mean iterative technique[186]
11. Rho filtered back projection[13,165]
12. Fourier reconstruction[67,76,164]
13. Summation of the projections after Hilbert transform of the derivative of the projection[24,60,85,172]

The problem of three-dimensional reconstruction can be simplified by performing a series of two-dimensional reconstructions from multiple one-dimensional projections, then stacking these sections along the rotation axis of the projection views to reconstitute the three-dimensional object (Fig. 2-20).

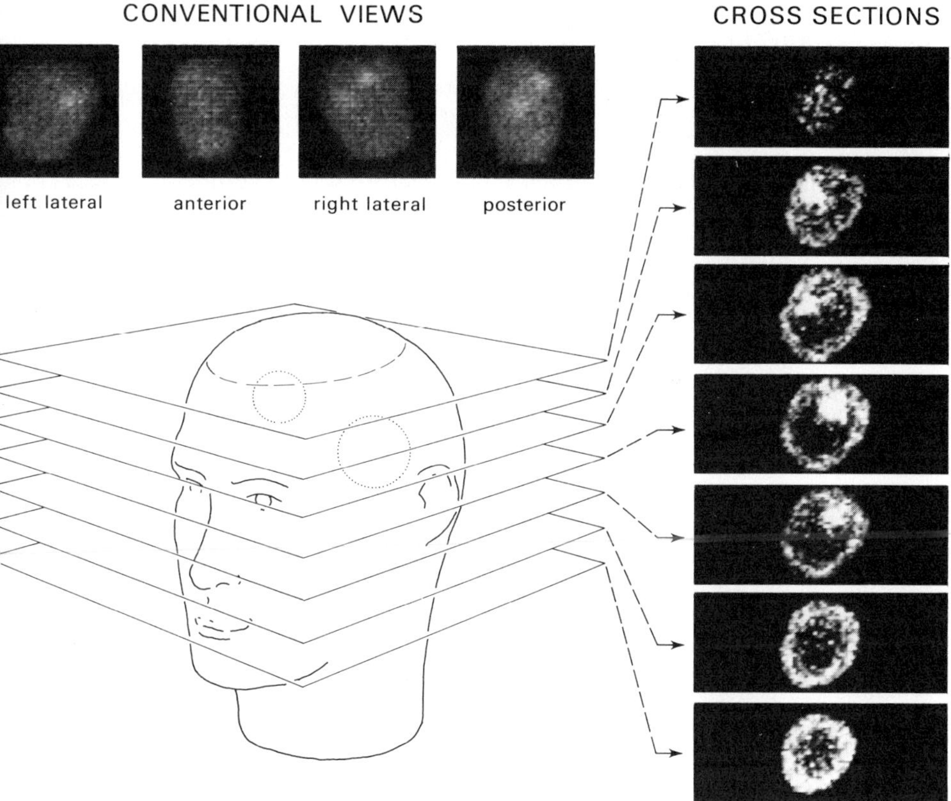

Fig. 2-20. Phantom study demonstrating the ability of least squares reconstruction technique to delineate the position of two hot spots from 18 conjugate views using the scintillation camera. One millicurie was used with a counting period for each view of 15 sec.

Matrix Inversion Techniques

Even today the large computers must toil endlessly and usually unsuccessfully with inversions of the size we are considering. However, the matrix approach should not be quickly discarded as techniques of the generalized inverse or pseudoinverse might some day be implemented to effect a direct solution by matrix multiplication. The problem can be formulated by requiring that an estimate of the set of values in a section $\{A(i,j)\}$ be a minimum to the least squares function

$$\Re(A) = \sum_{\theta} \sum_{k} \frac{(P_{k\theta} - R_{k\theta})^2}{\sigma_{k\theta}^2} \tag{53}$$

where the intensities $A(i,j)$ satisfy the relationship

$$P_{k(\theta)} = \sum_{(i,j)\in k(\theta)} A(i,j) \tag{54}$$

and $\sigma_{k\theta}$ is the standard deviation in the measured projection $P_{k(\theta)}$.* If $\Re$ is minimized, Eq. (53) becomes in matrix form

$$\hat{\mathbf{A}} = (\mathbf{\Psi}^t \mathbf{\Phi}^{-1} \mathbf{\Psi})^{-1} \mathbf{\Psi}^t \mathbf{\Phi}^{-1} \mathbf{P} \tag{55}$$

where $\mathbf{\Phi}^{-1}$ is the inverse of the covariance matrix and $\mathbf{\Psi}$ is an $m \times N^2$ matrix where row (k, θ) is composed of zeros and ones depending on whether the picture element (i, j) falls within a particular ray k (Fig. 2-10). The variable m is the total number of rays for all projections. Unfortunately we are limited in the number of views, and for a given problem the matrix $(\mathbf{\Psi}^T \mathbf{\Phi}^{-1} \mathbf{\Psi})$ is likely to be singular, thus threatening the existence of a solution to Eq. (55). This seemingly intractable problem might find for its solution the generalized inverse $\mathbf{\Psi}^+$ of the matrix $\mathbf{\Psi}$, which in the formulism of Boullion and Odel[30] gives the densities as

$$\hat{\mathbf{A}} = (\mathbf{\Psi}^t \mathbf{\Phi}^{-1} \mathbf{\Psi})^+ (\mathbf{\Psi}^t \mathbf{\Phi}^{-1} \mathbf{P}). \tag{56}$$

Once the generalized inverse has been determined, the estimate $\hat{\mathbf{A}}$ can be made by direct matrix multiplication. The generalized inverse is a function of the geometry of the object (imaging) space, the spatial change of the impulse response in this space, and photon attenuation. Thus in principle for a given imaging situation using projections at fixed but not necessarily equal angles, the generalized inverse matrix can be derived and used for

* The subscript $k(\theta)$ denotes a particular ray that passes through the particular $A(i, j)$'s that fall within the ray path; whereas the subscript $k\theta$ denotes the projection or the ensemble of ray sums belonging to a particular θ.

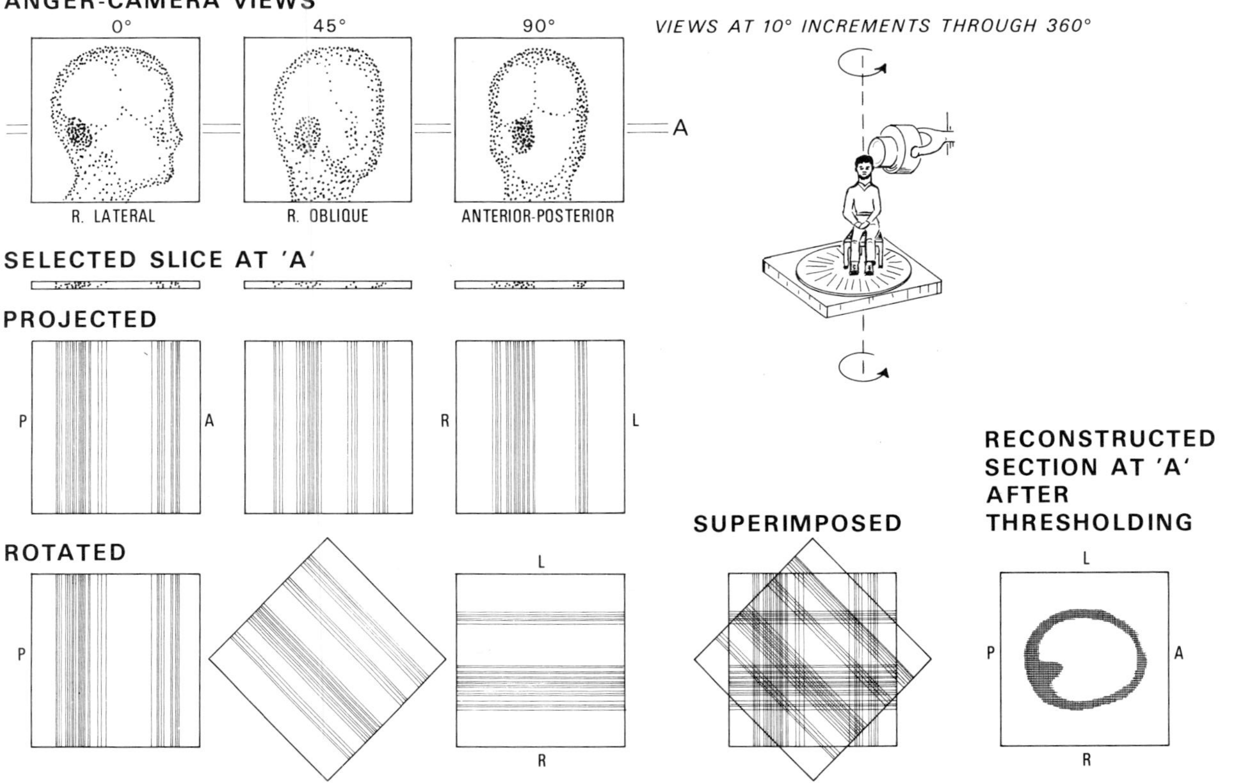

Fig. 2-21. Schematic demonstration of a technique of back projection or superposition from multiple camera or scanner views.

digital or electronic hard-wired multiplication of the projection data as per Eq. (56).

Back Projection or Superposition Technique

The simplest method of reconstructing a two-dimensional object from multiple views is to merely project the views back to a common object region as depicted in Figure 2-21. This technique has been explored extensively in nuclear medicine by Kuhl and Edwards since 1963 under the name "transverse section scanning."[125] Using rectilinear scanners, a profile corresponding to $P_{k\theta}$ in Figure 2-10 would be obtained at multiple angles and the section produced by film exposure summation to reorganize the scan data into a section picture (Fig. 2-22). More recently the Russian crystallographer Vainshtein[205] has explored the virtues of this back-projection technique of translating the one-dimensional function representing the projected density along the direction of the projections in electron microscopy. Though this technique is very simple, it can never give the true radionuclide concentration, but instead the distribution of isotope convoluted with $1/(x^2 + y^2)^{1/2} = 1/r$. This results from the fact that each point

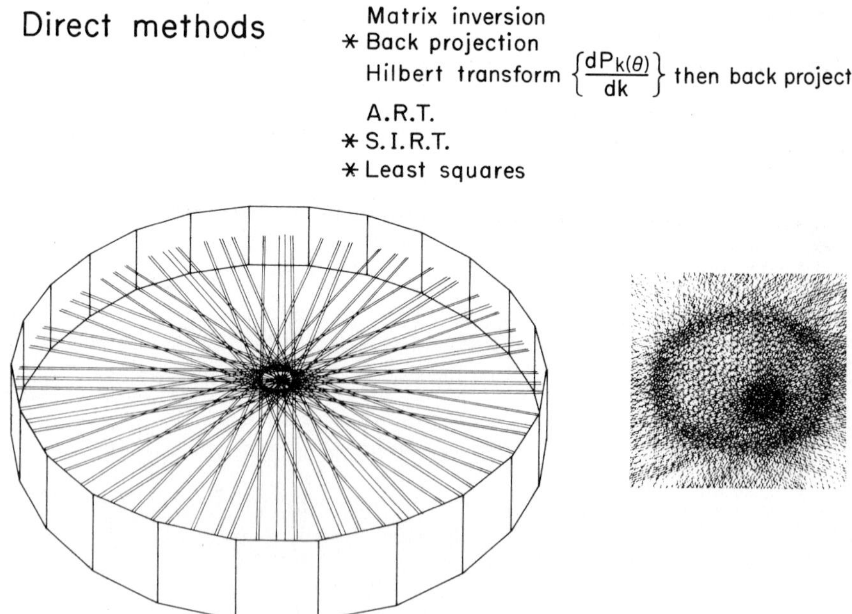

Fig. 2-22.   There are at least five direct methods that involve reconstruction from multiple views. The techniques compared in this chapter are designated by asterisks (*).

in an image reconstructed using back projection will be formed by the superposition of a set of straight lines corresponding to each projected ray from the true object. The superposition of a continuous set of lines around the point is equivalent to the rotation over a circumference of $2\pi r$ for the two-dimensional case and around a sphere of $4\pi r^2$ for the three-dimensional case. Thus, the blurring function is $1/r$ or $1/r^2$ for the two or three dimensional cases, respectively.

RELATIONS BETWEEN RAYS AND PICTURE ELEMENTS

The digital techniques of acquiring data and manipulating projections in order to obtain a two-dimensional reconstruction by any technique require some attention. In fact, a most important practical problem is finding the algorithms for determining the rays $k(\theta)$ which pass through a given picture element (Fig. 2-10), or alternatively, given any ray $k(\theta)$ we need a means of finding all pixels $(i,j) \in k(\theta)$ which intersect the ray. The development of the equations of the lines that define the rays and the distances of pixels from rays is illustrated in Figures 23a, b, and c for the three

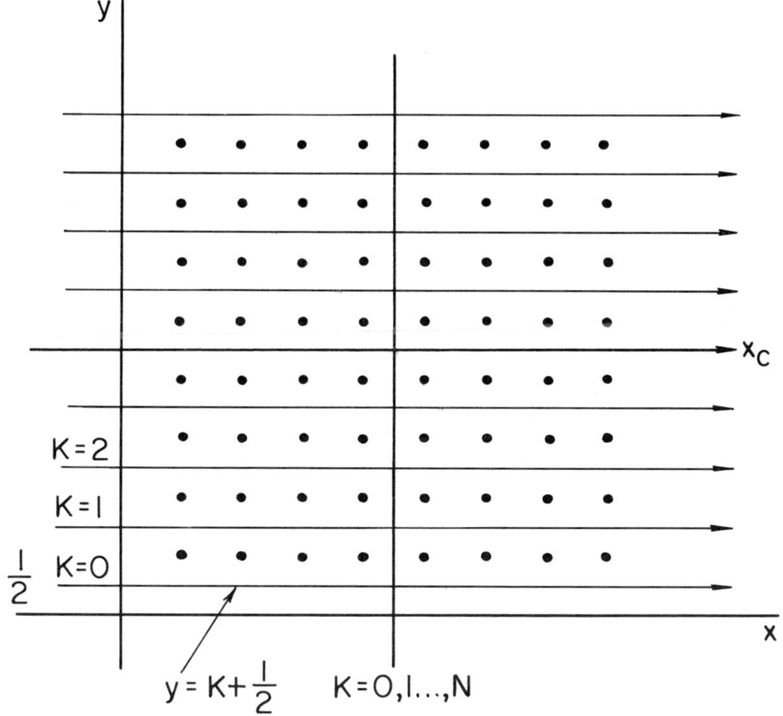

Fig. 2-23a.   The family of lines for the view at $\theta = 0$ or $90°$.

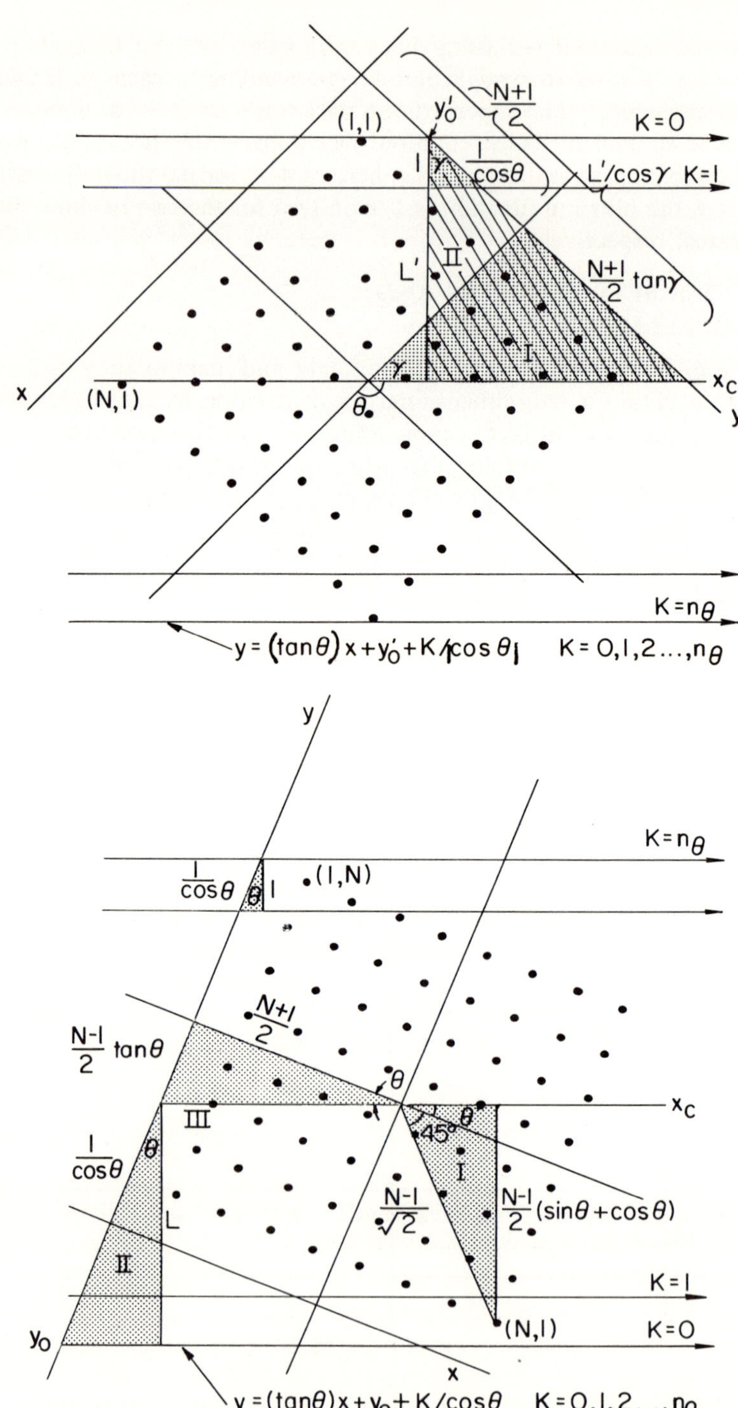

(1,1)
y'_0
N+1 / 2
K=0
1/cosθ
L'/cosγ K=1
L'
II
N+1 / 2 tanγ
x
(N,1)
θ
γ
I
x_c
y
K=n_θ
y = (tanθ)x + y'_0 + K/cosθ| K = 0,1,2...,n_θ
y
K=n_θ
1/cosθ
θ
(1,N)
N+1 / 2
N-1 / 2 tanθ
θ
III
θ
1/cosθ
θ
L
45°
x_c
N-1 / √2
N-1 / 2 (sinθ+cosθ)
I
II
K=1
y_0
(N,1)
K=0
x
y = (tanθ)x + y_0 + K/cosθ   K = 0,1,2...,n_θ

conditions of rotation $\theta = 0$, $\theta > 90°$, and $\theta < 90°$, respectively. The projection of rays passing through the plane remains fixed relative to the detector, while the coordinate system rotates within the field of these fixed rays. This is done so that the formulation corresponds to the actual experiments wherein an object or patient is rotated in front of a fixed camera and thus differs from other formulations (e.g., see Gordon, Bender, and Herman[88]). The practical results of these derivations are placed in convenient terms for the digital computer as follows:

Family of lines (rays)
For angles $\theta = 0°$, $180°$ the family of lines is

$$y = k + \tfrac{1}{2} \qquad k = 0, 1, 2, \ldots, N. \tag{57}$$

For all angles other than integral multiples of $\pi/2$

$$y = x \tan \theta + y_0 + k/|\cos \theta| \qquad k = 0, 1, 2, \ldots, n_\theta.$$

where

$$y_0 = \frac{N+1}{2} - \frac{L}{|\cos \theta|} - \frac{N+1}{2} \tan \theta$$

$$L = \begin{cases} \dfrac{N}{2} + INT\left\{\dfrac{N-1}{2}(|\sin\theta| + |\cos\theta| - 1) + \dfrac{1}{2}\right\} \\ \qquad\qquad\qquad\qquad \text{if } \{\ \} > INT\{\ \} \\[4pt] \dfrac{N}{2} + INT\left\{\dfrac{N-1}{2}(|\sin\theta| + |\cos\theta| - 1) + \dfrac{1}{2}\right\} - 1 \\ \qquad\qquad\qquad\qquad \text{if } \{\ \} = INT\{\ \} \end{cases}$$

$$n_\theta = \begin{cases} N + 2INT\left\{\dfrac{N-1}{2}(|\sin\theta| + |\cos\theta| - 1) + \dfrac{1}{2}\right\} \\ \qquad\qquad\qquad\qquad \text{if } \{\ \} > INT\{\ \} \\[4pt] N + 2INT\left\{\dfrac{N-1}{2}(|\sin\theta| + |\cos\theta| - 1) + \dfrac{1}{2}\right\} - 1 \\ \qquad\qquad\qquad\qquad \text{if } \{\ \} = INT\{\ \} \end{cases} \tag{58}$$

Using these equations, the minimum and maximum values for y or the j coordinates of the pixels that fall within a ray k (between lines k and

---

Figs. 2-23b and c.   Diagrams for the analytical method of determining the family of lines for projections corresponding to rotation greater than $90°$ but less than $180°$ (upper), and for projections between $0°$ and $90°$ (lower). See text for details and equations.

$k + 1)$ are determined for rays from all projection angles. Then between these bounds all the i coordinates are determined by solving the respective equations for x. This gives a set $\{(i, j) | (i, j) \in \text{ray } k(\theta)\}$ where the coordinate pairs belong to the kth ray of projection θ. If a coordinate pair falls on the line k, then the coordinate pair is placed in ray $k + 1$.

For each given projection angle θ, we determine the ray $k(\theta)$ that passes through a particular coordinate pair (i, j) using the following formula for the distance between the pixel represented by the coordinate pair (i, j) and the line $k = 0$:

$$D = \begin{cases} \left| L + \dfrac{(N + 1 - 2i)}{2} \right| |\sin \theta| + \left(\dfrac{2j - N - 1}{2} \right) |\cos \theta| \\ \qquad\qquad\qquad 0 < \theta < 90 \\ \qquad\qquad\qquad 180 < \theta < 270 \quad (59) \\[2em] \left| L' + \dfrac{(2i - N - 1)}{2} \right| |\sin \theta| + \dfrac{(2j - N - 1)}{2} |\cos \theta| \\ \qquad\qquad\qquad 90 < \theta < 180 \\ \qquad\qquad\qquad 270 < \theta < 360 \quad (60) \end{cases}$$

The integer value of $D + 1$ gives the ray number. Thus a one-statement operation for each projection θ will yield the kth ray for a given pixel. In the case of a simple back projection using Eq. (60), the number of calculations is 4096 (64 $\times$ 64 frame) times the number of projections; alternatively, the back-projection summation can be determined by assigning the value $P_{k(\theta)}$ to each pixel through which the ray passes, which means the number of calculations is the product of the number of projections, the 64 rays, and the number of pixels in each ray. The latter method might be more costly in time, because each ray must be bounded by a series of logical computer statements. This formulation does not take into account the fractional area of the pixel through which a ray passes. Incorporation of appropriate weighting factors to account for this problem is not essential if number of rays and fineness of the array are appropriately matched to the data.

Iterative Least Squares Technique

A technique of least squares approximation to the true image from multiple projections was suggested by Goitein[87] and explored by us for the application to nuclear medicine.[49] This method is a valid relaxation method of approximation and perhaps more acceptable from mathematical and statistical viewpoints than the previously tried methods (ART and SIRT) discussed below.

The derivation starts by rewriting Eq. (10) as

$$A^{n+1}(\eta, \xi) = R^n_{k(\theta)} - \sum_{i,j \in \text{ray } k(\theta)} A(i, j)\{1 - \delta(\eta, \xi)\} \tag{61}$$

where $R^n_{k(\theta)}$ is the estimated projected value of the kth ray for projection θ at iteration n and $[1 - \delta(\eta, \xi)]$ is the operator which excludes $A(\eta, \xi)$ from the summation of pixels $[i,j]$ that fall in ray k of projection θ.

The formal procedure is to minimize the difference between $R_{k(\theta)}$ and the observed projection $P_{k(\theta)}$ in a least squares sense, which gives

$$A^{n+1}(i, j) = A^n(i, j) + \left[\sum_\theta P_{k(\theta)} \Big/ \sigma^2_{k(\theta)} - \sum_\theta R^n_{k(\theta)} \Big/ \sigma^2_{k(\theta)}\right] \Big/ \sum_\theta 1 \Big/ \sigma^2_{k(\theta)}. \tag{62}$$

The standard deviation $\sigma_{k(\theta)}$ is chosen to be the square root of the observed data. Thus $\sigma^2_{k(\theta)}$ is just $P_{k(\theta)}$ and Eq. (62) can be rearranged as

$$\Delta A(i, j) = A^{n+1}(i, j) - A^n(i, j) = \left[\sum_\theta\left(1 - \frac{R^n_{k(\theta)}}{P_{k(\theta)}}\right)\right]\Big/ \sum_\theta \frac{1}{P_{k\theta}}. \tag{63}$$

The solution will oscillate at each iteration unless some damping is applied to $\Delta A^{n+1}(i, j)$, and this damping factor is also chosen in a least squares sense. Thus

$$\beta = \frac{\Sigma_\theta \Sigma_k[P_{k\theta} - R^n_{k\theta}][\Sigma_{(i,j) \in \text{ray } k(\theta)} \Delta A^n(i, j)]/P_{k\theta}}{\Sigma_\theta \Sigma_k[\Sigma_{(i,j) \in \text{ray } k(\theta)} \Delta A^n(i, j)]^2/P_{k\theta}}. \tag{64}$$

The new densities after each iteration $n + 1$ are

$$A^{n+1}(i, j) = \max[A^n(i, j) + \beta \Delta A^n(i, j); 0]. \tag{65}$$

An example of the results of this technique is shown for a head phantom with lesions of 2.5 and 4 cm filled with isotope concentration 2 times that of the background in Figure 2-20. A total of 1 mCi was used, and 18 conjugate views of 30-sec duration each were taken before a single gamma camera. A patient study is shown in Figure 2-24 where 18 conjugate views were taken 6 hr after 8 mCi was injected in a 14-year-old girl with a suspected brain lesion. In this case an extended tubular collimator was used to compensate for the distance between the camera and head occasioned by the patient's shoulder. Clinical trials with this technique have just now begun. In terms of accuracy of reconstruction this least squares method is superior to BP, ART, and SIRT as shown for phantom studies in Figures 2-25 and 2-26.

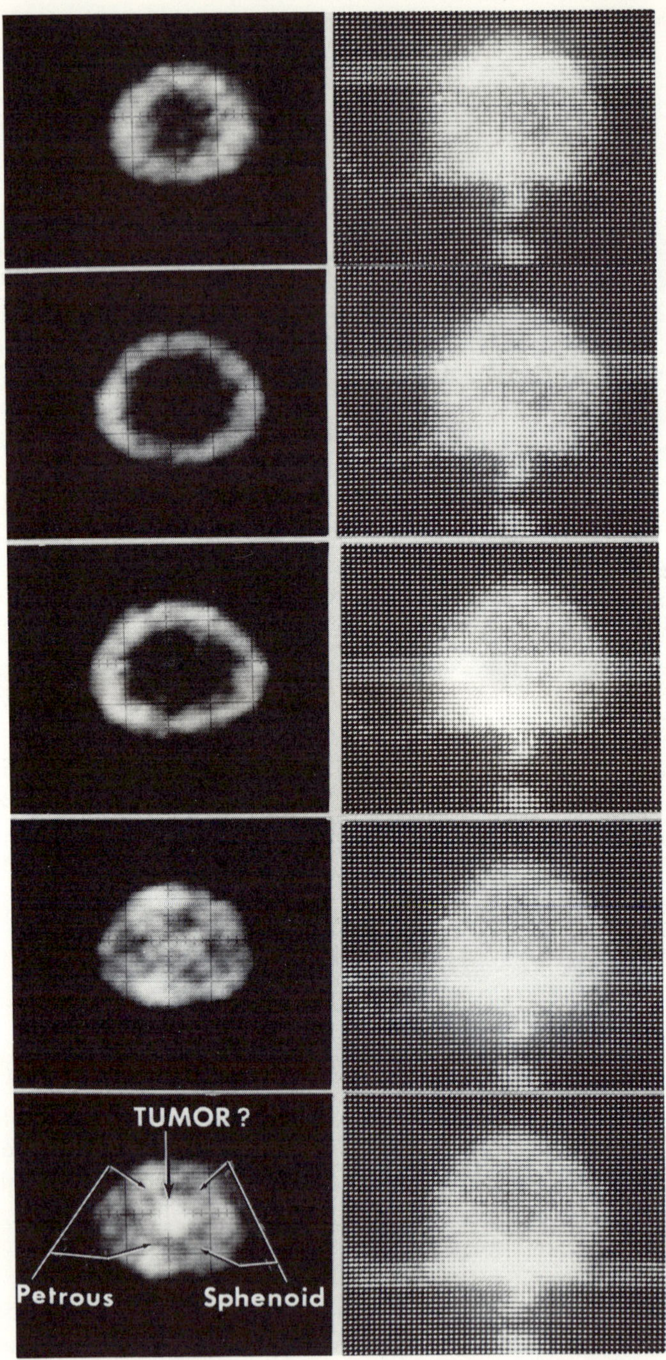

Fig. 2-24. Cross-sectional images produced by the ILST after 18 conjugate views of a 14-year-old patient's head 6 hr after 8 mCi ^{99m}Tc-pertechnetate. Suspected craniopharyngioma.

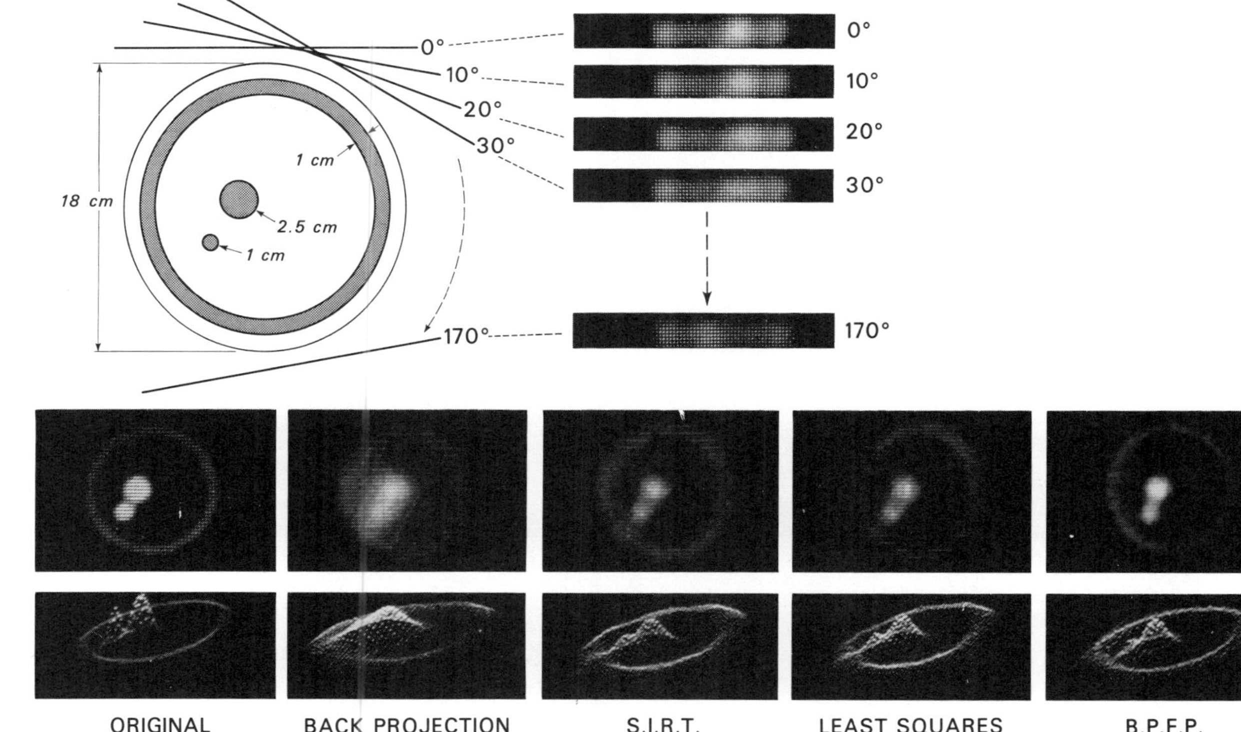

Fig. 2-25. Comparison of three techniques of three-dimensional reconstruction from 18 views taken at 10° increments on a ring phantom that has two hot spots. Note the ability to distinguish the 1-cm lesion, and the superiority of the least squares and SIRT techniques to the back-projection technique.

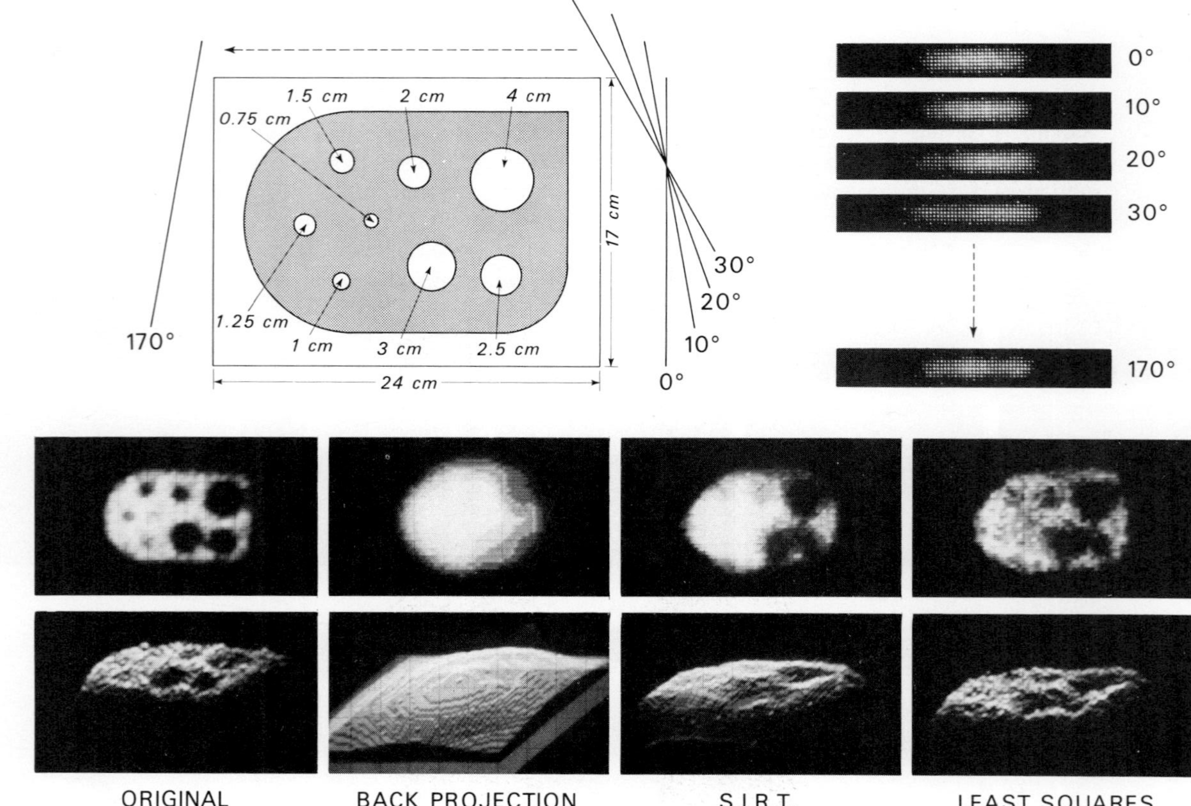

Fig. 2-26. Demonstration of the ability of three-dimensional reconstruction techniques to delineate holes in a liver phantom slice. The superiority of least squares over other techniques for this type of object is demonstrated here.

Other Iterative Techniques

In 1970, 3 years after the Fourier method was applied to strip integration in astrophysics[32] and the Fourier reconstruction technique was introduced by De Rosier and Klug,[67] algebraic reconstruction techniques (ART) called direct methods were introduced by Gordon, Bender, and Herman.[88] The direct technique (ART) was improved upon by Gilbert[83,84] who uses a simultaneous iterative reconstruction technique (SIRT), somewhat but not precisely similar in formulism to the iterative least squares technique discussed above.

Both ART and SIRT are less well fundamentally based than the least squares approach. The geometric mean technique developed independently by Schmidlin[185,186] is somewhat similar to the multiplicative SIRT of Gilbert.[83] The method of orthogonal tangent reconstruction recently proposed by Kuhl and co-workers[130,131] lies between the ART and SIRT procedures.

ART

The basic idea of the method developed by Gordon, Bender, and Herman[88] is the following. Starting with a blank picture, the projected ray values or sums $\{P_{k(\theta)}\}$ of Figure 2-10 are satisfied one after the other by distributing the difference between the desired ray sum and the actual ray sum equally among all the points in the ray. When ray sums of a particular projection are satisfied, however, the process will disturb the ray sums of the previously satisfied projections. The process is repeated and eventually all the projections will be nearly satisfied. Formally this procedure can be represented as

$$A^{n+1}(i, j) = \left(\frac{P_{k\theta}}{R_{k\theta}^n}\right) A^n(i, j). \tag{66}$$

Equation (66) is known as the direct multiplicative method. The direct) additive method is given as

$$A^{n+1}(i, j) = \max[A^n(i, j) + (P_{k(\theta)} - R_{k(\theta)}^n)/N_{k(\theta)}; 0] \tag{67}$$

where $N_{k(\theta)}$ is the number of points on a particular ray. It has been claimed[78] that for an $N \times N$ resolution ART requires approximately N equally spaced projections. This has been experimentally substantiated by Herman.[101] The techniques of ART have been analyzed and defended or debated by Bender, Bellman, and Gordon,[21] Crowther and Klug,[63] Bellman et al,[17] Frieder and Herman,[78] Herman and Rowland,[100] and Herman.[101]

SIRT

The simultaneous iterative technique (SIRT) proposed by Gilbert[83] is similar to ART, except that each iteration is performed by simultaneously evaluating the comparison between the calculated ray sums $R_{k\theta}$ and the measured projections $P_{k\theta}$ for all views. SIRT has two forms, one known as the multiplicative and the other the additive. The additive solution for the calculation of density for iteration $n + 1$ is given as

$$A^{n+1}(i, j) = \max \left[A^n(i, j) + \frac{\Sigma_\theta P_{k(\theta)}}{\Sigma_\theta L_{k(\theta)}} - \frac{\Sigma_\theta R^n_{k(\theta)}}{\Sigma_\theta N_{k(\theta)}}, 0 \right] \qquad (68)$$

where $L_{k(\theta)}$ is the length of the ray $k(\theta)$. The multiplicative SIRT algorithm is

$$A^{n+1}(i, j) = A^n(i, j) \times \left(\frac{\Sigma P_{k(\theta)} \cdot \Sigma N_{k(\theta)}}{\Sigma L_{k(\theta)} \cdot \Sigma R^n_{k(\theta)}} \right). \qquad (69)$$

These summations are over all projection points $P_{k\theta}$ to which the activity $A(i, j)$ contributes. The multiplicative SIRT method is somewhat similar to that proposed independently by Schmidlin,[186] and successfully applied to some nuclear problems. He calculates

$$A^{n+1}(i, j) = A^n(i, j) \times (\Pi(P_{k(\theta)}/R^n_{k(\theta)})^{\gamma-1}) \qquad (70)$$

where γ is the number of rays through $A(i, j)$. Thus on each iteration $A(i, j)$ is modified by the geometric mean of the ratio of the measured ray sums to the calculated ray sums. The technique of quantitative section scanning by Kuhl and co-workers,[130,131] known as the orthogonal tangent correction (OTC), involves using projections from orthogonal views and is an iterative technique analogous to SIRT. The comparison of SIRT after 20 iterations to the least squares technique shows it to be an inferior method for the objects examined (Figs. 2-25 and 2-26); however, it is much faster than the least squares method.

Integral Transform Techniques

Under this general heading one can group the Fourier three-dimensional reconstruction technique (FRT) pioneered by De Rosier and Klug[67] along with other methods that involve convolutions or integral transforms, such as the back projection of filtered projections,[32,173] the Hilbert transform of the first derivative,[24,60,85,172] and the high-pass filter of the back-projection image.[13,83–85] All of these techniques (Fig. 2-27) can be shown

Fourier transform
methods

$\mathscr{F}^{-1}\left\{\mathscr{F}\left(P_{k(\theta)}\right)\right\}$

$\mathscr{F}^{-1}\left\{|\vec{s}|\,\mathscr{F}\left(P_{k(\theta)}\right)\right\}$ then back project

$\mathscr{F}^{-1}\left\{|\vec{s}|\,\mathscr{F}\,(\text{back projection})\right\}$

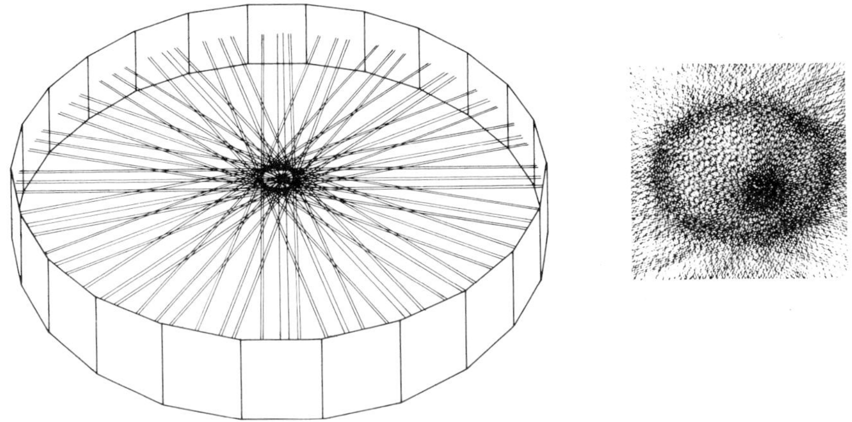

Fig. 2-27. Three reconstruction methods that employ the Fourier transform.

to be equivalent. For an infinite number of projections they will give the same results as the direct matrix inversion technique. Clues to the formal relation of these integral transform or convolution techniques to the least squares method (discussed above) can be found by examination of the relationship between least squares regression analyses and Fourier transform deconvolution techniques.[104] The relation of the integral transform techniques to the back-projection image is of fundamental importance, and is developed below.

DERIVATION OF THE TRUE IMAGE FROM THE BACK-PROJECTION IMAGE

The relationship of the densities in each picture element after back projection to the true densities is

$$B(x, y) = \iint \frac{A(x', y')}{[(x' - x)^2 + (y' - y)^2]^{1/2}}\, dx'\, dy'$$
$$-\infty < [(x - x')^2 + (y - y')^2]^{1/2} < +\infty. \quad (71)$$

Reconstruction techniques can be seen as an attempt to deconvolute $A(x', y')$ from the kernel in Eq. (71). The hope is to find a simple algorithm that will carry the back-projected image elements $[B(x, y)]$ into $[A(x, y)]$. One possibility mentioned in the discussion on matrix inversion techniques involves matrix multiplication by the generalized inverse matrix Eq. (56); however, this procedure has not been adequately implemented. It is possible to convert the back-projected image to the true image by applying a spatial frequency filter to the projected image. We can show[13,49,85] that the Fourier transform of the back-projected image $\{B(x, y)\} = \{B(r, \Phi)\}$ is related to the true image as

$$\mathfrak{F}[B(r, \Phi)] = \frac{1}{s}\, \mathfrak{F}[A(r, \Phi)] \tag{72}$$

where (r, Φ) are the cylindrical coordinates and s is the reciprocal space radius. Thus the true image can be derived from the back-projection image by the inverse transform of Eq. (72):

$$A(r, \Phi) = \mathfrak{F}^{-1}(|\mathbf{s}|\mathfrak{F}[B(r, \Phi)]). \tag{73}$$

An overview of the practical implementation of this technique will serve to clarify this derivation. First multiple views are obtained around some object. Next, the back-projection image is generated by computer, as suggested in Figure 2-27. This gives the array $B(r, \Phi)$. The third step consists of performing a two-dimensional Fourier transform, which gives

$$\mathfrak{F}[B(r, \Phi)] = \frac{1}{|\mathbf{s}|}\, \mathfrak{F}[A(r, \Phi)], \tag{74}$$

which is a complex array corresponding to Fourier coefficients spaced at frequency intervals of $1/2d$ where d is the real space sampling interval. To convert $\{B(r, \Phi)\}$ to $\{A(r, \Phi)\}$ two additional steps are required. The complex array is modified by multiplying each complex value by the frequency measure $|\mathbf{s}| \propto 1/r$ except for the zero-order term, which is left at its real value. Next perform the inverse Fourier transform of the complex array to give the true image.

$$A(r, \Phi) = \mathfrak{F}^{-1}[|\mathbf{s}|\mathfrak{F}\{B(r, \Phi)\}]. \tag{75}$$

Note that this procedure involves a ramplike high-pass filter in that the higher frequencies are amplified more than the low frequencies. This means noise will be amplified unless a cutoff frequency is applied near the point $|s| = N/2a$ where N is the number of samples along a. The cutoff should be rounded or smoothed to avoid ringing.

BACK PROJECTION OF FILTERED PROJECTIONS

This method and the iterative least squares method are the two techniques preferred by us. It involves modifying the projections by a convolution of the observed data with a function that in effect acts as a high-pass filter, and gives a result somewhat analogous to taking the first derivative of the projections before back projection. Recall the relation between the back-projection image and the true image data $A(x', y')$ [Eq. (71)]. Another way of writing Eq. (71) is

$$
\begin{aligned}
B(x, y) &= A(x, y)*\{x^2 + y^2\}^{-1/2} \\
B(r, \Phi) &= A(r, \Phi)*1/r
\end{aligned}
\tag{76}
$$

where $*$ denotes a convolution. The two-dimensional function (r^{-1}) can be considered the point spread function transforming the real data $A(r, \Phi)$ to the back-projection data B.

The Fourier convolution theorem and proper selection of the limits of integration[49] allow us to write

$$
A(r, \Phi) = \text{back projection of } \mathcal{F}^{-1}[|s|\mathcal{F}\{P_{k\theta}\}].
\tag{77}
$$

Reconstruction using Eq. (77) or its equivalent convolution form was first presented by Bracewell and Riddle,[32] and later explored by Ramachandran and Lakshminarayan[173,174] and Gilbert.[85] Peters,[165] Chesler,[55] and Budinger and Gullberg[49] have used this method for reconstruction of images from multiple gamma-camera views. The technique is faster than the least squares or the Fourier reconstruction technique (next section) and provides results similar to our least squares technique; however, this BPFP technique does not have the flexibility of the latter technique for incorporating attentuation and changes in the impulse response with object distance from the collimator.

The procedure for implementation of this method involves four steps. First the observed projections are Fourier transformed using the fast Fourier transform algorithm. This requires a time of 10 msec, 1 sec, or 60 sec, depending on whether the transform is made by a hard-wired system, FORTRAN, or a high level language such as BASIC or FOCAL.[44] Next the resultant spatial frequencies are modified by multiplying each amplitude by the magnitude of the frequency, which in effect is a high-pass filter.

Then the modified spatial frequency vectors are inverted to real space by an inverse Fourier transform, and the results of this operation are used as projections for back projection or superposition.

FOURIER TRANSFORM RECONSTRUCTION

This technique has received wide attention in electron microscopy and astrophysics. The early work of Bracewell,[31] De Rosier and Klug,[67] Tretiak et al,[204] and Crowther et al[62] is based on the Fourier projection theorem, which states that the Fourier transform of a projection of a two-dimensional object gives Fourier coefficients identical to the coefficients along a central radial line through the center of the Fourier transform of the two-dimensional object. This can be extended to three dimensions, in which case the Fourier coefficients of a two-dimensional section are identical to those in a central plane through the three-dimensional Fourier transform of the object and parallel to the projection plane.

This theorem can be proved readily.[76] The Fourier transform of the object $A(x, y, z)$ is

$$F(s_x, s_y, s_z)$$
$$= \iiint A(x, y, z) \exp [i2\pi(x \cdot s_x + y \cdot s_y + z \cdot s_z)] \, dx \, dy \, dz. \quad (78)$$

For $s_z = 0$ we have a central section of F:

$$F(x_x, s_y, 0) = \iint \{\int A(x, y, z) \, dz\} \exp [i2\pi(x \cdot s_x + y \cdot s_y)] \, dx \, dy \quad (79)$$
$$\equiv \iint P(x, y) \exp [i2\pi(x \cdot s_x + y \cdot s_y)] \, dx \, dy$$

$$\text{Q.E.D.}$$

where $P(x, y)$ is merely the projection along z.

We investigated this technique for nuclear medicine applications commencing in 1968. The time required for Fourier transformation of each projection followed by interpolation between known coefficients to fill Fourier space followed by two-dimensional transformation is greater than that needed for what in practice are equivalent integral transform techniques (see the sections on the derivation of the true image from the back-projection image, and the back projection of filtered projections). Application of this technique to medical imaging has been made on a limited basis to phantom studies by Peters et al,[164] Keyes et al,[117] and the group at the Cavendish Laboratory in Cambridge.[203a]

The projection theorem proved above and the properties of resolution, number of views, artifacts, and equivalence of methods are facets of fundamental importance to the science of three-dimensional reconstruction, and these can be analyzed conveniently by Fourier methods.

COMPARISON OF METHODS AND RESOLUTION

A comparison of the iterative least squares technique to SIRT and to the back projection is shown in Figure 2-25 for hot spot detection, and in Figure 2-26 for void detection. The superiority of 10 ILST iterations to 10 or 20 SIRT iterations can be seen in these comparisons. Another criterion of the capabilities of an algorithm is the root-mean-square deviation between the real object and the calculated reconstruction:

$$\frac{[\Sigma\Sigma_{i,j}(A'(i, j) - A^n(i, j))^2]^{1/2}}{[\Sigma\Sigma_{i,j}(A'(i, j) - A^0(i, j))^2]^{1/2}} \tag{80}$$

Here $\{A'(i, j)\}$ is the true object pixels, $\{A^0(i, j)\}$ is the mean and $\{A^n(i, j)\}$ represents the reconstruction. Using this criterion, the least squares technique was compared to the additive SIRT method (no constraints) at each iteration (Fig. 2-28).

If a reconstructed image is to be uniformly resolved to a resolution d of a completely unsymmetrical object, the number of discrete views must be at least

$$n \approx \pi D/d \tag{81}$$

where D is the dimension of the object.[62,120] Thus for a resolution of 1.5 cm in imaging a head 20 cm in diameter, we need 42 views. In practice less than 20 views are necessary for the class of objects of importance to nuclear medicine. An explanation for this discrepancy is that 42 projections would be required for an object that has no symmetry, and thus no regional correlation. Of course this is not true for an image, as there is great departure from complete randomness just in the fact that a recognizable image exists. Thus it is not surprising to find that the number of views required for reconstructing a two-dimensional distribution with a resolution distance of 1.5 cm is far less than the theoretical number for images of no symmetry. Another way of understanding the reason for the discrepancy is that in the class of objects of concern many different objects are essentially identical. The resolution and, to a great extent, appearance of artifacts are related to how close the axis of rotation is to a center of symmetry. For example, multiple views of a right cylinder taken around an axis that is displaced from the center of rotation will give a reconstruction that is distorted and contains "clutter" outside the object region.[165] Only a single view of the same right cylinder is necessary if the cylinder center is in the center of rotation for the reconstruction. However, no a priori assumption can be made regarding the topology of a cross section.

Whereas, the iterative least squares technique gives good resolution without artifacts, the techniques of back projection of filtered or compen-

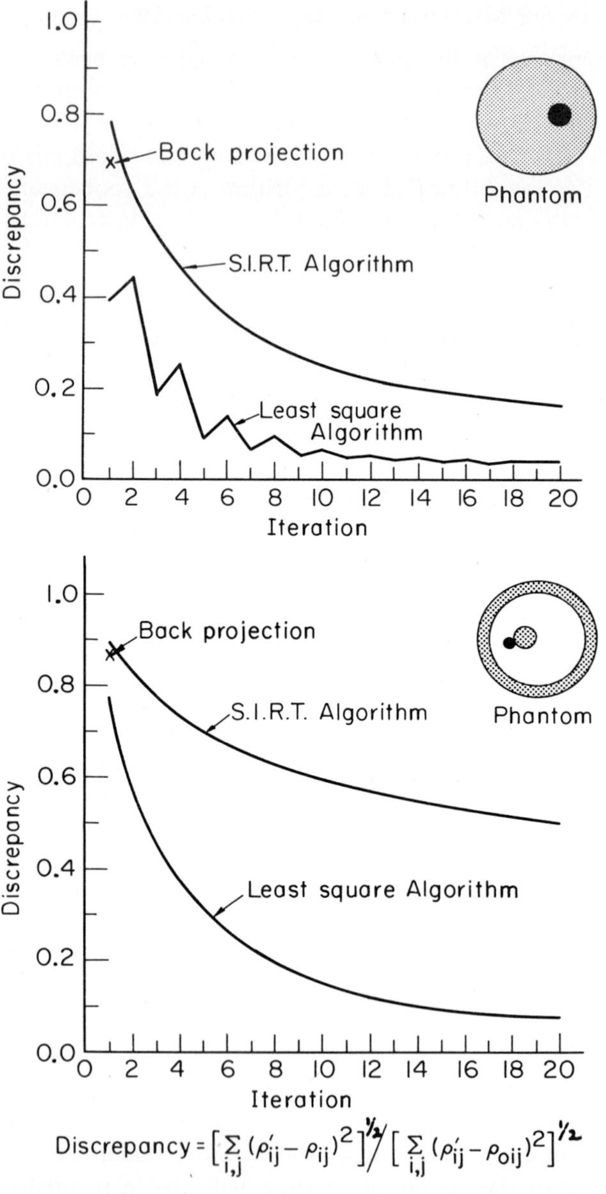

$$\text{Discrepancy} = \left[\sum_{i,j} (\rho'_{ij} - \rho_{ij})^2 \right]^{1/2} \Big/ \left[\sum_{i,j} (\rho'_{ij} - \rho_{oij})^2 \right]^{1/2}$$

Fig. 2-28. A comparison of the SIRT to the least squares algorithm for two objects. The deviation between the true object and the reconstructed object is less for the least squares algorithm than the SIRT algorithm. The least squares technique takes 20 min per plane on a small computer (HP-2100A).

sated projections are about 80 times faster. These latter techniques do not handle non-additive noise or attenuation, thus the least squares technique modified for photon attenuation[49] is the preferred quantitative technique for the gamma camera. Sections of 48×48 for 36 views are calculated in 25 minutes by the nuclear medicine computer system HP-5407[46] and in a few seconds by the CDC 6600 and CDC 7600. We have perfected a system of rapidly translating tape formats into and out of the CDC format so that the ultimate display and analysis of data can be done using the superior graphics of the smaller HP-5407 system.

Our results are similar to those of Kuhl and co-workers[125,127,128,130,131] who have pioneered in this work. The techniques differ in the mathematics of coping with noise and attenuation and the fact that we use the scintillation camera rather than the rectilinear scanner. Clinical trials have just now begun, but clearly show these techniques to be important advances in quantitative nuclear medicine. The mathematical algorithm is superior to that used for the EMI scanner (ART) and can be applied to transmission imaging as well as emission imaging.

QUANTITATIVE CARDIAC RADIOANGIOGRAPHY

Previous Qualitative Work

The qualitative assessment of radioangiograms in infants and adults is a very effective and useful adjunct to diagnosis of congenital and acquired hemodynamic defects that reflect heart pathology. The careful delineation of the time sequence of two-dimensional images by Kriss and co-workers (e.g., see Kriss and Matin,[121] Matin and Kriss,[154] and Wesselhoeft et al[211]) can lead to exact diagnoses without the attendant discomfort and morbidity of cardiac catheterization. This technique, which involves collection of the data from a flow study and examination of the time sequence of radionuclide movement through the heart chambers and outflow tract, has been used successfully by Wesselhoeft and co-workers[211] using the pinhole collimator to magnify the images from very small infants (see also Kriss et al[123] and Hurley et al[105]). An example of results from Kriss and co-workers is shown in Figure 2-29a, and a demonstration of the potential for noninvasive congenital heart disease diagnosis in premature infants[105,211] is shown in Figure 2-29b. The information comprising the images of Figure 2-29 can be used to glean precise quantitative measures about cardiac performance that in fact yield all the data now derived from right and left heart catheterization with the exception of blood gases and pressures.

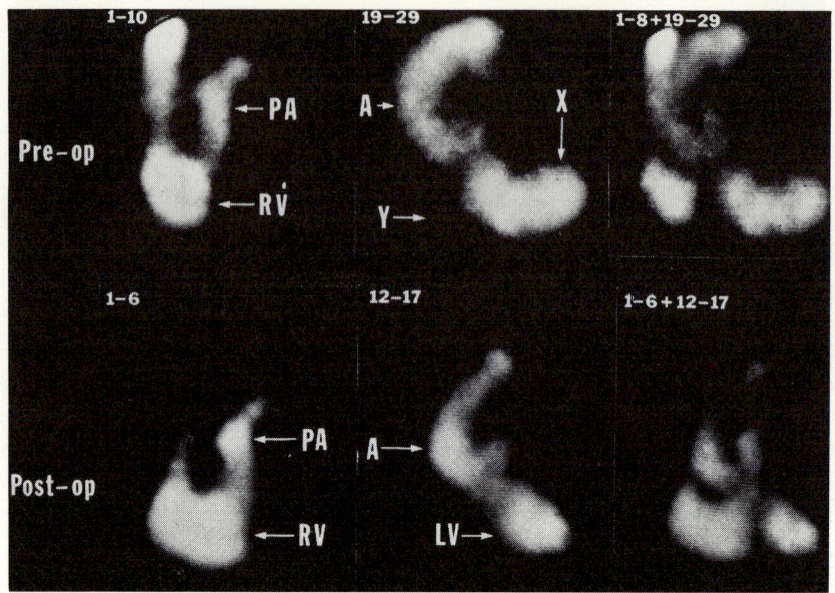

Fig. 2-29a. Quantitative flow study showing ventricular aneurysms at points X and Y on the image for the period 19 to 29 sec (upper). Lower set of figures shows a normal study after both aneurysms had been excised and the muscular walls patched. (With permission.[123])

Quantitative Work

Selective quantitative radiocardiography pioneered by Donato et al[72] offers the potentials of noninvasive, nonmorbid, and convenient outpatient evaluation of

    Cardiac output
    Stroke volume (CO/heart rate)
    Ejection fraction of right and left heart
    Ejection volume
    Right-to-left shunts
    Left-to-right shunts
    End-diastolic volume of right and left heart
    Mitral regurgitation
    Aortic regurgitation
    Combined mitral and aortic regurgitation
    Rate of volume changes
    Intracavitary transit times

The procedures involved in accomplishing these evaluations take approximately 5 min of patient time and $\frac{1}{2}$ to 4 hr of analysis, depending on the

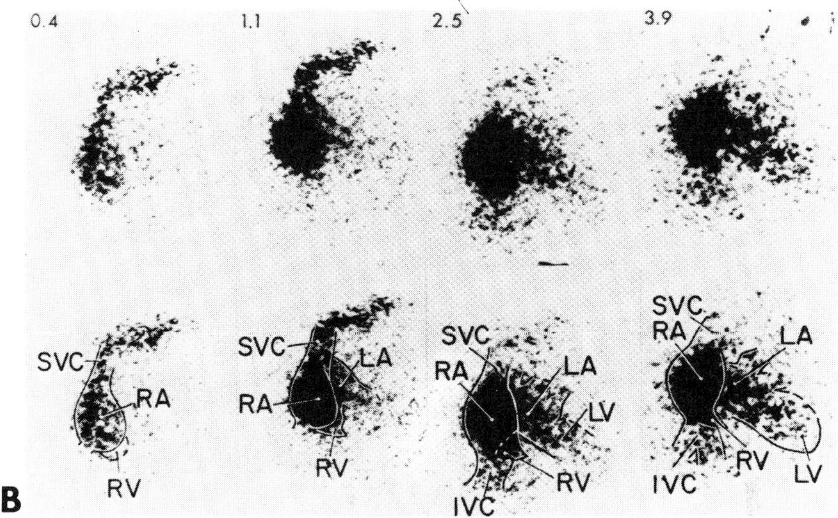

Fig. 2-29b. An anterior view demonstrating pulmonary atresia in a 6-month-old, 6.2-kg child. There is reflux from the right atrium (RA) into the inferior vena cava (IVC); the right ventricle (RV) and pulmonary artery (PA) are never well seen. The left ventricle (LV) filled early due to an intra-atrial shunt and the left ventricle fills only after left atrium (LA). (With permission.[105])

analysis algorithms and associated computing hardware. The above can be done by a single camera view and one or two isotope injections. The view accepted by many investigators and clinicians is the modified left anterior oblique (Fig. 2-30) because the longitudinal rotation axis in this view of the detector is parallel to the ventricular septum. This view allows resolution of the right and left sides of the heart and better separation of the atria from the ventricles. Most evaluations of left end-diastolic volume are from the right anterior oblique view (RAO).

CARDIAC OUTPUT AND STROKE VOLUME

The cardiac output is calculated by observing the time–activity curves of the isotope movement through the left ventricle in the anterior or modified left anterior oblique view. The data are acquired by flagging the region of the left ventricle using a computer system, or alternatively by selecting the field of interest on video playback using a photodiode or PMT to transfer the activity data to a strip chart recorder.[26,207] The cardiac output is given by

$$\text{CO} = \frac{C_{eq} \times \text{blood volume}}{A + B} = \frac{\text{total amount}}{\int C(t)\, dt} \tag{82}$$

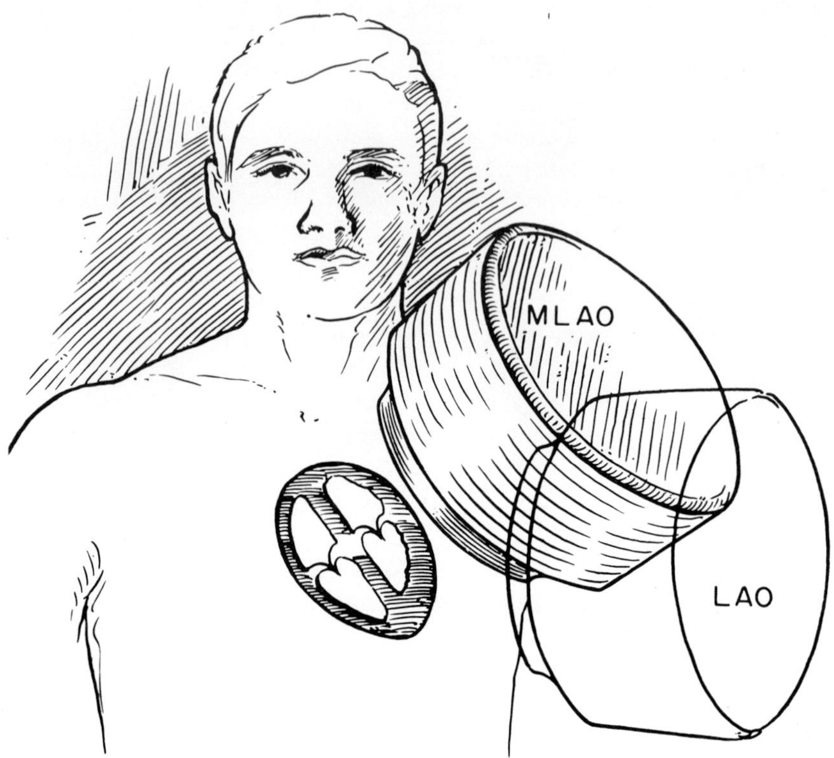

Fig. 2-30. The LAO and MLAO gamma camera views. (With permission.[29])

where C_{eq} is the count rate at equilibrium and area $A + B$ represents the area under the uptake–washout curve. B is an extrapolated portion of the curve (Fig. 2-13). When using a strip chart recorder, the practical implementation of this equation is given as

$$\text{CO (l/min)} = \frac{\text{(curve height at equilibrium)}\,\text{(chart speed)} \times \text{(blood vol.)}}{\text{area}}.$$

In practice it has not been easy to obtain the area under the recirculation curve of Figure 2-13; however, as discussed in the section on left-to-right and right-to-left shunts, this problem can be overcome and automated using the gamma variate fit to the time–activity curve.[197] Cardiac output can be determined by this technique using either gamma camera or collimated scintillation probe, as has been explored by MacIntyre et al,[147] Shreiner et al,[189] Glick et al,[86] Razzak et al,[176] and more recently by Dr. Van Dyke and associates at Donner Laboratory and Drs. Jackson and Scheibe at Stanford. The scintillation probe provides a convenient portable means of evaluating cardiac output at the patient's bedside; however, the position of probe placement relative to the left ventricle is critical in most situations, and the selected area compatibility of the camera would seem to be preferred if a small portable camera with area integration capabilities were available. No such device exists at present, although technically and economically a portable instrument 14 cm in diameter could perform most of the needed cardiac analyses.

Once the cardiac output is known, the stroke volume is calculated from

$$\text{stroke volume} = \text{CO/heart rate.} \tag{83}$$

Using the stroke volume, it is straightforward to calculate the end-diastolic volume (EDV) from a measure of ejection fraction (EF) discussed in the next section:

$$\text{EDV} = \text{stroke volume/EF.} \tag{84}$$

EJECTION FRACTION

The fraction of left ventricle blood ejected through the aortic valve is the forward ejection fraction. It is the difference between the end-diastolic volume and end-systolic volume (ESV) divided by the end-diastolic volume.

$$\text{EF} = \frac{\text{EDV} - \text{ESV}}{\text{EDV}}. \tag{85}$$

Ejection fraction can be determined by external monitoring using either of two methods. The first is by calculation of the ratio of the volume at end-diastole to the volume at end-systole.[45,199,215] The method of Zaret, Strauss, and co-workers is as follows: ^{99m}Tc-albumin is injected intravenously with the patient in the RAO view, and images of the heart at end-systole and end-diastole are obtained using a scintillation camera and an electronic gate triggered by the patient's electrocardiogram. Each image is composed of 300,000 counts, representing a summation of 200 to 400 heartbeats at end-systole and end-diastole (Fig. 2-31). An outline of the left ventricle free wall is drawn from each gated image. The position of the aortic and mitral valve planes is determined using a radionuclide angiogram obtained at the time of tracer injection. Left ventricle ejection fraction is calculated from the area and length of the long axis of the ventricular outline at end-systole and end-diastole.

A second technique involves the measurement of the peak to valley, count difference of the undulating activity curve as the isotope moves into and out of the left ventricle.[119,161,207,210] This technique can be employed

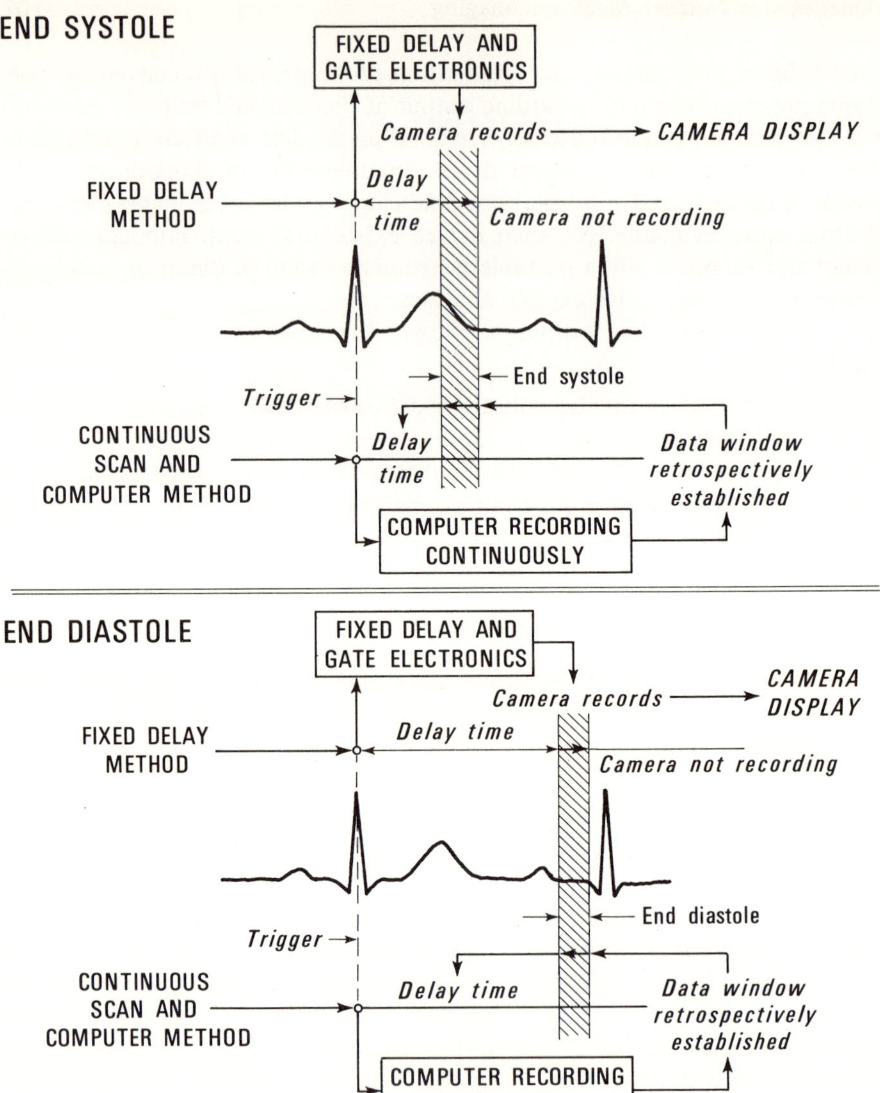

Fig. 2-31. Schematic diagram illustrating techniques of gating the gamma camera to record images of the activity in the left ventricle during end-systole and end-diastole.

with a high-speed camera–computer system or a single-crystal probe and strip chart recorder.

This latter method requires the area of interest to be as large as the ventricle in end-diastole; however, unwanted activity from the right ventricle, left atrium, aorta, and tissue blood pool contributes significantly to the time–activity curve of the left ventricle. Thus the ejection fraction must be calculated from

$$EF = \frac{\text{diastole counts} - \text{systole counts}}{\text{diastole counts} - \text{BACKGROUND}}. \tag{86}$$

The magnitude of this background or cross-talk contribution must be determined to describe the effective baseline for the peak to background measurement (Fig. 2-32). Two methods have been used. The baseline can be established by placing a ring or annular region of interest around the left ventricle (LV) area of interest. This new time–activity curve is used

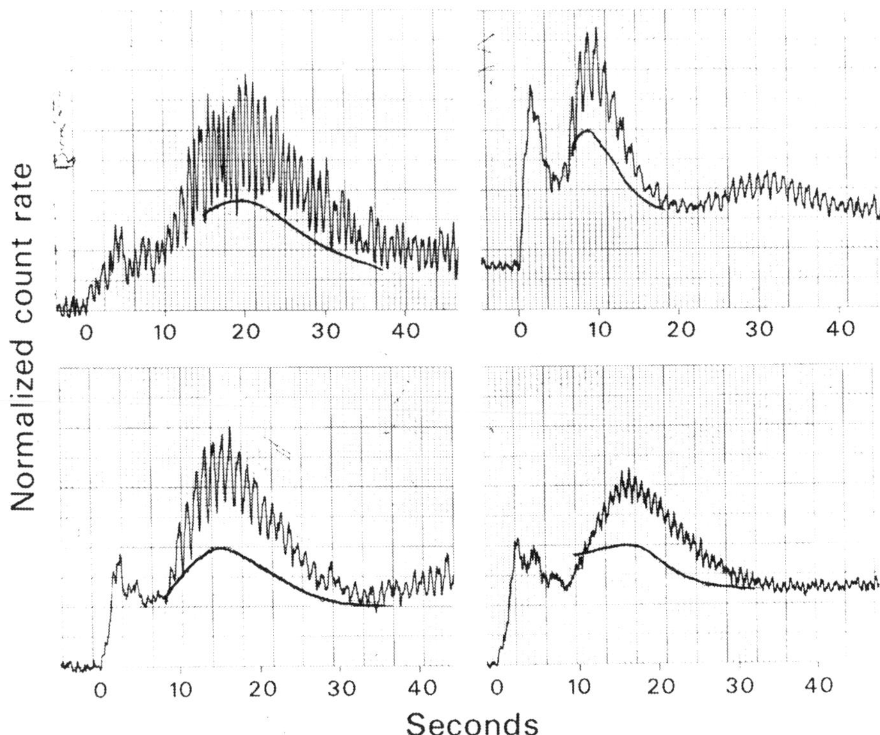

Fig. 2-32. Strip chart recordings of the change in activity with each heartbeat over the left ventricle for four separate studies. The solid line indicates the background correction curve; cf. test for details. (With permission.[207])

to compensate for background. Usually the area of the annulus is chosen to be the same as that for the left ventricle.[207,210] The background curve is adjusted such that its activity is the same as that at the nadir of the LV curve, but before the beginning of recirculation, as shown by the solid lines in Figure 2-32. The technique can be applied in the anterior, MLAO, LAO, or RAO views. In the latter view Kirch and co-workers[119] use an ellipse rather than an annulus to avoid atria and great vessels. The second method[161] of background subtraction has a good anatomical basis in that the background time–activity curve is derived by the contributions from the area where the ventricle is during diastole, but not during systole. Thus the computer forms an image of diastole minus systole, and within the region that was flagged as the left ventricle, the computer is programmed to select the picture element with the maximum activity in the subtraction image. Then any element within the previously defined LV area of interest which has half this activity or greater is selected for a new area of interest The BACKGROUND area of interest is thus defined. Both procedures give good correlation with ejection fraction determined from LV contrast cineangiography.

The ejection volume of the right ventricle can be determined from the exponential washout slope of the time–activity curve of the right ventricle. The EF is merely the cardiac output divided by the rate of decay constant ($EF_{rv} = CO/\lambda = CO \times$ mean time). This attractive procedure cannot be applied to the left ventricle because the washout does not follow a single exponential; however, the most likely rate constant could be derived from $\Sigma A(t)/\Sigma A(t)t$ after the washout curve is analytically extended, as given in the section on quantitative information from a single view.

VENTRICULAR VOLUMES

Assessment of left ventricular volumes can be made from single or biplane radioangiocardiography using the gamma camera and techniques similar to those for contrast cineangiography. The isotope techniques do not have any discomfort or morbidity; further, these techniques do not interfere with heart function, as is true for contrast dye studies. The right anterior oblique view is preferred because this projection is perpendicular to the long axis of the left ventricle during diastole, and there is less foreshortening in this plane than in either the anteroposterior or lateral projections. From measurements of Sandler and Dodge[183a] the heart movement during systole results in a foreshortened left ventricular axis for the RAO position, and thus the calculation of end-systolic volume is likely to be too small if done from the RAO position; nevertheless, calculation of volumes from a single view gives accurate results if the values are corrected by a calibration factor based on comparison between single and biplane studies or model phantom studies.

The biplane technique pioneered by Dodge et al[71] for contrast studies was first applied to radioangiography by Mullins et al,[157] who obtained two orthogonal views (anterior and lateral) of the flow of ^{99m}Tc-pertechnetate through the canine heart after direct intercavitary injections. Volume estimates for end-diastole were calculated by performing three measurements on the outline of the left ventricle for the two views. The assumption made is that the left ventricle at end-diastole can be approximated by solid ellipsoid whose volume is

$$V = \tfrac{4}{3}\pi(l/2)bc, \tag{87}$$

where l is the major axis and b and c are the minor semi-axes of the ellipsoid. These minor axes are determined from the planimetered area X of the outline from each view; thus

$$b = 2X_{ant}/\pi l, \qquad c = 2X_{lat}/\pi l_s$$

where l_s is the shorter of the two long axes. Substitution of these equations into Eq. (87) gives a concise expression for ventricular volume:

$$V = \frac{0.849 X_{ant} \cdot X_{lat}}{l_s}. \tag{88}$$

This biplane technique has not been actively pursued, perhaps because of the need for two injections for the two views.

The left ventricular volume can be calculated from one view by two methods. Sullivan and co-workers[200] demonstrated that a single RAO view gave sufficient information for calculation of the volume using the longest axis for l and the widest axis perpendicular to l for $2b$ and $2c$. In this case Eq. (87) becomes

$$V = \tfrac{4}{3}\pi(l/2)bc = \tfrac{4}{3}\pi(l/2)(w/2)^2 = (\pi/6)lw^2 \tag{89}$$

where w is the widest measurement perpendicular to the long axis l. The correlation of results from this technique with those of LV cineangiography is impressive. The data in this case are from average isotope distribution in LV systole and diastole.

Volumes at end-diastole and end-systole can be calculated from gated studies wherein summation images of the heart at end-diastole and end-systole are obtained by collecting data in specified time intervals relative to the EKG (cf. previous section). The end-systolic recording interval is the last 40 msec of the T wave and the end-diastolic record is obtained during 60 msec before each R wave (Fig. 2-31). A somewhat similar method is retrospective gating using the change in amount of isotope present; this procedure gives similar or superior results to the other techniques, and can be performed in 15 sec (Fig. 2-14). The volume of end-systole and end-diastole can be calculated quite accurately using a modified Simpson's rule:

$$V = \frac{\pi t}{3}\left[\frac{1}{4}\left(d_0^2 + d_{2n}^2\right) + \sum_i d_i^2 + \frac{1}{2}\sum_j d_j^2\right] \tag{90}$$

where t is the thickness of an even number of strips placed perpendicular to the axis, d_i denotes the odd diameters, and d_j denotes the even diameters surrounding the strips.

An indirect method of determining volume arises from the relation

$$V_i = FT_i = CO\ T_i \tag{91}$$

where T_i is the time constant determined by parameter fit to the Laplace transform transfer function as described in the section on the application of transfer function theory. This technique, proposed by Ishii and MacIntyre,[109] gives good results as long as there is no regurgitation.

The five methods of LV volume measurement outlined above are

1. EDV = stroke volume/EF.
2. EDV by Eq. (87) or (88).
3. LV by Eq. (89).
4. EDV by Eq. (90).
5. Vol. by Eq. (91).

LEFT-TO-RIGHT AND RIGHT-TO-LEFT SHUNTS

Using the pulmonary time–activity curve, Maltz and Treves[152] have presented a clever method for determining the pulmonary-to-systemic ratios (Qp/Qs) which reflect quantitatively the degree of left-to-right shunts. Their method involves fitting the pulmonary curve to a gamma variate of the form

$$A(t) = t^\alpha e^{-t/\beta} \tag{92}$$

using a simple least squares technique. Here α and β are arbitrary constants. The fit is made to data from about the last 10 percent of the uptake portion to 70 percent from the maximum on the washout slope of the pulmonary time–activity curve. The complete calculated curve is then sub-

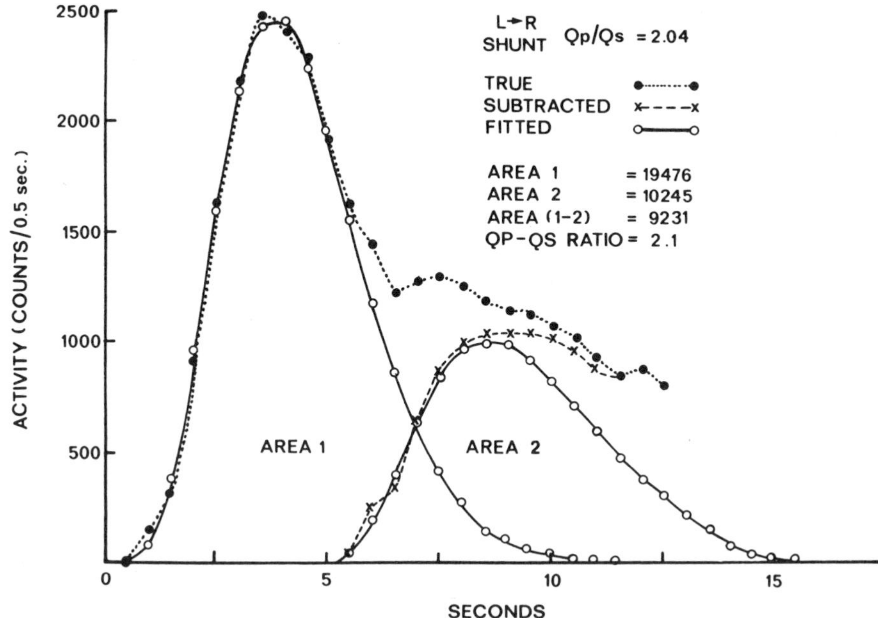

Fig. 2-33a.   Technique of quantitating left-to-right shunts using the gamma variate function for extraction of area information from the pulmonary uptake–washout curves after intravenous isotope injection. (With permission.[152])

tracted from the observed uptake–washout curve and the resulting curve again fitted by the gamma variate. The areas under these two curves were used to calculate the Qp/Qs ratio, as illustrated in Figure 2-33a. This method can separate those shunts with Qp/Qs greater than 1.2 and can quantitate the amount of shunting when Qp/Qs is between 1.2 and 3.0.

Another method of analyzing the presence of left-to-right shunts using the radionuclide pulmonary time–activity curve[3,75,124a,175] involves a simple ratio of the activity C_2 on the down slope curve corresponding to a time increment between the maximum activity C_1 and the first appearance of isotope as illustrated in Figure 2-33b. This technique relies heavily on the correct determination of the appearance time and time of maximum concentration. Nevertheless this method has been useful in clinical evaluations.

Another technique that allows quantitative evaluation of both left-to-right and right-to-left shunts involves comparison of the time–activity curves from two isotope injections, ^{133}Xe and ^{99m}Tc, and is based on the fact that Xe is almost completely washed out in the lungs before returning to the left heart unless there exists an intercavitary shunt.[29] The patient is positioned in the MLAO oblique position (Fig. 2-30) and ^{133}Xe in saline solution is injected intravenously first, followed about 1 min later by

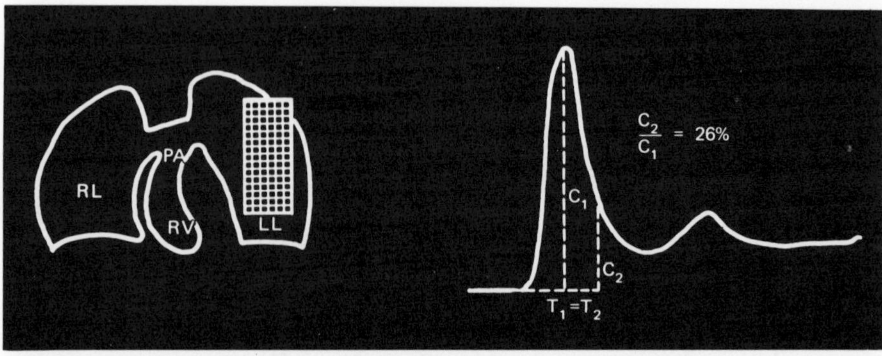

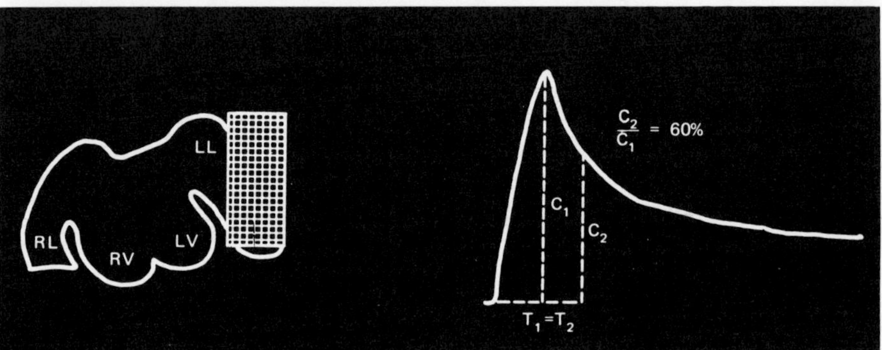

Fig. 2-33b.   Technique of detection of left-to-right shunts using uptake–washout curves after intravenous injection by simple parameter extraction from the pulmonary dilution curves. (With permission.[3,91])

[99mTc]-sulfur colloid without moving the patient. The data are collected and stored for each injection. The flow pattern of [99mTc]-sulfur colloid gives visualization of the heart chambers, and is used for selecting regions of interest over various heart chambers during the playback of the data for generation of time–activity curves for both [99mTc] and [133Xe] flow series since the patient remains stationary for the two injections. The normal [99mTc] time–activity curve will show a single-peaked curve over either the right heart or the left heart (Fig. 2-34). The normal [133Xe] curve will be a single-peaked curve for the right heart only as all the Xe ejected from the right ventricle will be cleared by the lungs before reaching the left ventricle unless, of course, there is a right-to-left shunt (Fig. 2-34). In left-to-right intracardiac shunts the [133Xe] in saline curve will be normal, but the [99mTc]-sulfur colloid curve will show a characteristic double-peaked curve over the right heart (Fig. 2-34). Quantitative work using this technique is limited due to camera speed and the change in the spatial impulse response with isotope energy.[220]

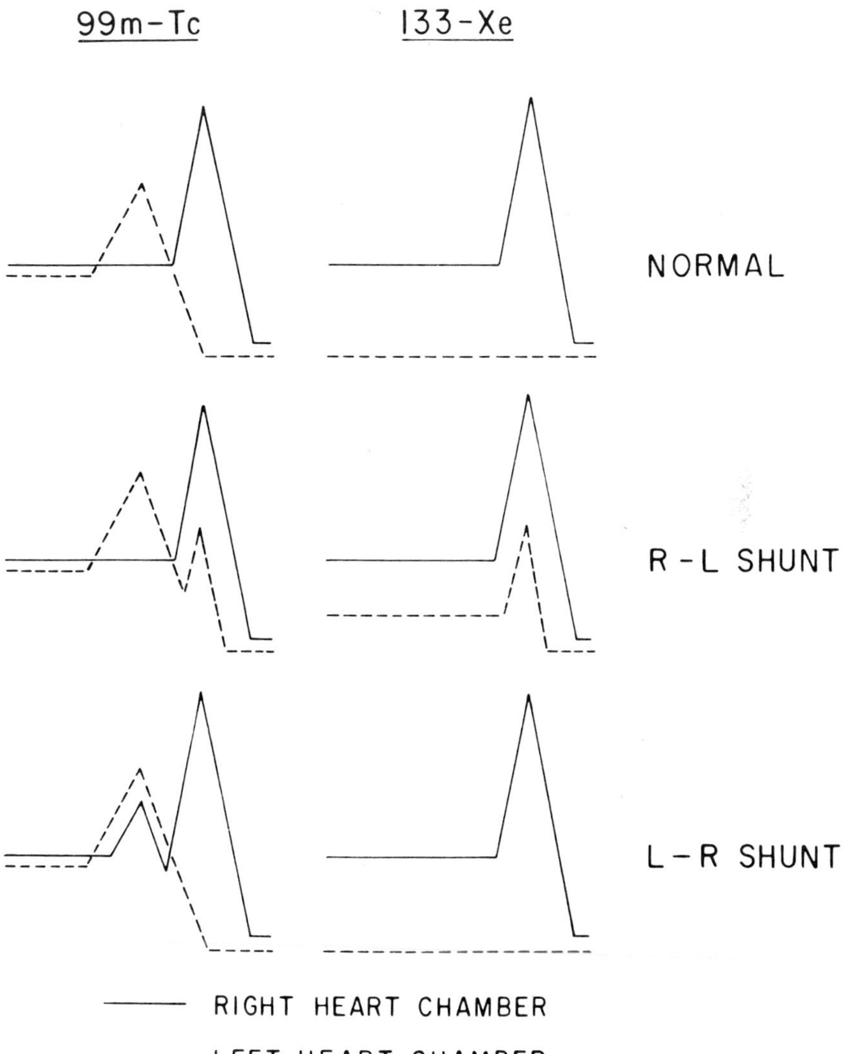

Fig. 2-34. Dual isotope technique of detecting right-to-left and left-to-right shunts; see text for details. (With permission.[29])

Left-to-right or regurgitant shunting can also be determined by calculating the variation in the time constant T_i of Eq. (35).[77] Recall [Eq. (34)] that for the nonregurgitant, cascade model the activity in the left ventricle is

$$A(t) = \frac{F}{V_i}\left[\int_0^t A_{i-1}(t - \tau_i)\, dt - \int_0^t A_i(t)\, dt \right]$$

or

$$\frac{F}{V_i} = \lambda(t) = \frac{A(t)}{\int_0^t A_{i-1}(t - \tau_i)\, dt - \int_0^t A_i(t)\, dt} \tag{93}$$

where $\lambda(t)$ is constant. If regurgitant flow exists, then $\lambda(t)$ will not be constant and this variation of λ is a measure of regurgitant flow (right-to-left shunts are not regurgitant).

Yet another technique can be used to measure shunting by evaluating the discrepancy between diastolic volume calculated by the area–length technique, Eq. (89), and the ventricular volume from the stroke volume, Eq. (84). Weber and co-workers[210] give the quantitative estimate of fraction regurgitated as

$$\frac{\text{volume by area} \cdot \text{EF} - \text{stroke volume}}{\text{volume by area} \cdot \text{EF}}.$$

AORTIC AND MITRAL REGURGITATION

The problem of regurgitation from the aortic or mitral valves has been dealt with successfully recently by Kirch, Steele, and Metz,[119] who have analyzed the pulsatile movement of isotope in the left atrium and left ventricle using a single view in the RAO ($40°$) position with the scintillation camera. Previous attempts to solve this problem using the Laplace transform approach were not successful because the Laplace transform does not adequately describe the pulsatile flow of the heart. Their technique consists of solving a set of difference equations, which involve four parameters that describe flow into and out of the two chambers—left atrium and left ventricle. The solution is facilitated by the Z transform, and is easily implemented using the left atrial and left ventricular time–activity curves obtained from injection of approximately 12 mCi of technetium from a Swan-Ganz catheter in the pulmonary wedge position.

The forward ejection fraction for the two chambers and the regurgitant fractions for two valves on the left side of the heart have been determined in approximately 30 cases with very good correlation to findings from the left ventricular conventional cineangiography studies.

The regurgitant flow on the right side of the heart can be determined in a similar fashion, but now with the catheter in the superior vena cava.

The background is removed by using a semiannular (ellipse) region of interest surrounding the heart, but excluding the atria and great vessels. The statistics are adequate for these studies, and the only problem encountered is that in the early phases of the study there is not complete mixing, and this might lead to some difficulty in detecting combined mitral and aortic regurgitation.[119]

RECENT ADVANCES LEADING TO QUANTITATIVE NUCLEAR MEDICINE OF CLINICAL IMPORTANCE

The present ability to acquire, store, manipulate, and then display scintillation camera and whole-body scanner data coupled with the advanced application of mathematical physics to these data leads to some new frontiers in clinical applications. For example, the combination of the high resolution of 2 mm (full width half-maximum) and high efficiency of the liquid xenon multiwire chambers[66] with techniques of motion extraction or gating and three-dimensional reconstruction from either multiple views or multiple cameras can give a definitive picture of the flow through cardiac chambers and the myocardium. Much of the new instrumentation and new techniques involved in these developments rely heavily upon the availability of new isotopes such as rubidium-81 for myocardial imaging,[47] ^{123}I (Myers, Chapter 3), and other relatively short-lived isotopes or radiopharmaceuticals such as iodinated fatty acids.[168]

The development of quantitative whole-body scanning discussed in an earlier section can now provide with ease, for the first time, accurate dosimetry in an organ by organ basis for all the isotopes and radiopharmaceuticals used in nuclear medicine. Further, digital whole-body scanning allows the investigation of electrolyte, fatty acid, cholesterol, and sugar metabolism pathophysiology for both research and clinical aid to the patients we serve.

ACKNOWLEDGMENTS

The new work from Donner Laboratory on the computer interfaces, quantitative whole-body scanning, three-dimensional reconstruction, and quantitative radiocardiology cited in this chapter was done under the sponsorship of the US Atomic Energy Commission and the encouragement of John H. Lawrence, M.D., James L. Born, M.D., and James McRae, M.D. Ph.D. The work on computer systems was done with Frank T. Upham, Victor P. Elischer, John Harpootlian, and William D. Hogan. The whole-body quantitation is being done with James McRae, M.D. Ph.D. and Mary Lou Nohr. Three-dimensional reconstruction is being done with Grant Gullberg, M.S., and continued work as it relates to myocardial perfusion is being done with Yukio Yano and James McRae, M.D. Ph.D. Further technical assistance of Marcy Wales, Brian Moyer, and John Flambard is gratefully acknowledged. The author has benefited from association with the research progress in projects of quantitative radioangiography from other contributors in the Bay Area: namely, H. Anger, Sc.D., M. Goris, M.D. Ph.D., J. Kriss, M.D., H. Parker, M.D. Ph.D., and D. Van Dyke, M.D.

Nathaniel Alpert, Ph.D., S. R. Amtey, Ph.D., William Ashburn, M.D., L. W. Bennett, M.D., A. B. Brill, M.D. Ph.D., D. A. Chesler, Ph.D., Gerald Freeman, M.D., Marvin Goodman, Ph.D., Ron Huseman, Ph.D., Dennis Kirch, M.S., David Kuhl, M.D., Burns Macdonald, Ph.D., William MacIntyre, Ph.D., Lucien Mathieu, M.D., Norman Poe, M.D., Myron Pollycove, M.D., Eugene Saenger, M.D., James Sorenson, Ph.D., William Strauss, M.D., S. Treves, M.D., Henry Wagner, Jr., M.D., Paul Weber, M.D., and Saul Winchell, M.D. Ph.D. contributed to parts of the discussion of this chapter indirectly through generous sharing of ideas during the past 2 years.

REFERENCES

1. Adam WE, Schenck P, Kampmann H, Lorenz WJ, Schneider WG, Ammann W, Bilaniuk L: Investigation of cardiac dynamics using scintillation camera and computer, in Medical Radioisotope Scintigraphy, vol 2, Proceedings of a Symposium, Salzburg, 1968. Vienna, IAEA, 1969, pp 77–91

2. Adams R, Zimmerman D: Methods for calculating the dead time of Anger camera systems. J Nucl Med 14:496–498, 1973

3. Alazraki NP, Ashburn WL, Hagan A, Friedman WF: Detection of left-to-right cardiac shunts with scintillation camera pulmonary dilution curve. J Nucl Med 13:142–147, 1972

4. Alpert J, Garcia del Rio H, Lassen NA: Diagnostic use of radioactive xenon clearance and a standardized walking test in obliterative arterial disease of the legs. Circulation 34:849–855, 1966

5. Alpert NM, Burnham CA, Hoop B Jr, Brownell GL, Deveau LA, Correll JE, Chesler DA, Ahluwalia B, Greene R, Potsaid MS, Kazemi H: Clinical and research application of a multiprogrammed computer system, in Proceedings of the Third Symposium on Sharing of Computer Programs and Technology in Nuclear Medicine. Miami, Florida, USAEC, Conf. 730627, 1973, pp 64–76

6. Ambrose J, Hounsfield G: Computerized transverse axial tomography. Proc Br Inst Radiol 46:148–149, 1973

7. Anger HO: Whole-body scanner Mark II. J Nucl Med 7:331–332, 1966

8. Anger HO: Tomographic gamma-ray scanner with simultaneous readout of several planes, in Gottschalk A, Beck RN (eds): Fundamental Problems in Scanning. Springfield, Illinois, Charles C Thomas, 1968, pp 195–211

9. Ashburn WL, Moser KM, Guisan M: Digital and analog processing of Anger camera data with a dedicated computer-controlled system. J Nucl Med 11:680–688, 1970

10. Atkins HL, Klopper JF, Eckelman WC, Richards P: Technetium-99M-DTPA renal study, in Medical Radioisotope Scintigraphy, vol 2, Symposium, Monte Carlo, 1972. Vienna, IAEA, 1973, pp 251–262

11. Barrett HH: Fresnel zone plate imaging in Nuclear Medicine. J Nucl Med 13:382–385, 1972

12. Barrett HH, DeMeester GD, Wilson DT, Farmelant MH: Recent advances in Fresnel zone-plate imaging, in Medical Radioisotope Scintigraphy, vol 1, Symposium, Monte Carlo, 1972. Vienna, IAEA, 1973, pp 269–284

13. Bates RHT, Peters TM: Towards improvements in tomography. NZ J Sci 14:883–896, 1971

14. Beck RN: A theory of radioisotope scanning systems, in Medical Radioisotope Scanning, vol I. Vienna, IAEA, 1964, pp 35–36

15. Beck RN, Zimmer LT, Charleston DB, Hoffer PB: Aspects of imaging and counting in nuclear medicine using scintillation and semiconductor detectors. IEEE Trans Nucl Sci NS-19:173–178, 1972

16. Bell RL, DeNardo GL: Enhanced scintigraphic information display using computer-generated ratio techniques. J Nucl Med 11:655–659, 1970

17. Bellman SH, Bender R, Gordon R, Rowe JE Jr: ART is science being a defense of algebraic reconstruction techniques for three-dimensional electron microscopy. J Theor Biol 32:205–216, 1971

18. Bender MA, Blau M: Data presentation in radioisotope scanning: contrast enhancement, in Knisely RM, Andrews GA, Harris CC (eds): Progress in Medical Radioisotope Scanning. Oak Ridge, Tennessee, USAEC, 1962, pp 105–110

19. Bender MA, Moussa-Mahmoud L, Blau M: Quantitative radiocardiography with the digital autofluoroscope, in Medical Radioisotope Scintigraphy, vol 2, Proceedings of a Symposium, Salzburg, 1968. Vienna, IAEA, 1969, pp 57–61

20. Bender M, Blau M, Bakshi S, Steinback J: Value of radioisotope scanning for detection of pancreatic tumors. Canr Bull 22:113, 1970

21. Bender R, Bellman SH, Gordon R: ART and the ribosome: a preliminary report on the three-dimensional structure of individual ribosomes determined by an algebraic reconstruction technique. J Theor Biol 29:483–487, 1970

22. Benua RS, Weber DA, Kenny PJ, Laughlin JS: Digital scanning compared with photoscanning in liver examination. J Nucl Med 9:135–139, 1968

23. Berman M, Shahn E, Weiss MF: The routine fitting of kinetic data to models: a mathematical formalism for digital computers. Biophys J 2:275–287, 1962

24. Berry MV, Gibbs DF: The interpretation of optical projections. Proc R Soc Lond A 314:143–152, 1970

25. Bitter F, Adam WE: A data acquisition and processing system for rapid dynamic investigations with a scintillation camera, in Medical Radioisotope Scintigraphy, Symposium, Monte Carlo, 1972. Vienna, IAEA, 1973, vol I, pp 443–457

26. Bitter F Besch W, Schäfer N, Sigmund E: Integrierte HerzKreislaufanalyse mit Hilfe der quantitativen Funktionsszintigraphie, in Horst W (ed): Frontiers of Nuclear Medicine. Berlin, Springer-Verlag, 1971, p 250–261

27. Blanquet P, Beck C, Pigneux J, Hecquet MF: Intérêt et limites de la scintigraphie pancréatique, in Medical Radioisotope Scintigraphy, vol 2, Proceedings of a Symposium, Salzburg, 1968. Vienna, IAEA, 1969, pp 707–719

28. Blaufox MD, Potchen EJ, Merrill JP: Measurement of effective renal plasma flow in man by external counting methods. J Nucl Med 8:77–85, 1967

29. Bosnjakovic VB, Bennett LR, Greenfield LD, Vincent WR: Dual-isotope method for diagnosis of intracardiac shunts. J Nucl Med 14:514–521, 1973

30. Boullion TL, Odell PL: Generalized Inverse Matrices. New York, Wiley, 1971

31. Bracewell RN: Strip integration in radio astronomy. Aust J Phys 9:198–217, 1956

32. Bracewell RN, Riddle AC: Inversion of fan-beam scans in radio astronomy. Astrophys J 150:427–434, 1967

33. Brill AB, Erickson JJ, Lindahl CE: Digital systems for data acquisition and storage, in Kenny PJ, Smith EM (eds): Quantitative Organ Visualization in Nuclear Medicine. Coral Gables, Florida, University of Miami Press, 1971, pp 339–379

34. Brill AB, Erickson JJ: Factors affecting the collection and analysis of radiotracer images. Semin Nucl Med 3:285–300, 1973

35. Britton KE, Brown NJG: Clinical Renography. London, Lloyd-Luke, 1971, 298 pp

36. Brown DW: Digital computer analysis and display of the radioisotope scan. J Nucl Med 5:802–806, 1964

37. Brown DW, Kirch DL, Ryerson TW, Throckmorton AJ, Kilbourn AL, Brenner, NM: Computer processing of radioisotope scans using Fourier and other transformations. J Nucl Med 12:287, 1971

38. Brownell GL, Callahan AB: Transform methods for tracer data analysis. Ann NY Acad Sci 108:172–181, 1963

39. Brownell GL, Berman M, Robertson JS: Nomenclature for tracer kinetics. Int J Appl Radiat Isot 19:249, 1968

40. Brownell GL, Burnham CA, Hoop B Jr, Bohning DE: Quantitative dynamic studies using short-lived radioisotopes and positron detection, in Dynamic Studies with Radioisotopes in Medicine, Proceedings of a Symposium, Rotterdam, 1970. IAEA–SM-136/126. Vienna, IAEA, 1971, pp 161–172

41. Bruno FP, Brookeman VA, Williams CM: A digital computer data acquisition display and analysis system for the gamma camera. Radiology 96:658–661, 1970

42. Budinger TF, Howerton RJ: Characterization of the time variations of reproductive processes in living cells. Nature 214:397–399, 1967

43. Budinger TF: Transfer function theory and image evaluation in biology: applications in electron microscopy and nuclear medicine. PhD Thesis, Lawrence Berkeley Laboratory Ms 565, 1971, 232 pp

44. Budinger TF: Rapid manipulation and display of counts vs time curves by hardware and software, in Proceedings of the Second Symposium on Sharing of Computer Programs and Technology in Nuclear Medicine, Oak Ridge, Tennessee, 1972. USAEC Report CONF-720430, 1972, pp 305–324

45. Budinger TF: High counting rate performance of the Anger scintillation camera. Lawrence Berkeley Laboratory Report No 2145, 1973, 17 pp

46. Budinger TF: Clinical and research quantitative nuclear medicine system, in Medical Radioisotope Scintigraphy, vol 1, Symposium, Monte Carlo, 1972. Vienna, IAEA, 1973, pp 501–555

47. Budinger TF, Yano Y, McRae J: Rubidium-81 used as a myocardium imaging agent. Lawrence Berkeley Laboratory Report No 2157, Gesellshaft für Nuklearmedizin, 1973, Athens, Greece, Schattaver-Verlag, Stuttgart, 1974

48. Budinger TF, Macdonald B: Fresnel hologram reconstruction by digital computer algorithm. Lawrence Berkeley Laboratory Report LBL-2147, 1973

49. Budinger TF, Gullberg GT: Three-dimensional reconstruction in nuclear medicine by iterative least squares and Fourier transform techniques. Lawrence Berkeley Laboratory Report No 2146, 1974

49a. Burdine JA, Murphy PH, Alagarsamy V, Ryder LA, Carr WN: Functional pulmonary imaging. J Nucl Med 13:933–938, 1972

50. Burke G, Halko A, Peskin G: Determination of cardiac output by radioisotope angiography and the image-intensifier scintillation camera. J Nucl Med 12:112–116, 1971

51. Callahan AB, Pizer SM: The applicability of Fourier transform analysis to biological compartmental models, in Pattee HH, Edelsack EA, Fein L, Callahan AB (eds): Natural Automata and Useful Simulations. Washington, Spartan Books, 1966, p 149–177

52. Carlson JC: Matching gray scale display programs to various film types, in Proceedings of the Second Symposium on Sharing of Computer Programs and Technology in Nuclear Medicine, Oak Ridge, Tennessee, 1972. USAEC Report CONF-720430, 1972, pp 207–213

53. Chang S-K, Chow CK: The reconstruction of three-dimensional objects from two orthogonal projections and its application to cardiac cineangiography. IEEE Trans Comput C-22:18–25, 1973

54. Charleston DB, Beck RN, Eidelberg P, Schuh MW: Techniques which aid in quantitative interpretation of scan data, in Medical Radioisotope Scanning, vol 1, IAEA Symposium, Athens, 1964. Vienna, IAEA, 1964, pp 509–525

55. Chesler DA: Positron tomography and three-dimensional reconstruction technique, in Freedman GS (ed): Tomographic Imaging in Nuclear Medicine. New York, Society of Nuclear Medicine, 1972, pp 176–183

56. Chesler DA, Hoop B Jr, Brownell GL: Transverse section imaging of myocardium with $^{13}NH_4$. J Nucl Med 14:623, 1973

57. Clarke JM, Deegan T, McKendrick CS, Herbert RJT, Kulke W: Technetium-99m in the diagnosis of left-to-right shunts. Thorax 21:79–82, 1966

58. Cormack AM: Representation of a function by its line integrals, with some radiological applications. J Appl Phys 34:2722–2727, 1963

59. Cormack AM: Representation of a function by its line integrals, with some radiological applications, II. J Appl Phys 35:2908–2913, 1964

60. Cormack AM: Reconstruction of densities from their projections, with applications in radiological physics. Phys Med Biol 18:195–207, 1973

61. Cox JR Jr, Hill RL III: Design considerations for interfacing computers to gamma-ray cameras, in Kenny PJ, Smith EM (eds): Quantitative Organ Visualization in Nuclear Medicine. Coral Gables, Florida, University of Miami Press, 1971, pp 465–489

62. Crowther RA, De Rosier DJ, Klug A: The reconstruction of a three-dimensional structure from projections and its application to electron microscopy. Proc R Soc Lond A 317:319–340, 1970

63. Crowther RA, Klug A: ART and science or conditions for three-dimensional reconstruction from electron microscope images. J Theor Biol 32:199–203 1971

64. De Grazia JA, Scheibe PO, Jackson PE, Lucas ZJ, Fair WR, Vogel JM, Blumin LJ: Clinical applications of a kinetic model of hippurate distribution and renal clearance. J Nucl Med 15:102–114, 1974

65. Delaloye B, Delaloye-Bischof A: L'exploration rénale séquentielle, régionale et quantitative, in Medical Radioisotope Scintigraphy, Symposium, Monte Carlo, 1972. Vienna, IAEA, 1973, vol II, pp 237–249

66. Derenzo SE, Budinger TF, Smits RG, Zaklad H, Alvarez LW: Liquid xenon filled wire chambers for medical imaging applications, in Symposium on Advanced Technology Arising from Particle Physics Research, Argonne National Laboratory, 1973. Lawrence Berkeley Laboratory Report LBL-2092, 1973

67. De Rosier DJ, Klug A: Reconstruction of three-dimensional structures from electron micrographs. Nature 217:130–134, 1968

68. De Rosier DJ, Moore PB: Reconstruction of three-dimensional images from electron micrographs of structures with helical symmetry. Mol Biol 52:355–369, 1970

69. Desgrez A, Razafindramamba V, de Saint-Laurent J Kellershohn C: Étude théorique et expérimentale de la soustraction de deux images scintigraphiques: Application à la mise en évidence du pancréas, in Medical Radioisotope Scintigraphy, vol 2, Proceedings of a Symposium, Salzburg, 1968. Vienna, IAEA, 1969, pp 677–694

70. Deutsch R: Estimation Theory. Englewood Cliffs, New Jersey, Prentice Hall, 1965, 269 pp

71. Dodge HT, Sandler H, Ballew DW, Lord JD Jr: The use of biplane angiocardiography for the measurement of left ventricular volume in man. Am Heart J 60:762–776, 1960

72. Donato L, Giuntini C, Lewis ML, Durand J, Rochester DF, Harvey RM, Cournand A: Quantitative radiocardiography: 1. Theoretical considerations. Circulation 26:174, 1962

73. Esser PD, Bradley-Moore PR, Atkins HL, Robertson JS, Ansari AN: Small computer-assisted analysis of camera renograms, in Proceedings of the Third Symposium on Sharing of Computer Programs and Technology in Nuclear Medicine. Miami, Florida, USAEC, Conf. 730627, 1973, pp 113–122

74. Evans RC: Radium poisoning: II. The quantitative determination of the radium content and radium elimination rate in living persons. Am J Roentgenol 37:368, 1937

75. Folse R, Braunwald E: Pulmonary vascular dilution curves recorded by external detection in the diagnosis of left-to-right shunts. Br Heart J 24:166–172, 1962

76. Frank J: Computer processing of electron micrography, in Koehler JK (ed): Advanced Techniques in Biological Electron Microscopy. New York, Springer-Verlag, 1973, pp 215–274

77. Freedman G, Dwyer A, Berman M, Wolberg J: Time variation in cardiac flow/volume—and index of shunting and regurgitation. J Nucl Med 14:395, 1973

78. Frieder G, Herman GT: Resolution in reconstructing objects from electron micrographs. J Theor Biol 33:189–211, 1971

79. Gaarder NT, Herman GT: Algorithms for reproducing objects from their x-rays. Comput Graph Image Process 1:97–106, 1972

80. Gabor HT: Two direct methods for reconstructing pictures from their projections: a comparative study. Comput Graph Image Process 1:123–144, 1972

81. Garcia EV, Amtey SR: Determination of the unknown three-dimensional radionuclide distribution in a scattering medium. Q Bull Am Assoc Phys Med 7:105, 1973

82. Genna S: Analytical methods in whole-body counting, in Clinical Uses of Whole-Body Counting, Proceedings of a Panel, Vienna, 1965. Vienna, IAEA, 1966, p 37–63

83. Gilbert PFC: Iterative methods for the three-dimensional reconstruction of an object from projections. J Theor Biol 36:105–117, 1972

84. Gilbert PFC: An iterative method for three-dimensional reconstruction from electron micrographs. Proceedings of the Fifth European Congress on Electron Microscopy, Manchester, England, 1972, pp 602–604

85. Gilbert PFC: The reconstruction of a three-dimensional structure from projections and its application to electron microscopy. II. Direct methods. Proc R Soc Lond B 182:89–102, 1972

86. Glick G, Schreiner BF Jr, Luria MN, Yu PN: Determination of cardiac output by means of radioisotope dilution technique. Prog Cardiovasc Dis 4:586–615, 1962

87. Goitein M: Three-dimensional density reconstruction from a series of two-dimensional projections. Nucl Instrum Methods 101:509–518, 1972

88. Gordon R, Bender R, Herman GT: Algebraic reconstruction technique (ART) for three-dimensional electron microscopy and x-ray photography. J Theor Biol 29:471–481, 1970

89. Goris M, De Roo MJK, Vanderschueren G: An approach to a storage and data handling procedure in static and dynamic scintigraphy. J Belge Radiol 52:168–189, 1969

90. Greenberg EJ, Weber DA, Pochaczevsky R, Kenny PJ, Myers WPL, Laughlin JS: Detection of neoplastic bone lesions by quantitative scanning and radiography. J Nucl Med 9:613–620, 1968

90a. Gustaffson T, Todd-Pokropek AE: Filters with variable shape in radioisotope image processing, in The Data Processing and Data Handling of Radioisotope Scans. Proceedings of a symposium, Hannover, 1971 (in press)

91. Hagan AD, Friedman WF, Ashburn WL, Alazrak N: Further applications of scintillation scanning techiques to the diagnosis and management of infants and children with heart disease. Circulation 45:858–868, 1972

92. Halko A, Burke G, Sorkin A, Enenstein J: Computer-aided statistical analysis of the scintillation camera ^{131}I-hippuran renogram. J Nucl Med 14: 253–264, 1973

93. Hamamoto K, Torizuka K, Mukai T, Kosaka T, Suzuki T, Honjyo I: Usefulness of computer scintigraphy for detecting liver tumor with ^{67}Ga-citrate and the scintillation camera. J Nucl Med 13:667–672, 1972

94. Handmaker H, McRae J, Buck EG: Intravenous radionuclide voiding cistography (IRVC)—an atraumatic method of demonstrating vesicoureteral reflux. Radiology 108:703–707, 1973

95. Harbert JC, Ashburn WL: Selection of Polaroid film for scintiphotography. J Nucl Med 10:127–132, 1969

96. Harper PV: The three-dimensional reconstruction of isotope distributions, in Gottschalk A, Beck RN (eds): Fundamental Problems in Scanning. Springfield, Illinois, Charles C Thomas, 1968, pp 191–194

97. Haybittle JL: The quantitative analysis of cerebral scintiscans. Phys Med Biol 11:474–475, 1966

98. Heiss W-D, Prosenz P, Roszuczky A, Tschabitscher H: Die Verwendung von Gamma-Kamera und Vielkanalspeicher zur Messung der gesamten und regionalen Hirndurchblutung. Nucl Med 7:297–318, 1968

99. Heiss W-D, Prosenz P, Roszuczky A: Technical considerations in the use of a gamma camera 1600-channel analyzer system for the measurement of regional cerebral blood flow. J Nucl Med 13:534–543, 1972

100. Herman GT, Rowland S: Resolution in ART. An experimental investigation of the resolving power of an algebraic picture reconstruction technique. J Theor Biol 33:213–223, 1971

101. Herman GT: Two direct methods for reconstructing pictures from their projections: a comparative study. Comput Graph Image Process 1:123–144, 1972

102. Hoop B Jr, Ojemann RG, Brownell GL: A stochastic model of regional cerebral circulation. J Nucl Med 12:540–546, 1971

103. Hundeshagen H, Creutzig H, Henskes DTh, Geisler S: Computerized dual-isotope pancreas function scintigraphy with a multicrystal scanner, in

Medical Radioisotope Scintigraphy, vol 2, Symposium, Monte Carlo, 1972. Vienna, IAEA, 1973, pp 193–199

104. Hunt BR: An improved technique for using the fast Fourier transform to solve convolution-type integral equations, in Mathematics and Computers. Los Alamos Scientific Laboratory Report No LA-4515-MS, 1970, 22 pp

105. Hurley PJ, Wesselhoeft H, James AE Jr: Use of nuclear imaging in the evaluation of pediatric cardiac disease. Semin Nucl Med 2:353–372, 1972

106. Iinuma TA, Nagai T: Image restoration in radioisotope imaging systems. Phys Med Biol 12:501–509, 1967

107. Iinuma TA: Image enhancement by the iterative approximation method, in Kenny PJ, Smith EM (eds): Quantitative Organ Visualization in Nuclear Medicine. Coral Gables, Florida, University of Miami Press, 1971, pp 550–580

108. Inkley SR, MacIntyre WJ: Measurement of regional area gas exchange by perfusion and clearance of ^{133}Xe from the lung. J Nucl Med 14:490–495, 1973

109. Ishii Y, MacIntyre WJ: Measurement of heart chamber volumes by analysis of dilution curves simultaneously recorded by scintillation camera. Circulation 44:37–46, 1971

110. Ivančević D, de Vernejoul P, Kellershohn C: Right and left ventricular volumes in atrial septal defect studied by radiocardiography, in Dynamic Studies with Radioisotopes in Medicine, Proceedings of a Symposium, Rotterdam, 1970. Vienna, IAEA, 1971, pp 675–688

111. Jackson PE, Scheibe PO: Computer-aided renogram interpretation, in Third Asilomar Conference on Circuits and Systems. Western Periodicals, N. Hollywood, CA, 1969, pp 20–28

112. Jones RH, Bates BB: Gamma camera performance characteristics for dynamic quantitative radionuclide studies. J Nucl Med 14:413, 1973

113. Kaihara S, Natarajan TK, Wagner HN Jr, Maynard CD: Construction of a functional image from regional rate constants. J Nucl Med 10:347, 1969

114. Kasser IS, Kennedy JW: Measurement of left ventricular volumes in man by single-plane cineangiocardiography. Invest Radiol 4:83–89, 1969

115. Kawin B, Huston FV, Cope CB: Digital processing/display system for radioisotope scanning. J Nucl Med 5:500–514, 1964

116. Kety SS: The theory and applications of the exchange of inert gas at the lungs and tissue. Pharmacol Rev 3:1–41, 1951

117. Keyes JW Jr, Kay DB, Simon W: Digital reconstruction of three-dimensional radionuclide images. J Nucl Med 14:628–629, 1973

118. Kirch DL, Brown DW: Recent advances in digital processing static and dynamic scintigraphic data. Proceedings of the Second Symposium on Sharing of Computer Programs and Technology in Nuclear Medicine, Oak Ridge, Tennessee, 1972. USAEC Report CONF-720430, 1972, pp 27–54

119. Kirch DL, Steele PP, Metz CE: Quantitative radioisotope angiocardiography, in Proceedings of the Third Symposium on Sharing of Computer Programs and Technology in Nuclear Medicine. Miami, Florida, USAEC, Conf. 703627, 1973, pp 16–30

120. Klug A, Crowther RA: Three-dimensional image reconstruction from the viewpoint of information theory. Nature 238:435–440, 1972

121. Kriss JP, Matin P: Diagnosis of congenital and acquired cardiovascular diseases by radioisotopic angiocardiography. Trans Assoc Am Physicians 82:109–120, 1969

122. Kriss JP: Diagnosis of pericardial effusion by radioisotopic angiocardiography. J Nucl Med 10:233–241, 1969
123. Kriss JP, Enright LP, Hayden WG, Wexler L, Shumway NE: Radioisotopic angiocardiography. Wide scope of applicability in diagnosis and evaluation of therapy in diseases of the heart and great vessels. Circulation 43:792–808, 1971
124. Kriss JP, Enright LP, Hayden WG, Wexler L, Shumway NE: Radioisotopic angiocardiography: findings in congenital heart disease. J Nucl Med 13:31–40, 1972
124a. Kuchař O, Krč I, Vyhnálek J: Zur Verwendung der Szintillations-kamera in der Diagnostik von intrakardialen Shunts. Nucl Med 12:138–147, 1973
125. Kuhl DE, Edwards RQ: Image separation radioisotope scanning. Radiology 80:653–661, 1963
126. Kuhl DE, Edwards RQ: Perforated tape recorder for digital scan data store with grey shade and numeric readout. J Nucl Med 7:269–280, 1966
127. Kuhl DE, Pitts FW, Sanders TP, Mishkin MM: Transverse section and rectilinear brain scanning with ^{99m}Tc-pertechnetate. Radiology 86:822–829, 1966
128. Kuhl DE, Edwards RQ: Reorganizing data from transverse section scans of the brain using digital processing. Radiology 91:975–983, 1968
129. Kuhl DE, Sanders TD, Edwards RQ, Makler PT Jr: Failure to improve observer performance with scan smoothing. J Nucl Med 13:752–757, 1972
130. Kuhl DE, Edwards RQ, Ricci AR, Reivich M: Quantitative section scanning, in Medical Radioisotope Scintigraphy, Symposium, Monte Carlo, 1972. Vienna, IAEA, 1973, vol I, pp 347–353
131. Kuhl DE, Edwards RQ, Ricci AR, Reivich M: Quantitative section scanning using orthogonal tangent correction. J Nucl Med 14:196–200, 1973
132. Ladefoged J: Measurements of the renal blood flow in man with the ^{133}xenon washout technique. Scand J Clin Lab Invest 18:299, 1966
133. Lake JA: Reconstruction of three-dimensional structures from electron micrographs: the equivalence of two methods, in Arceneaux CJ (ed): Proceedings of the Electron Microscopy Society of America, 29th Annual Meeting. Baton Rouge, Louisiana, Claitor's Publications Division, 1971, pp 90–91
134. Lange RC, Freedman GS, Treves S: Analysis of maximum frame rates for gamma-ray camera-computer systems. Phys Med Biol 17:624–629, 1972
135. Larsen OA: Xenon-133 methods for determining peripheral blood flow and blood pressure in patients with occlusive arterial disease. Angiology 23:153–162, 1972
136. Laughlin JS, Weber DA, Kenny PJ, Corey KR, Greenberg E: Total body scanning. Br J Radiol 37:287–296, 1964
137. Laughlin JS, Weber DA, Benua RS, Kenny PJ, Ritt F: Quantitative storage, analysis and display in digital scanning, in Gottschalk A, Beck R (eds): Fundamental Problems in Scanning. Springfield, Illinois, Charles C Thomas, 1968, pp 267–274
138. Laughlin JS, Ritter FW, Dwyer AJ, Mayer K, Greenberg EJ, Dimich AB, Hasan S, Rothschild E, Myers WPL: Development and applications of quantitative and computer-analyzed counting and scanning. Cancer 25:395–405, 1970
139. Lindbjerg IF: Leg muscle blood flow measured with ^{133}Xenon after ischaemia periods and after muscular exercise performed during ischaemia. Clin Sci 30:399–408, 1966

140. Llaurado JG: Relationship between kinetics of inflow and outflow as the basis of a computer simulation for solving compartmental models: example of electrolyte transfers in cardiovascular tissues, in Dynamic Studies with Radioisotopes in Medicine, Proceedings of a Symposium, Rotterdam, 1970. Vienna, IAEA, 1971, pp 13–26

141. Loken MK, Linnemann RE, Kush GS: Evaluation of renal function using a scintillation camera and computer. Radiology 93:85–94, 1969

142. Loken MK, Ponto RA, Bache R, Burchell H: Intravenous radioisotope angiography with computer processing of data. Am J Roentgenol Radium Ther Nucl Med 112:682–690, 1971

143. Lorenz WJ, Georgi P, Meder HG, Pistor P, Walch G, Wiebelt H: Interactive Processing and displaying of digital scintigrams, in Medical Radioisotope Scintigraphy, vol 1, Symposium, Monte Carlo, 1972. Vienna, IAEA, 1973, pp 613–633

144. Love WD, Romney RB, Burch GE: A comparison of the distribution of potassium and exchangeable rubidium in the organs of the dog, using rubidium-86. Circ Res 2:112–122, 1954

145. Love WD, Burch GE: Estimation of the rates of uptake of ^{86}Rb by the heart, liver, and skeletal muscle of man with and without cardiac disease. Int J Appl Radiat Isot 3:207–216, 1958

146. Love WD, Smith RO, Pulley PE: Mapping myocardial mass and regional coronary blood flow by external monitoring of ^{42}K or ^{86}Rb clearance. J Nucl Med 10:702–707, 1969

147. MacIntyre WJ, Storaasli JP, Krieger H, Pritchard W, Friedell HL: ^{131}I-labeled serum albumin: its use in the study of cardiac output and peripheral vascular flow. Radiology 59:849–857, 1952

148. MacIntyre WJ, Rejali AM, Christie JH, Gott FS, Houser TS: Techniques for the visualization of internal organs by an automatic radioisotope scanning system. Int J Appl Radiat Isot 3:193–206, 1958

149. MacIntyre WJ: In vivo tracer studies by external γ-ray counting, in Hine GJ (ed): Instrumentation in Nuclear Medicine, vol 1. New York, Academic Press, 1967, pp 351–379

150. MacIntyre WJ, Inkley SR: Functional lung scanning with ^{133}Xe. J Nucl Med 10:355, 1969

151. MacIntyre WJ, Inkley SR, Roth E, Drescher WP, Ishii Y: Spatial recording of disappearance constants of xenon-133 washout from the lung. J Lab Clin Med 76:701–712, 1970

152. Maltz DL, Treves S: Quantitative radionuclide angiocardiography. Determination of Qp:Qs in children. Circulation 47:1049–1056, 1973

153. Marcus ML, Schuette WH, Whitehouse WC, Bailey JJ, Glancy DL: An automated method for the measurement of ventricular volume. Circulation 45:65–76, 1972

154. Matin P, Kriss JP: Radioisotopic angiocardiography: Findings in mitral stenosis and mitral insufficiency. J Nucl Med 11:723–730, 1970

155. McHenry PL, Knoebel SB: Measurement of coronary blood flow by coincidence counting and a bolus of ^{84}RbCl. J Appl Physiol 22:495–500, 1967

156. Metz CE: A mathematical investigation of radioisotope scan image processing. PhD. Thesis, University of Pennsylvania, 1969

157. Mullins CB, Mason DT, Ashburn WL, Ross J Jr: Determination of ventricular volume by radioisotope-angiography. Am J Cardiol 24:72–78, 1969

158. Myers MJ, Kenny PJ, Laughlin JS: Quantitative analysis of data from scintillation camera. Nucleonics 24:58–61, 1966

159. Natarajan TK, Wagner HN Jr: "Functional imaging" of regional ventilation and perfusion of the lungs. J Nucl Med 13:456, 1972

160. Oberhausen E, Romahn A: Bestimmung der Nierenclearance durch externe Gamma-Strahlenmessung, in Kreislaufforschung und Kreislaufdiagnostik, 5, Jahrestagung der Ges. f. Nuclearmedizin, Vienna, 1967. Stuttgart, Schattauer-Verlag, 1968, p 323

160a. Oppenheim BE: Method using digital computer for reducing respiratory artifact on liver scans made with a camera. J Nucl Med 12:625, 1971

161. Parker JA, Secker-Walker R, Hill R, Siegel BA, Potchen EJ: A new technique for the calculation of left ventricular ejection fraction. J Nucl Med 13:649–651, 1972

162. Patton J, Brill AB, Erickson J, Cook WE, Johnston RE: A new approach to mapping three-dimensional radionuclide distributions. J Nucl Med 10:363, 1969

163. Patton DD, Cutler JE: Gamma camera dynamic flow studies on a single film by color coding and time proceedings. Fifteenth Annual Technical Symposium, Anaheim, California, 1970, Soc. Photo-optical Instr. Engineers, pp 237–242

164. Peters TM, Smith PR, Gibson RD: Computer-aided transverse body-section radiography. Br J Radiol 46:314–317, 1973

165. Peters TM: Image reconstruction from projections. PhD Thesis, University of Canterbury, Christchurch, New Zealand, 1973

166. Pizer SM, Vetter HG: Processing radioisotope scans. J Nucl Med 10:150–154, 1969

167. Planiol Th, Garnier G, Itti R, Brochier M: La triscintigraphie cardiaque. J Biol Méd Nucl 25:3–11, 1971

168. Poe ND, Robinson GD, MacDonald NS: Myocardial extraction of variously labeled fatty acids and carboxylates. J Nucl Med 14:440, 1973

169. Pollycove M, Mortimer R: The quantitative determination of iron kinetics and hemoglobin synthesis in human subjects. J Clin Invest 40:753–782, 1961

170. Ponto RA, Loken MK, Payne JT: Dual-isotope renal studies using a scintillation camera. J Nucl Med 14:441, 1973

171. Potchen EJ, Bentley R, Gerth W, Hill RL, Davis DO: A means for the scintigraphic imaging of regional brain dynamics. Regional cerebral blood flow and regional cerebral blood volume, in Medical Radioisotope Scintigraphy, vol 2. (Proc. Symp. Salzburg, 1968), Vienna, IAEA, 1969, pp 577–583

172. Radon J: Über die bestimmung von funktionen durch ihre integralwerte längs gewisser Mannigfultigkieten. Ber Verh Süchs Akad 69:262–278, 1917

173. Ramachandran GN, Lakshminarayanan AV: Three-dimensional reconstruction from radiographs and electron micrographs: application of convolutions instead of Fourier transforms. Proc Natl Acad Sci USA 68:2236–2240, 1971

174. Ramachandran GN, Lakshminarayanan AV: Three-dimensional reconstruction from radiographs and electron micrographs: Part III. Description and application of the convolution method. Indian J Pure Appl Phys 9:997–1003, 1971

175. Ramirez de Arellano AA, Hetzel PS, Wood EH: Measurement of pulmonary blood flow using the indicator–dilution technic in patients with a central arteriovenous shunt. Circ Res 4:400–405, 1956

176. Razzak MA, Botti RE, MacIntyre WJ, Pritchard WH: Consecutive determination of cardiac output and renal blood flow by external monitoring of radioactive isotopes. J Nucl Med 11:190–195, 1970

177. Rhodes BA, Porter VL, Natarajan TK: Functional imaging of the distribution of arteriovenous anastomoses. J Nucl Med 14:444–445, 1973

178. Rigo P, Strauss HW, Pitt B: Left ventricular function in acute myocardial infarction determined by gated cardiac blood pool scans. J Nucl Med 14:445, 1973

179. Roberts GW, Larson KB, Spaeth EE: The interpretation of mean transit time measurements for multiphase tissue systems. J Theor Biol 39:447–475, 1973

180. Rogers WL, Han KS, Jones LW, Beierwaltes WH: Application of a Fresnel zone plate to gamma-ray imaging. J Nucl Med 13:612–615, 1972

181. Rollo FD, Schulz AG: Effect of pulse-height selection on lesion detection performance. J Nucl Med 12:690–696, 1971

182. Ross RS, Ueda K, Lichtlen PR, Rees JR: Measurement of myocardial blood flow in animals and man by selective injection of radioactive inert gas into the coronary arteries. Circ Res 15:28–41, 1964

183. Runczik I, Černoch V, Vavrejn B: Hybrid simulation—a new method for comparison of scintigraphic devices, in Medical Radioisotope Scintigraphy, vol 1, Symposium, Monte Carlo, 1972. Vienna, IAEA, 1973, pp 691–704

183a. Sandler HS, Dodge HT: The use of single plane angiocardiograms for the calculation of left ventricular volume in man. Am Heart J 75:325–334, 1968

184. Schepers H, Winkler C: An automatic scanning system, using a tape perforator and computer techniques, in Medical Radioisotope Scanning, vol 1, Symposium, Athens, 1964. Vienna, IAEA, 1964, pp 321–329

185. Schmidlin P: Iterative separation of sections in tomographic scintigrams. Nucl Med 11:1–16, 1972

186. Schmidlin P: The method of iterative section separation in tomoscintigraphy, in Metz CE, Pizer SM, Brownell GL (eds): Third Int. Conf. Data Handling and Image Processing in Scintography. Boston, 1973

186a. Schmidlin P, Palmtag H, Clorius J: Correction of organ motion by filtering techniques, in Proceedings of the Third Symposium on Sharing of Computer Programs and Technology in Nuclear Medicine. Miami, Florida, USAEC, Conf. 730627, 1973, pp 53–63

187. Shames DM, Weber PM: A general logical structure for quantitative analysis of radiocardiographic data. Clin Res 20:210, 1972

188. Sheppard CW: Stochastic models for tracer experiments in the circulation. III. The lumped catenary system. J Theor Biol 33:491–515, 1971

189. Shreiner BF, Lovejoy FW, Yu PN: Estimation of cardiac output from precordial dilution curves in patients with cardiopulmonary disease. Circ Res 7:595–601, 1959

190. Silber J, Sorenson JA: On-line data recording and analysis systems, in Hine GJ (ed): Instrumentation in Nuclear Medicine, vol 2. New York, Academic Press, 1974, Chapter 7

191. Silverman JF, Obrez I, Kriss JT: Coronary artery fistula, diagnosis and evaluation by selective contrast and radioisotopic coronary arteriography. Personal communication, 1974

192. Smith EM, Brill AB: Progress with computers in nuclear medicine. Nucleonics 25:64–71, 1967

193. Smith RO, Love WD, Lehan PH, Hellems HK: Delayed coronary blood flow detected by computer analysis of serial scans. Am Heart J 84:670–677, 1972

194. Šnaider J, Erjavec M, Kernel G: Data processing in liver scintigraphy, in Medical Radioisotope Scintigraphy, vol 2, Symposium, Monte Carlo, 1972. Vienna, IAEA, 1973, pp 97–108

195. Sorenson JA: Methods for quantitating radioactivity in vivo by external counting measurements. PhD Thesis, University of Wisconsin, Madison, 1971

196. Staab EV, Babb OA, Klatte EC, Brill AB: Pancreatic radionuclide imaging using electronic subtraction technique. Radiology 99:633–640, 1971

197. Starmer CF, Clark DO: Computer computations of cardiac output using the gamma function. J Appl Physiol 28:219–220, 1970

198. Stewart GN: Researches on the circulation time and on the influences which affect it. IV: The output of the heart. J Physiol 22:159–183, 1897

199. Strauss HW, Zaret BL, Hurley PJ, Natarajan TK, Pitt B: A scintiphotographic method for measuring left ventricular ejection fraction in man without cardiac catheterization. Am J Cardiol 28:575–580, 1971

200. Sullivan RW, Bergeron DA, Vetter WR, Hyatt KH, Haughton V, Vogel JM: Peripheral venous scintillation angiocardiography in determination of left ventricular volume in man. Am J Cardiol 28:563–567, 1971

201. Tauxe WN, Chaapel DW, Allan CS: Contrast enhancement of scanning procedures by high-speed digital computer. J Nucl Med 7:647–656, 1966

202. Tauxe WN, Broadbent JC, Thorsen HC: Disappearance of iodoalbumin from pericardial sac in a patient with myxedema. J Nucl Med 11:554–558, 1970

202a. Thompson HK Jr, Starmer CF, Whalen RE, McIntosh HD: Indicator transit time considered as a gamma variate. Circ Res 14:502–515, 1964

203. Tkocz H-J, Oberhausen E, Glöbel B: Measurement of liver clearance rate with partially shielded whole body counter, in Dynamic Studies with Radioisotopes in Medicine. Vienna, IAEA, 1971, p 409–418

203a. Todd-Propropek, AE: Personal communication, 1973

204. Tretiak OJ, Eden M, Simon W: Internal structure from x-ray images. Eighth International Conference, Medical Biology Eng., Chicago, Session 12-1, 1969

205. Vainshtein BK: Finding the structure of objects from projections. Sov Phys—Crystallog 15:781–787, 1971

206. Van Breemen JFL, Van Bruggen EFJ, Eikelenboom JC, Wiebenga EH: Three-dimensional reconstruction from electron micrographs of tilted objects. Proceedings of the Fifth European Congress on Electron Microscopy, Manchester, England, 1972, pp 600–601

207. Van Dyke D, Anger HO, Sullivan RW, Vetter WR, Yano Y, Parker HG: Cardiac evaluation from radioisotope dynamics. J Nucl Med 13:585–592, 1972

208. Wagner HN Jr, Natarajan TK, Knowles L, McEwan CE: Practical applications of the computer in radionuclide imaging, in Medical Radioisotope Scintigraphy, vol 1, Symposium, Monte Carlo, 1972. Vienna, IAEA, 1973, pp 459–484

209. Waltz AG, Wanek AR, Anderson RE: Comparison of analytic methods for calculation of cerebral blood flow after intracarotid injection of ^{133}Xe. J Nucl Med 13:66–72, 1972

210. Weber PM, Dos Remedios LV, Jasko IA: Quantitative radioisotopic angiocardiography. J Nucl Med 13:815–822, 1972

211. Wesselhoeft H, Hurley PJ, Wagner HN Jr, Rowe RD: Nuclear angiocardiography in the diagnosis of congenital heart disease in infants. Circulation 45:77–91, 1972
212. ˙ zum Winkel K, Jost H, Motzkus F, Golde G: Review paper. Renal function studies with radioisotopes, in Dynamic Studies with Radioisotopes in Medicine, Symposium, Rotterdam, 1970. Vienna, IAEA, 1971, pp 229–251
213. Winkler C: Datenverarbeitung in der Nuklearmedizin im Klinikum der Universität Bonn (ed 2). Nürnberg, Siemens Aktiengesellschaft, 1971
214. Wood EH: Diagnostic applications of indicator-dilution techniques in congenital heart disease. Circ Res 10:531–568, 1962
215. Zaret BL, Strauss HW, Hurley PJ, Natarajan TK, Pitt B: Left ventricular ejection fraction and regional myocardial performance in man without cardiac catheterization. Circulation 42 (Suppl 3): 120, 1970
216. Zaret BL, Strauss HW, Hurley PJ, Natarajan TK, Pitt B: A noninvasive scintiphotographic method for detecting regional ventricular dysfunction in man. N Engl J Med 284:1165–1170, 1971
217. Zaret BL, Strauss HW, Martin ND, Wells HP Jr, Flamm MD Jr: Noninvasive regional myocardial perfusion with radioactive potassium. Study of patients at rest, with exercise and during angina pectoris. N Engl J Med 288:809–812, 1973
218. Zierler KL: Equations for measuring blood flow by external monitoring of radioisotopes. Circ Res 16:309–321, 1965
219. Zierler KL: The cardiovascular system, in Bergner P-EE, Lushbaugh CC (eds): Compartments, Pools and Spaces in Medical Physiology. Wash DC, USAEC Division of Technical Information, 1967, pp 265–281
220. Zimmerman RE, Holman BL: Modulation transfer function for the Pho/Gamma III and Pho/Gamma HP scintillation cameras using ^{99m}Tc and ^{133}Xe. J Nucl Med 13:481–482, 1972

William G. Myers

3

Radioiodine-123 for Medical Research and Diagnosis

EARLY APPLICATIONS OF IODINE-123

The first scintiphotographic image obtained with ^{123}I is shown in Figure 3-1A. It is the image of the thyroid gland of a large dog which was made in December 1961[2] about 2 hr after ^{123}I-iodide (plus [124]I contaminant) had been injected intravenously. The pinhole scintillation camera[30,38] was equipped with a 0.25 $\times$ 8-in. NaI(Tl) crystal. The 13.0-hr ^{123}I had been generated about 2 to 3 half-lives earlier by bombarding natural antimony with 30-MeV He-4 ions[20] in the Crocker medical cyclotron.[21] Hence, it was accompanied by several percent of 4.2-day [124]I, and the "hard" radiation from the latter caused "edge penetration" of the pinhole and deterioration of the image.

An image of the author's thyroid gland, which was formed with a rectilinear scanner in 1965,[1] is shown in Figure 3-1B. It was made about 6 hr after ingesting 100 μCi of ^{123}I-iodide. The ^{123}I kindly was furnished by The Oak Ridge National Laboratory, where it had been generated in the [123]Te(p,n)[123]I reaction.[2,3] It was estimated that the resultant radiation exposure, involved in obtaining this excellent image of my thyroid was only about 1 to 2 percent of what it would have been had the common scanning dosage of 100 μCi of Iodine-131 been used instead.[1,2,4-11,13-16,18,94]

The image in Figure 3-1C was made similarly about 6 hr after ingesting 100 μCi of the ^{123}I-iodide. This first patient was a girl who was referred because of the low radiation exposure from [123]I.[8] A 24-hr thyroid uptake study with ^{131}I about 2 months previously had given results in the normal range. But the endocrinologist suspected that the accumulation would not

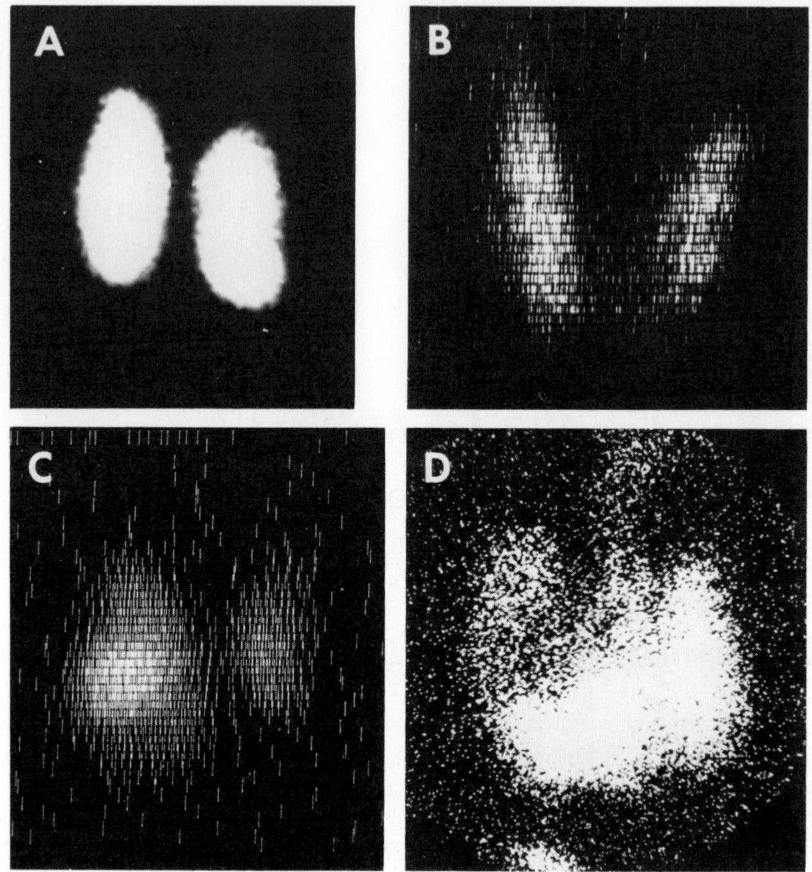

Fig. 3-1. (A) Scintiphoto image of the thyroid gland of a dog made in 1961 about 2 hr after ^{123}I-iodide (contaminated with several percent of ^{124}I) was injected intravenously.[2] A pinhole scintillation camera was used, which had a 0.25 × 8-in. NaI(TI) crystal. "Edge penetration" by the hard radiation of the contaminating ^{124}I degraded the quality of the image. (B) Rectilinear scan of the author's thyroid made in 1965 by means of 159-keV gamma rays about 6 hr after ingesting 100 μCi of ^{123}I-iodide. It is estimated[1] that this excellent image involved a radiation exposure no greater than would have resulted from a dose of only 1 to 2 μCi of ^{131}I-iodide. (C) Rectilinear scan of a girl's thyroid gland made in 1966 6 hr after she had swallowed about 100 μCi of ^{123}I-iodide. Note the inhomogeneous accumulation, despite a normal uptake of ^{131}I about 2 months previously. (D) Scintiphoto image made 6 hr after 200 μCi of ^{123}I-iodide; 16,000 counts in 5 min. The multinodular gland had markedly decreased accumulation in the upper two-thirds of the right lobe and smaller areas in the bases of both lobes. The pyramidal lobe is visualized clearly here by means of the 159-keV γ-rays of ^{123}I. The results of uptake studies were in the euthyroid range despite the heterogeneity of distribution. Because of the low radiation exposure from ^{123}I, this inconsistency makes routine ^{123}I "evaluation" studies desirable to supplant only partially informative "uptake" studies.

be uniform were the gland to be scanned. However, he was reluctant to do this on a young girl with 100 μCi of ^{131}I-iodide because of the large radiation exposure from the ^{131}I as compared to that from the same dose of ^{123}I-iodide.[14] The image in Figure 3-1C confirmed his suspicion of a heterogeneous distribution, and at an exposure equivalent to that from only 1 to 2 μCi of ^{131}I, an amount so small as to preclude making an image with [131]I.[13,15,16]

The scintiphoto image in Figure 3-1D was obtained with a Nuclear-Chicago Pho/Gamma-III pinhole scintillation camera 6 hours after the patient swallowed 2 capsules each containing 100 μCi of ^{123}I-iodide.* Sixteen thousand counts accumulated in 5 min. The image shows an enlarged multinodular goitrous gland having markedly decreased concentration of ^{123}I in the upper two-thirds of the right lobe and smaller areas in the bases of both lobes. Of particular note is the clarity of visualization of the pyramidal lobe, which is resolved rarely when ^{131}I is used for imaging. The uptake at 6 hr was 12 percent and at 24 hr, 22 percent, each of which is in the euthyroid range, in this laboratory.[17] The heterogeneity of ^{123}I distribution, despite the normal uptakes, demonstrates clearly the desirability of routinely imaging the gland with ^{123}I for nuclear-medical "evaluation" studies to supplant only partially informative "uptake" assays.[18]

Figure 3-2 shows four scintiphoto images of thyroid glands. The patients had swallowed a capsule containing approximately 100 μCi of ^{123}I-iodide* 4 to 6 hr before the images were made with a Nuclear-Chicago pinhole scintillation camera.[18]

In Figure 3-2A, the ^{123}I did not accumulate in a large defect that is delineated sharply in the lateral part of the left lobe. Resolution actually is adequate to discern the extension of decreased uptake to the medial aspect of the lobe. A broad defect in the inferior part of the left lobe is seen as well. Uptake of ^{123}I was 24 percent, which falls within the normal range. However, the striking inhomogeneity in distribution seen in the image furnishes a third illustration of how images provide important additional information to supplement simple uptake studies.[18]

The image in Figure 3-2B not only demonstrates clearly that I-123 was taken up only along the medial aspect of the left lobe, but that it did not accumulate uniformly in the lower half of the right lobe as well.

Except for a small area of ^{123}I accumulated in the upper right part of the isthmus, the image in Figure 3-2C depicts a morphologically normal thyroid gland.

The ^{123}I in image D (Figure 3-2) furnished adequate resolution to demonstrate a developmental anomaly in the right lobe which extends upward from the superior end of the lobe.

* Furnished by Medi + Physics, Emeryville, California.

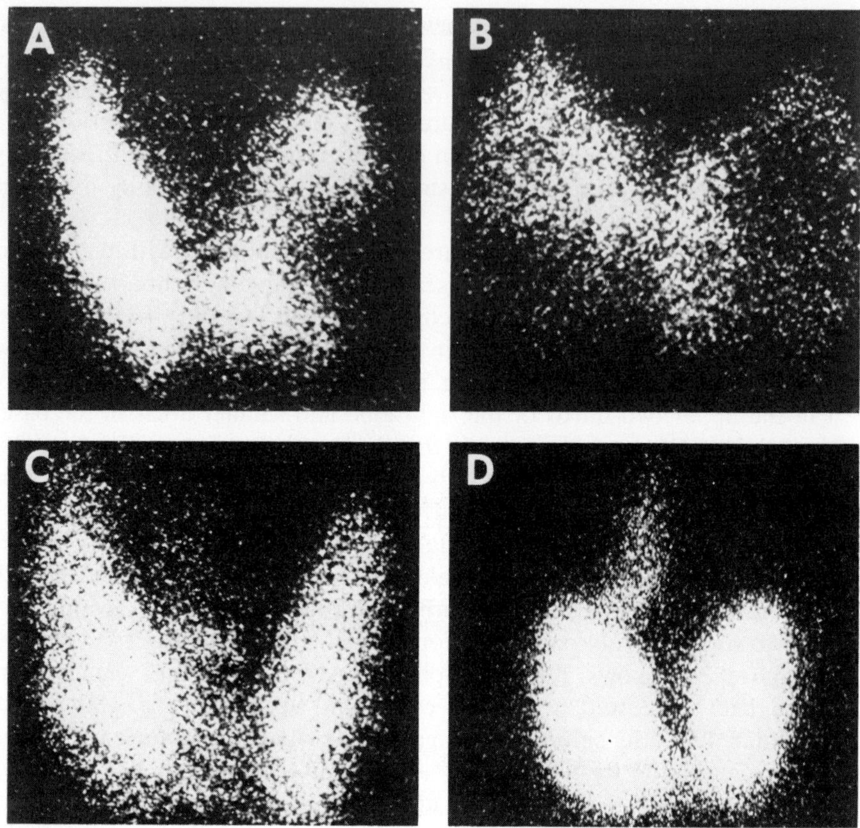

Fig. 3-2. Four scintiphoto images of thyroid glands made by means of the 159-keV γ-rays of 13.0-hr iodine-123, with a Nuclear-Chicago Pho/Gamma-III pinhole scintillation camera. The patients had swallowed a capsule containing about 100 μCi of ^{123}I-iodide about 4 to 6 hr previously. (A) Iodine-123 did not accumulate in a large defect that is delineated sharply in the lateral part of the left lobe. Resolution is adequate to discern extension of the decreased uptake to the medial aspect of the lobe. A broad defect along the inferior edge of the left lobe also can be seen. (B) The image demonstrates clearly that ^{123}I was taken up only along the medial border of the left lobe. Also, it did not accumulate uniformly in the lower half of the right lobe. (C) Except for a small area of ^{123}I accumulated in the upper right part of the isthmus, this image depicts a morphologically normal thyroid gland. (D) The ^{123}I furnished resolution adequate to demonstrate a developmental anomaly in the right lobe that extends upward from the superior end of the lobe.

The excellence of the images made with ^{123}I stems from the advantageous physical properties that make "[123]I fulfill the criteria of our ideal gamma isotope for in situ and in vivo diagnostic procedures more closely than any other of the 28 radionuclides of iodine."[1]

RADIOIODINE-123: HALF-LIFE = 13.0 HR

This γ-nuclide* of iodine was generated first in 1949[20] in the $^{121}_{51}\text{Sb}(^{4}_{2}\text{He},2\text{n})^{123}_{53}\text{I}$ nuclear reaction by bombarding antimony with ^{4}He ions in the 60-in. medical cyclotron[21,22] at Berkeley. The half-life was found to be 13 hr and γ-rays and conversion electrons of 150 ± 15 keV (kiloelectron-volts) were demonstrated. Observation of the 13-hr activity of ^{123}I was reported almost simultaneously from another laboratory[23] where the γ-ray was found to have an energy of 159 keV. It is this 159-keV γ-ray that gives to ^{123}I its prime significance and importance in biomedicine.

The pertinent physical properties now known about [123]I[24-26] and of interest to us are depicted in Figure 3-3; they are categorized in Table 3-1 for convenience of analysis. Many of the "output data" in the figure and table kindly were furnished by Dillman.[27,28] Intercomparisons of them with criteria listed in Table 3-2 for an "ideal" γ-nuclide to minimize radiation for in vivo diagnostic applications demonstrate that ^{123}I is indeed the γ-nuclide of choice for most such uses.[1]

Decay Mode and Rate

Iodine-123 is "neutron deficient"[20] by 4 in comparison with the 74 neutrons in stable [127]I, of which there are only about 30 mg in a 70-kg "standard" man. Iodine-123 decays solely by electron capture. Therefore, it emits *no* undesirable (in diagnosis) high-energy, short-range, beta particles as does ^{131}I and many other iodine radionuclides. This highly significant advantage, combined with the 13.0-hr half-life and the predominant 159-keV γ-ray, make ^{123}I the "ideal"[1] iodine γ-nuclide, in accordance with the criteria in Table 3-2.[2,4,8,18]

Half-Life of Iodine-123

This has been reported by various investigators to lie between 13 and 13.5 hr. The decay was followed carefully for 7 days (13 half-lives) and analyzed by two methods to give values of 13.00 ± 0.016 and

* A γ-nuclide is designated[19] as a nuclide that emits penetrating gamma rays (γ-rays) regardless of other types of emission that may accompany its disintegrations. It is used for brevity to avoid the awkward term "gamma-ray-emitting" nuclide.

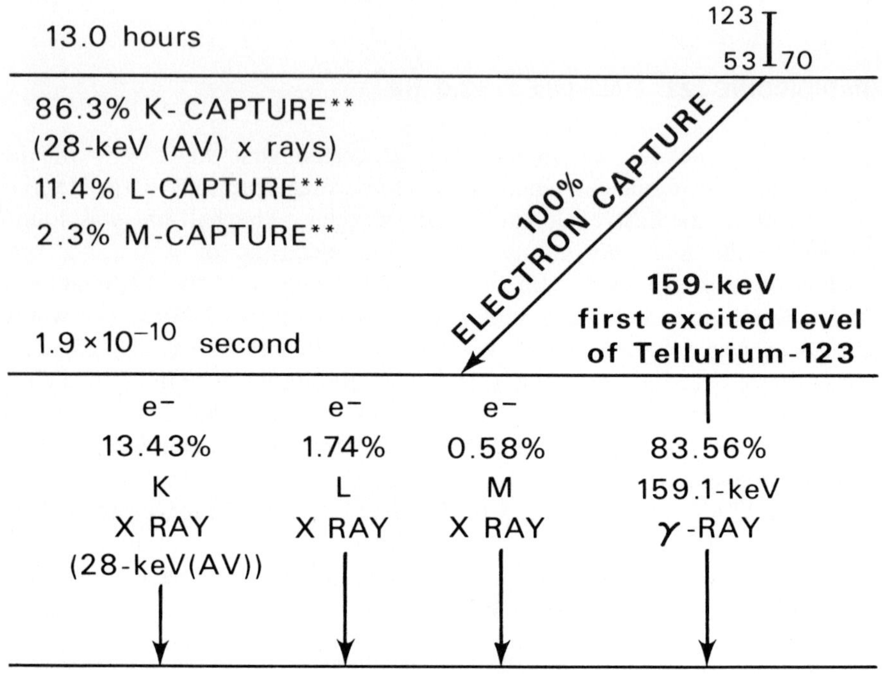

Fig. 3-3.   *This decay scheme has been simplified to account for $\sim$97 percent of the modes of decay of iodine-123 which are principally of interest in biomedicine. Actually, there are 13 additional γ-rays, with energies in the 184 to 784 keV range, but they aggregate only 2.3 percent of the γ-ray emissions.

**These values for electron capture abundances kindly were calculated by Dillman[27] on the basis of theory.

13.04 $\pm$ 0.018 hr. The average value was 13.02 $\pm$ 0.02 hr.[3] A rounded value of 13.0 hr is used here in Figure 3-3 and Table 3-3. The reciprocal values are included in this table for convenience, to indicate increasing volumes of solutions containing ^{123}I which are required to provide a given initial activity, as a function of time of decay.

The 13.0-hr half-life provides most of the advantages listed in Table 3-4. For example, should a physician wish to repeat a thyroid study by

Table 3-1

Physical Properties of Iodine-123 of Interest in Biomedicine

A.	Decay mode		

100% Electron capture [K = 86.3%; L = 11.4%; M = 2.3%]*

B. Decay rate

Half-life = 13.0 hr;[3] average life = 18.8 hr

C. Principal photons

	K x-rays	γ-ray
K x-rays, or γ-ray (keV)	28 (av)	159.1 keV
K x-rays, or γ-ray (%)	86.71%†	83.56†
Half-thicknesses in water (cm)	1.7 cm‡	4.7 cm‡
Half-thicknesses in lead (cm)	0.0016	0.037
Half-thicknesses in NaI (cm)	0.020	0.37
Photopeak efficiency in		
0.5-in. NaI(Tl)	99%	87.4%§
1.0-in. NaI(Tl)	99%	96.6%
2.0-in. NaI(Tl)	99%	98.0%

D. Analysis of the characteristic K x-rays†

	keV	Percent
K-α1 x-rays	27.4	47.15
K-α2 x-rays	27.2	24.19
K-β1 x-rays	30.9	12.73
K-β2 x-rays	31.8	2.64
Total		86.71

E. Other photons

13 High-energy γ-rays	2.31%	183.7–784.4 keV†
"Soft" L x-rays	13.32%	3.7 keV†

F. Particulate emissions from iodine-123

		Percent†	keV†
(i)	Internal conversion electrons		
	K conversion	13.43	127.2
	L conversion	1.74	154.5
	M conversion	0.58	158.2
	Total conversion	15.75	
	Weighted average/conversion electron		131.4‡
	Average energy/159-keV γ-ray		24.8‡
(ii)	Auger electrons		
	KLL Augers	8.77	22.6
	KLX Augers	3.70	26.4
	KXY Augers	0.59	30.1
	LMM Augers	92.42	2.9
	MXY Augers	218.64	0.8
	Total Auger electrons	324.12	
	Weighted average/Auger electron		2.33‡
(iii)	Total particle energy/100 disintegrations		2826‡
	Total particle energy/159-keV γ-ray		34.4‖

* Kindly calculated from theory by Dillman.[27]
† Obtained from Dillman[28] in advance of publication.
‡ Values calculated by the author.[2,4,8,18]
§ Myers et al,[18] from Anger and Davis.[29]
‖ Includes energy from L x-rays.

Table 3-2
Properties of an "Ideal" γ-Nuclide to Minimize Radiation
Exposures from *In Situ* and *In Vivo* Diagnostic Applications

---

1. The energy of the γ-rays should assure
    (a) adequate tissue penetration, with minimum scatter
    (b) maximum photoelectric interactions in readily manipulatable detectors, having minimum background sensitivities
    (c) maximum directionality, for highest resolution
    (d) minimum collimator penetration, to maximize the umbra

2. It should have the shortest practicable physical half-life so that the average life closely matches the physiological phenomenon under study

3. It should give a minimum of useless radiation from beta particles, conversion and/or Auger electrons, and low-energy photons following electron capture and/or internal conversion

4. It should have the maximum "γ-ray merit ratio" = usable γ-ray signal/ useless locally absorbed energy

---

means of ^{123}I, he may do so in as little as 3 days since a maximum of only 2 percent of a previous dose could then remain (Table 3-3). Thus, rapid physiological processes or changes induced pharmacologically readily are evaluated.

The average life of 18.8 hr closely approaches the time of assay in the popular 24-hr uptake study of labeled iodide ion by the thyroid gland. This is in contrast to the 15-fold longer 279-hr average life of ^{131}I, which unnecessarily and undesirably prolongs radiation exposures to patients long after the information the clinician seeks has been obtained.[1,4,8,18] This large difference in residual exposure is a major factor in greatly reducing radiation exposures to patients when ^{123}I supplants ^{131}I in forms that enter the iodide pool.

Diminished Interference with Other Radionuclide Procedures

About 30 percent of all patients admitted to The Ohio State University Hospital now have γ-nuclides administered to them for in vivo diagnostic studies.[17] In many cases repetitive procedures are carried out with a given radionuclide, and frequently two or more γ-nuclides may be given at different times. Consequently, the use of γ-nuclides of relatively short half-life greatly facilitates such sequential studies because these γ-nuclides are rapidly "self-scavenging" and diminishing interference occurs from any residual radioactivity from a previous study.

Table 3-3
Cyclotron-Generated Radioiodine-123
Half-Life = 13.0 hr. Average Life = 18.8 hr

Time *Hours*	Percent remains	Recip-rocal	Time *Hours*	*Days*	Percent remains	Recip-rocal
0	100.0	1.000	6	0.25	72.6	1.377
1	94.8	1.055	12	0.50	52.7	1.896
2	89.9	1.113	18	0.75	38.3	2.611
3	85.2	1.173	24	1.00	27.8	3.595
4	80.8	1.238	30	1.25	20.2	4.951
5	76.6	1.306	36	1.50	14.7	6.817
6	72.6	1.377	42	1.75	10.7	9.388
7	68.9	1.452	48	2.00	7.74	12.93
8	65.3	1.532	54	2.25	5.62	17.80
9	61.9	1.616	60	2.50	4.08	24.51
10	58.7	1.704	66	2.75	2.96	33.75
11	55.6	1.798	72	3.00	2.15	46.48
12	52.7	1.896	96	4.00	0.60	167.1

Also, the nuclear-medical physician enjoys the convenience of γ-nuclides that die away rapidly because he is relieved of concern for contaminated glassware, instruments, and hood; and, frequently, the facilities he needs can be simpler than those required to work safely with long-lived γ-nuclides.

Improved Statistics; Brief Imaging Intervals

Studies of rapid dynamic processes depend upon very high γ-ray flux densities momentarily to provide statistical significance during short time increments. This is especially the case when a scintillation camera is used to provide several scintiphotos sequentially within a few minutes, each of which may require 25,000 to 100,000 γ-rays to be recorded within seconds.[30,31] Obviously, intolerable radiation exposures might occur unless a γ-nuclide such as ^{123}I is used which has a relatively short half-life, or unless a γ-nuclide is used in the form of "γ-ray carrier"[32-35] compounds having short biological half-periods. It is anticipated that many such ^{123}I compounds quickly will come into widespread use when ^{123}I becomes available in large quantities.

An example has been observed recently where imaging intervals only half as long were required 24 hr postdose when ^{123}I replaced ^{131}I in studies of thyroid disease.[11] Shortened imaging times should be advantageous especially with children, or even essential with hyperactive or uncooperative patients.

Principal 159-keV γ-Rays

These are emitted from the ^{123}I nucleus in 84 percent of the disintegrations (Table 3-1).

The calculated 4.7-cm half-thickness of the 159-keV γ-rays in water provides adequate penetration, even from structures lying deep within the body (Table 3-2). For example, in comparing isotopes for scanning, Matthews[36] concluded that ^{123}I-HSA or ^{99m}Tc would be superior to ^{131}I-HSA for brain tumor localization. Indeed, ^{123}I-HSA was the first substance, other than iodide ion, to be labeled with ^{123}I; and it was used successfully for brain tumor scanning.[9] Beck et al[37] also found that, when scattering is taken into account for detecting midline brain lesions, a 150-keV γ-ray gave the best figure of merit per unit concentration of radioactivity.

The half-thickness of the 159-keV γ-ray in lead is less than 0.4 mm so that directionalization effectively is simplified and resolution is improved greatly in clinical practice in comparison with [131]I.[1,8,10,11,18,19] Collimator septa can be thinner and dosages need be less because of the improved efficiency resulting from the availability of the larger area of the crystal for interaction with the γ-rays. Conversely, a given dosage leads to decreased scanning time,[11] which often may be a major consideration clinically.

The half-thickness is less than 0.4 cm (Table 3-1) in the sodium iodide crystals of scintillation detectors. Thus, the NaI(Tl) crystals may be thinner, lighter, and cheaper, and they have lower background counting rates. Of special importance is the high probability of photoelectric interaction with the 0.5-in.-thick NaI(Tl) crystal of The Anger Camera. Accordingly, studies were initiated in 1961[2] to explore these advantageous features of ^{123}I while developmental improvements in the early scintillation cameras[38] were in progress.

The photoelectric efficiency of 87 percent (Table 3-1) for the 159-keV γ-rays in the scintillation camera is about three-fold greater than it is for the principal 364-keV γ-ray of [131]I.[18] This permits lowered dosages to be used, or it leads to decreased scanning time.[11]

Principal 28-keV (Average) X-Rays

These characteristic K x-rays resulting from the rapid deexcitation of the [123]Te daughter (Fig. 3-3), which have energies in the 27.2 to 31.8 keV range, are emitted from the atom in 87 percent of the decays.

The energies are identical to the x-rays emitted by [125]I.[1] The half-thickness of 28-keV x-rays in water is 1.7 cm (Table 3-1). This makes them adequately penetrating for many applications as was demonstrated initially[45] with ^{125}I in this laboratory[1,4,39-44] and then confirmed quickly by other investigators.[46-55]

Especially in the case of ^{123}I where the 28-keV x-rays (87 percent) and 159-keV γ-rays (84 percent) are emitted about equally abundantly, one has opportunities to use these rays conjointly because of the large differences in absorption in overlying tissues. Advantages have been taken of these differences in two ways in this laboratory. First, the locations of ^{123}I beneath surfaces of absorbing media as a function of depth were found by comparison with curves of decreasing x-ray/γ-ray ratios determined experimentally.[1,8,56-58] Secondly, two images of my thyroid gland were made by means of energy discriminators tuned to the photons separately[1] or simultaneously.[58] The latter method has advantages over the use of ^{125}I and [131]I[59] together, to achieve the same objective.

Other Photons

Improved instrumentation recently has led to the finding[24-26,28] that ^{123}I emits 13 additional γ-rays, with energies in the 184 to 784-keV range (Table 3-1). However, they occur in a total of only 2.3 percent of the disintegrations; and the most abundant of them is emitted with 529-keV energy in only one percent of the decays. Since these higher energy γ-rays are emitted so infrequently, they are not included in the simplified decay scheme shown in Figure 3-3 and they are indicated in Table 3-1 merely for completeness.

Additionally, 13 percent of the 3.7-keV (average) L x-rays are emitted from the ^{123}I atoms. But these are so "soft" as to be absorbed principally photoelectrically quite near their points of emission in tissues, and thus they may be related to the particulate radiations.

Particulate Radiations

The mode of decay of ^{123}I is solely by electron capture, and therefore ^{123}I emits *no* beta particles. However, short-range particles are present in the form of internal conversion electrons and Auger electrons. The average energy of these is calculated to be 34.4 keV for each 159-keV γ-ray emitted from the ^{123}I atom. This is only ~14 percent of the 232 keV emitted as localized particulate radiations per 364-keV γ-ray in 82 percent of the decays of ^{131}I, based on calculations made from values in Lederer et al.[60]

Thus it becomes apparent that the ~15-fold shorter average life of ^{123}I, together with the ~sevenfold lesser energy absorbed from short-range particles combine to reduce radiation exposures to at most only a few percent of those from ^{131}I in procedures completed during the first day after administering labeled iodide ion.[1,2,4,5,8–10,13–16,18,19]

IODINE-123 PRODUCTION

Antimony Targets

When natural antimony ([121]Sb, 57.25 percent; [123]Sb, 42.75 percent) was bombarded with [4]He ions,[20] [123]I was generated by transmutation. Several other iodine radionuclides were produced simultaneously, including 2.1-hr [121]I, 3.5-min [122]I, 4.2-day [124]I, 60-day ^{125}I, and 13.0-day [126]I. And, of course, the same contaminants were present when we bombarded natural antimony with [4]He ions in the Crocker medical cyclotron.[2,21] Antimony-124 soon became troublesome because of its abundance and longer half-life. But when a target enriched in [121]Sb to 99.4 percent was bombarded to generate ^{123}I in the [121]Sb([4]He,2n)[123]I reaction, there was only slight initial contamination with [124]I.[2]

When it became feasible to accelerate [3]He ions in the cyclotron at The Ohio State University, they were used to bombard natural antimony at incident energies of about 18 MeV. Average yields of 2.1 μCi of ^{123}I and 3.6 μCi of [121]I per microampere-hour (μA-hr) were obtained in four bombardments, and little [124]I was produced.[57] We then tried to produce "pure" [123]I by bombarding 99+ percent [121]Sb in the [121]Sb([3]He,n)[123]I reaction, with subsequent "purification by aging" to permit the decay of the [121]I which was made simultaneously in the [121]Sb([3]He,3n)[121]I reaction. But, only [121]I was made in copious amounts and almost no ^{123}I was found.[61,62] This led us to feel that the ^{123}I generated by bombarding natural antimony with [3]He occurred in the [123]Sb([3]He,3n)[123]I reaction. This conclusion was reached independently by Richards at The Brookhaven National Laboratory.[63]

Were highly-enriched [123]Sb to be bombarded with [3]He ions at 1 to 2 day intervals, it is our impression that practicable amounts of ^{123}I would be generated in adequate purity for use in biomedicine before the relative amounts of 4.2-day [124]I, made simultaneously in the [123]Sb([3]He,2n)[124]I reaction, would become limiting.[57]

Tellurium Targets

The first studies of thyroid metabolism in situ in man, which were carried out in 1939–40[64,65] by means of interactions of γ-rays emitted from within the gland with an external detector, involved principally the use of 8.06-day [131]I. It was made by bombarding tellurium with 8-MeV deuterons from the Berkeley cyclotron[22] and was contaminated initially with a mixture of several other identified iodine radionuclides.[66]

However, since the target contained the eight stable nuclides of tellurium, it seems probable that the mixture also contained 13.0-hr ^{123}I as well as 60-day ^{125}I, both of which had not been discovered yet![4] And when in situ assays were made soon after bombardment and administration, the 159-keV γ-rays of ^{123}I produced in the [122]Te(d,n)[123]I reaction almost certainly activated the Geiger-Müller tube placed against the neck over the thyroid isthmus.[67]

The suggestion was made that ^{123}I might be generated in the [123]Te(p,n)[123]I reaction.[2] However, [123]Te comprises only 0.87 percent of natural tellurium so that only targets that are highly enriched in it may be used. This is essential to minimize the production of several contaminants simultaneously, such as [124]I in the [124]Te(p,n)[124]I reaction. Obviously, were much 4.2-day [124]I to be present initially, its emission of positrons and very high-energy γ-rays would quickly vitiate the advantages of ^{123}I because the eight-fold longer half-life of the [124]I contaminant causes the ^{123}I/[124]I ratio to decrease rapidly.

When [123]Te enriched to 79.2 percent was bombarded with 185 μA of 15.5-MeV protons in a cyclotron at The Oak Ridge National Laboratory for a few hours,[3] hundred-millicurie amounts of ^{123}I were generated. It was contaminated initially with 0.88 percent [124]I, 0.075 percent ^{125}I, and 0.24 percent [126]I. Some of this product was used to make the images shown in Figures 3-1B and 3-1C.

Iodine-123 from Commercial Suppliers

Iodine-123 is now being produced on both coasts in small cyclotrons by manufacturers of radioindicators.[68] One of these* uses [122]Te enriched to greater than 95 percent to make ^{123}I in the [122]Te(d,n)[123]I reaction. At calibration time the radionuclidic composition is more than 98 percent [123]I[69] and the contaminants are: I-124 ($\sim$0.3 percent); [126]I ($\sim$0.15 percent); [130]I ($\sim$1.0 percent); and [131]I ($\sim$0.15 percent).

Scintiphoto images made 4 to 6 hours after administering $\sim$100 μCi of this product[18] are shown in Figures 3-1D and 3-2 and demonstrate excellent resolution and detail in the thyroid gland that we had not observed previously with [131]I.

Radiation absorbed by the thyroid from this amount of the ^{123}I, together with the contaminants, was estimated not to have exceeded 6 rads,

* Medi + Physics, 5855 Christie Avenue, Emeryville, California.

with only 20 mrads to the whole body. The comparable radiation exposures from 100 μCi of ^{131}I were estimated to be approximately 150 rads to the thyroid and 200 mrads to the whole body.[5] Thus the radiation exposures from the mixture are only about 4 and 10 percent, respectively, of those from [131]I. Had the ^{123}I lacked the contaminating iodine radionuclides, 100 μCi of "pure" [123]I would have exposed the thyroid to 1.6 rads and the whole body to only about 4 mrads,[5] or to about one-fourth as much radiation.

Iodine-123 Production Indirectly Through Decay of Xenon-123

A discoverer of [123]I[20] suggested to me[70] that the best route to the "pure" nuclide would be indirectly by first generating 2.1-hour Xenon-123 and collecting the ^{123}I from it as the [123]Xe decayed, chiefly by positron emission. This would avoid entirely the [124]I we had been encountering[2] when we followed his original method[20] for making ^{123}I and several other iodine radionuclides by bombarding antimony with [4]He ions. Professor Perlman suggested the use of highly enriched Tellurium-122 targets for the [122]Te([4]He,3n)[123]Xe reaction and that a system easily might be contrived to pump off the [123]Xe continuously during bombardment. Although the cross section was not known, he estimated it might be $\sim$0.2 barn as an average for $\sim$60-MeV [4]He ions incident on a highly purified [122]Te target of thickness sufficient to degrade the energy to $\sim$30 MeV. His estimate was that several Curies of ^{123}I might be generated continuously by bombardment to saturation, should the target withstand a 100-μA beam of 60-MeV [4]He ions.[70]

Sodd and co-workers[71-77] carefully evaluated this and other reactions for generating [123]Xe to obtain ^{123}I indirectly, as well as the relative yields and contaminants from a half-dozen direct transmutation reactions to produce [123]I. Investigators at The Brookhaven National Laboratory[78-83] recently have confirmed that Perlman's indirect method through decay of [123]Xe is a practical way to make ^{123}I that is free of other iodine radionuclides, except for a slight contamination by $\sim$0.1 to 0.2 percent of 60-day [125]I. For imaging this is of no consequence since the 27.2 to 35.4-keV photons emitted by [125]I[1,39-55] fall well below the 159-keV γ-ray of [123]I.[56]

The [127]I(p,5n)[123]Xe reaction has been used recently[84,85] to produce ^{123}I through the [123]Xe indirect method also. The only contaminant was 0.1 percent of [125]I. The yield was 3 mCi/μA $\cdot$ hr, which was tenfold greater than was obtained by Sodd et al[77] when they used Perlman's[2,70] method with a gas-flow target. This method for making ^{123}I, with only slight contamination by ^{125}I, presently is limited by the requirement for accelerators of protons to about 60 MeV. However, it is projected to have the potential to generate ^{123}I at rates of a few Curies per hour of bombardment with beams of $\sim$180 μA of $\sim$65-MeV protons.[86]

Recognition of the significance of ^{123}I is reflected in the support by governmental agencies,[1-3,74,75,78,86-91,106] chiefly at national laboratories, to make it available in this country. Similarly, there has been much effort abroad to prepare it in sufficient purity for clinical use.[92-94]

Potential Iodine-123 Production. Indirect Method; Xenon-124 Target

The great potential usefulness of ^{123}I, when it becomes available in large quantities,[87] justifies studies of variants of the indirect method of Professor Perlman[2,70] to try to make it from very highly-enriched [124]Xe[95] in [124]Xe(,)[123]Xe reactions.[96] Thus, cross-sections might well be studied of reactions such as (γ,n), $(n,2n)$, (p,d), (d,t), and $(^3He,^4He)$ with a very pure [124]Xe target. Although the Coulomb barrier for the [124]Xe(^{3}He, ^{4}He)[123]Xe reaction will be $\sim$16 MeV,[97] it may prove to be an especially interesting one since the Q-value is strongly positive at 10 MeV[97] and $(^3He,^4He)$ reactions often have high cross sections.[97,98] The [124]Xe already has been enriched $\sim$600-fold to 60 percent, from its low natural abundance of only 0.096 percent.[95] Studies involving some of these reactions with natural Xenon have been proposed and initiated previously.[75,99,100]

Iodine-123 for Studies of Thyroid Metabolism

Aside from a few initial studies with I-123[1,2,4,9,89] including those shown in Figure 3-1, the scarcity of this radionuclide (and contamination chiefly by 4.2-day [124]I) until recently has discouraged the use of it, despite early recognition by others[89] of its advantageous properties.

Wellman and co-workers have been especially active in their assiduous efforts to exploit the advantages of [123]I.[101-105] These experiences were incorporated[10] into intercomparisons of ^{123}I with ^{125}I, ^{131}I, and [132]I in respect to radiation dosimetry, imaging resolution, and production.[74-76] The conclusion was that the contamination by [124]I at that time limited the utilization of ^{123}I despite its having the best combination of physical properties.

An interesting way to circumvent much of the distortion due to [124]I contamination of ^{123}I, which was produced in the [121]Sb(^{4}He,2n)[123]I reaction,[20] was demonstrated in phantom studies that showed the usefulness of a computer to compensate for deterioration of images induced by the presence of [124]I.[94]

Iodine-123 having a purity greater than 99.995 percent was used in a recent objective clinical intercomparison with [131]I.[11] A rectilinear scanner equipped with a variety of collimators, and a scintillation camera were used 24 hr after a dose of 100 μCi of ^{123}I, followed later by the same dose of [131]I. The ^{123}I not only gave images of better quality, but also halved the scanning time. And, of course, the ^{123}I gave a radiation exposure that was markedly lower.[1,2,4,10,13,14,18,76,78,87,89,90,105]

Atkins et al[107,108] intercompared ^{123}I with ^{99m}Tc for imaging the thyroid glands of a large number of patients. They used Professor Perlman's indirect method[2,70] to generate the ^{123}I in high purity,[78,79,81–83] where the only contaminant was 0.2 percent of ^{125}I, and there was no [124]I. Patients were given 2 to 3 mCi of ^{99m}Tc-pertechnetate intravenously and a pinhole scintillation camera was used to obtain images of the gland 30 min later. Then ^{123}I-iodide was given orally in dosages of 100 to 350 μCi (only 60–75 μCi in some instances), and scintiphotographic images were obtained 18 hr later. The superiority of the images obtained with the ^{123}I was attributed to the very high thyroid/non-thyroid ratio, with consequent reduction in background counts. These authors concluded also that[1] "Iodine-123 is a nearly 'ideal' radionuclide for thyroid imaging."

Isotope Effect

It was postulated previously[18] that, because ^{123}I is "neutron deficient"[20] by 4 in comparison with the $\sim$30 mg of stable [127]I atoms in standard man, whereas ^{131}I has 4 neutrons more than [127]I, biochemical differences might be discovered that are due to "isotope effects," based on the 6.3 percent difference in mass.

A preliminary impression[109] is that the rate of uptake of ^{123}I by the thyroid gland is higher than that of [131]I. Data to support this stemmed from the finding in a series of patients of higher median uptake rates of ^{123}I than of ^{131}I at 1, 2, 4, and 24 hr.[110] The median percent uptake of ^{123}I in 44 patients at 4 hours was 31 percent, whereas for ^{131}I in 22 patients at 4 hours it was 16 percent, or only about one-half. In both series, the labeled iodide was ingested in liquid form and not in capsules. Hence, the differences in uptake rates could not have arisen from the method of administration.[111] Although the number of subjects was not indicated in another study,[94] uptake curves showed a strikingly higher rate for ^{123}I than for ^{131}I during the first 12 hr. Contrariwise, other investigators[11] found comparable uptake values of the two nuclides in the same patients.

Should additional uptake data, or other criteria, indicate that ^{123}I/[131]I "isotope effects" indeed become discernible, then fundamental researches might reveal opportunities to exploit them in developing new methods to study thyroid disease, as well as variants in glandular function induced physiologically or pharmacologically. Studies are contemplated in this laboratory that are designed to test these hypotheses.

Short-Term Uptake Gradient Studies with Iodine-123

The $\sim$2-fold higher uptake rate of ^{123}I in comparison with ^{131}I at 4 hr found in the preliminary studies of Verdon[110] indicates that one might use ^{123}I to intercompare gradients of uptake rates during the first few hours to establish criteria of disease.[4,40] The method of accumulating counts serially, or continuously, has the advantage that the patient serves as his own control during the evaluation. This was explored in this laboratory in 1960 with doses of ^{125}I as small as 0.1 μCi. The radiation exposure to my thyroid was only $\sim$100 mrads. During a few hours after ingesting the ^{125}I-iodide, a small scintillation detector repeatedly was placed in a reproducible position close to my thyroid. The net counts per second were then plotted as a function of time to give a line that was essentially straight during the first few hours.

Since then, instrumentation has improved greatly to the point that conceivably a miniaturized detector and circuit could be attached in a manner to give a constant geometry.* Telemetry might be incorporated to relay the counts from the patient located anywhere in a hospital, or even from distant points in a city, to a central receiver and plotter, for the analysis. Not only would this relieve some of the congestion found in busy nuclear-medicine services but it would also be more physiological than the present cumbersome system.

The physical properties of ^{123}I (Table 3-1) would greatly simplify the assembly of such a system. Since the geometry would be constant, the detector crystal could be very light because it would need to be no more than a few millimeters thick[39] to interact efficiently with the 27.2 to 31.8 keV x-rays of ^{123}I, and to an appreciable extent also with the 159-keV γ-rays.

The ^{123}I dosage would need to be only $\sim$1 μCi, *or less,* because of the excellent geometry, and radiation exposure to the thyroid would be less than $\sim$3 mrads in standard man.[14] Such evaluations would be especially appropriate when diagnostic studies were deemed desirable in children[14] or during pregnancy because of the relatively trifling radiation. Even the newborn would receive 278 mrads[14] ($\sim$ twice the annual natural background radiation) were the dose to be as large as 1 μCi of ^{123}I.

Also, since x-rays in this energy region tend to be inherently directional because almost half of them are absorbed in soft tissues by the "all-or-none" photoelectric process,[39,45] the region of interest during the assay

---

* Such an instrument should find many additional applications in nuclear medicine, e.g., with ^{121}I[1,61], ^{125}I[4,40] and ^{99m}Tc. After attachment over sites of potential interest (liver, head, bone, etc.), the optimal time for imaging would be indicated as the plotter approached a maximum rate asymptotically.

will be less distorted by scattered radiation coming from outside the thyroid.

Among the many advocates of various methods to study the rate of accumulation of labeled iodide by the thyroid are investigators[112–116] who feel that only those methods designed to evaluate the avidity soon after administration are maximally advantageous in avoiding distortions induced by significant loss of label from the gland in the form of the compounds synthesized by it.

Particularly noteworthy was a method[116] in which 2.3-hr ^{132}I was used because the short half-life greatly reduced radiation exposures in comparison with 8-day ^{131}I. This necessitated the development of an automatic counting procedure that resulted in uptake curves that differentiated among euthyroids, hyperthyroids, and hypothyroids 100 min after administration of the ^{132}I.*

^{123}I-Labeled Compounds and Substances

Early efforts to label Rose Bengal with ^{123}I by exchange when ^{123}I-iodide became available to me[2] were thwarted by the ^{124}I contaminant which soon became limiting during the time required to do the chemistry and purification. However, the lability of the ^{127}I-carbon bond lends itself to the facile labeling of many compounds by simple exchange, not only with ^{123}I but even with 2.1-hr ^{121}I also.[1]

The scarcity of ^{123}I in adequate purity until recently has prevented the use of it extensively for labeling compounds. As mentioned earlier ^{123}I-HSA[9] was the first substance to be labeled with ^{123}I and it was used in brain tumor scanning.

----

* *2.1-hr Iodine-121 versus 2.3-hr Iodine-132.* It seems appropriate to insert here as a footnote a brief intercomparison of these two iodine radionuclides, which decay with almost the same half-lives, because the physical properties of ^{121}I[20,28,61] would be highly advantageous over those of ^{132}I for the short-term studies under consideration. Iodine-121 decays principally by electron capture in 87 percent of the decays and by emitting 1.13-MeV (maximum) positrons in 13 percent of the disintegrations.[28] Iodine-132 decays by emitting beta particles, most of which have high energies.[28] Iodine-121 emits ~85 percent of 28-keV (average) x-rays and ~91 percent of 214-keV γ-rays in addition to the 26 percent of 511-keV "annihilation" photons.[1,28,61] The same detector system indicated above obviously would be almost equally effective with ^{121}I as with ^{123}I. Contrariwise, many of the γ-rays emitted by ^{132}I have such high energies as to make detection inefficient and directionalization unsatisfactory.

Iodine-121 can be generated readily in large amounts with a small cyclotron.[1,57,61,62] Short-term thyroid assays by means of 2.1-hr ^{121}I might be performed conveniently, and with minuscule radiation exposures, in the several medical centers in which cyclotrons now are installed.[87,117–122]

But now one may even anticipate the preparation of triiodothyronine and thyroxine labeled with [123]I.[1] The low radiation exposures will provide new opportunities not only to study their metabolism, per se, in vivo but to take advantage of it in devising new diagnostic procedures, e.g., for evaluation of liver function.[123,124] Conceivably the low radiation exposures from ^{123}I-iodide (or [121]I-iodide) may also permit in vivo studies of gastric function in health and disease.[125,126]

Wellman et al[127] made ^{123}I-hippuran by exchange labeling *o*-iodohippurate with ^{123}I-iodide. They found it to be useful for dynamic quantitative renal imaging with a scintillation camera. Counting rates were 10 to 20 times higher for radiation that was approximately equal to that from ^{131}I-hippuran. This gave excellent statistics and permitted sequential images to be made rapidly so that superior delineation of renal and outflow tract morphology was obtained. They feel that new normal ranges will become established when more extensive use is made of ^{123}I-hippuran for quantitative renography.

Extensive experiences in this laboratory during 25 years of working with iodine monochloride as an iodinating agent, labeled with ^{131}I by simple exchange, indicates the general applicability[128] of it for the de novo synthesis of compounds[33] labeled with ^{123}I or [121]I. Especially advantageous opportunities to label many compounds with ^{123}I in high specific activity will stem from the discovery of the preparation of high-purity no-carrier-added ^{123}I-iodine monochloride (80).

At Service Hospitalier Frederic Joliot d'Orsay it was found that the firmness of the bond between ^{123}I and albumin gave results that were superior to labeling with Technetium-99m when the labeled protein was used in the form of macroaggregates in studies of cardio-pulmonary dynamics.[129]

[123]I-Streptokinase was labeled by the iodine monochloride method.[130] When its distribution was studied in vivo in mice and dogs, rapid accumulation of radioactivity occurred in the liver, followed by deiodination. This finding limits the potential usefulness as a "clot-detecting agent."

Fibrinogen, labeled either with ^{125}I or ^{131}I, has been used extensively for detecting sites of thrombi, especially in the deep veins in the legs. Were the label to be changed to ^{123}I instead, then estimation of the depth by the x-ray/γ-ray ratio method[1,8,56–58] described above might be feasible.

Iodine-125[39] now is used extensively in radioimmunoassay methods.[131,132] In procedures carried out during a few hours, opportunities to increase the sensitivity up to ~100-fold arise by substituting 13-hr ^{123}I for 60-day [125]I.[18]

Welch[133] cleverly labeled albumin with ^{123}I by freezing it in an ampoule along with [123]Xe that he had generated in the [122]Te(^{3}He,2n)[123]Xe reaction. During decay of 2-hr [123]Xe into ^{123}I, the recoil energy was adequate to attach the ^{123}I to the albumin. This "recoil" method has the potential to label compounds of biological interest in extremely high specific activity since no carrier [127]I is involved.

Low-Energy Particles from Electron-Capture Nuclides

The sum of the LMM (2.9 keV) and MXY (0.8 keV) Auger electrons is 311 per 100 disintegrations of [123]I (Table 3-1). The aggregate energies of these very low-energy electrons is calculated to be only ~17 percent of the total energy of the conversion and the Auger electrons plus the L x-rays, in the case of [123]I.

There are those who feel these low-energy electrons that accompany the decay of nuclides by electron capture may have an unusually high relative biological effectiveness (RBE). This may be due to differences in the mode of energy transfer to give rise to qualitatively disproportionately large biological effects.[134-138]

The ranges of these low-energy Auger electrons from [123]I([121]I, ^{125}I, etc.) in water are of the order of approximately only 0.1 to 0.3 μm[139] and any enhanced effects may occur "as a result of the vacancy cascade which gives rise to extensive internal electron transfer and multi-center coulombic repulsion of the many positive charge centers which build up on the molecule."[140] More data are required to assess any significance of this "Auger effect" in the use of [123]I.

REDUCED RADIATION TO PATIENTS

Whenever a physician introduces a radionuclide into his patient to aid in diagnosis, he prudently strives to make his measurements with least radiation (Tables 3-2 and 3-4). In doing so he embraces conclusions that "all steps designed to minimize irradiation of human populations will act to the benefit of human health" and that "even the smallest amounts of radiation are liable to cause deleterious genetic, and perhaps also somatic, effects"[141] and he is guided by the strong recommendation "that every effort be made to reduce exposures to all types of ionizing radiations to the lowest possible level."[142] Continuing concern regarding additional exposures, which stem from the rapidly increasing employment of in vivo nuclear-medical procedures, has been expressed in the literature.[143-145]

The current availability now of iodine-123 has demonstrated our capacity to meet the challenge to "ensure that full advantage is taken of all techniques which lead to reduction of patient dose in diagnostic exami-

Table 3-4
Advantages of Cyclotron-Generated Radioiodine-123

---

1. *Reduced radiation exposures to patients*
   (a) Especially significant in children and during pregnancy
   (b) 18.8-hr average life is highly appropriate; matches closely the common 24-hr thyroid "uptake"
   (c) Thus, little residual exposure after the desired diagnostic information has been derived

2. Studies repeatable at intervals as short as only 3 days
   (a) to evaluate physiological or pharmacological changes
   (b) for confirmation when initial study is equivocal

3. Improved resolution and statistics; briefer imaging times

4. Diminished interference with other radionuclide procedures

5. Decreased radiation self-decomposition of labeled substances

6. Dies away promptly; radiation ceases quickly; rapidly "self-scavenging." Usually simplifies handling and facilities

7. Radiation readily shielded; decreased exposures to personnel

---

nation . . . and give every encouragement to the new developments in engineering and physics which will allow smaller and smaller doses of radiation to be used."[146]

The advent of the commercially fabricated "biomedical cyclotron"[19,87,117–122] with which to generate the ^{123}I that is now reducing radiation,[1,2,8,11,18] as well as the scintillation camera[18,19,30,31,34,38,147,148] with which to image its distribution in vivo, represent but two of the many advances "in engineering and physics" which now effectively support this view.

In his address at the dedication of The Biomedical Cyclotron at UCLA[87] Professor Seaborg (co-discoverer of [131]I[66]) said:

Perhaps one of the most important medical isotopes this cyclotron will be making is iodine-123, an isotope with a half-life of 13.3 hours. The short half-life of this isotope compared with the half-lives of other readily available iodine isotopes, makes it the iodine isotope of choice for an increasing number of diagnostic procedures; further, the energies of the photons emitted are ideal for scanning purposes.

It is expected, therefore, that many of the diagnostic tests based on use of iodine-131 in various forms and compounds will be reevaluated with iodine-123. The dose commitment to the patient from the test will be much smaller and tests can be repeated if necessary after much shorter waiting periods. If iodine-123 works out as expected, perhaps iodine-131 will in large part be reserved for therapy and those circumstances where the radiopharmaceutical must be shipped fair distances or where transportation is uncertain. With its 13.3 hours half-life, there is time to transport iodine-123 for local use or, if it is needed farther away, to ship it by air.

There is no question about the utility of iodine-123. The question is whether enough can be produced in the present target-cyclotron configuration and then rapidly extracted for conversion into pharmaceutically suitable forms. If this alone can be accomplished, AEC's investment of men, machines, and time shall have been a major success.

HISTORICAL EPILOGUE

The story of ^{123}I is an especially interesting one, historically. The intuition of Professor Ernest Lawrence was the beginning of nuclear medicine in his recognition in 1934, within 6 months after the discovery of man-made radioactivity, of the applicability of radionuclides created in large quantities in his cyclotron.[149] "In the biological field radio-sodium has interesting possibilities that hardly need be emphasized here."

And it was he again who indicated this cognizance by designating his new 60-in. Crocker cyclotron as a "medical" cyclotron, in 1939.[21] During the next several years, ^{123}I unknowingly was being generated[4] with it in the $^{122}Te(d,n)^{123}I$ reaction, a way it is now being made commercially.[18]

A decade later the same Crocker "medical" cyclotron was used in the discovery of ^{123}I in the $^{121}Sb(^{4}He,2n)^{123}I$ reaction.[20] And the author had the pleasure of generating ^{123}I for biomedical applications,[2] also in this way in the same instrument.

When the 88-in. cyclotron became operational at The Lawrence Berkeley Laboratory, the 60-in. Crocker cyclotron was dismantled in 1962 and transferred to the Davis campus of The University of California. There, after modernizing alterations, the energies of proton beams were greatly increased. Hence, it became possible recently[84,85] to generate ^{123}I in the highest yields and purity in the same Crocker "medical" cyclotron[21] by a variation of the indirect method[2,70] of a discoverer of ^{123}I[20] in the $^{127}I(p,5n)^{123}Xe \rightarrow ^{123}I$ reactions.

REFERENCES

1. Myers WG: Radioisotopes of iodine, in Radioactive Pharmaceuticals, AEC Symposium Series 6, Proceedings of a Symposium, Oak Ridge Institute of Nuclear Studies, November 1–4, 1965, USAEC CONF-651111, Chapter 12, pp 217–243
2. Myers WG, Anger HO: Radioiodine-123. J Nucl Med 3:183, 1962

3.   Hupf HB, Eldridge JS, Beaver JE: Production of iodine-123 for medical applications. Int J Appl Radiat 19:345–351, 1968

4.   Myers WG: Comparisons of I^{131}, I^{125}, and I^{123} for in vivo and in vitro applications in diagnosis, in Transactions of the Seventh International Congress of Internal Medicine, Munich, 1962, vol 2. Stuttgart, Georg Thieme Verlag, 1963, pp 858–863

5.   Hine GJ, Johnston RE: Absorbed dose from radionuclides. J Nucl Med 11:468–469, 1970

6.   Vennart J, Minski M: Radiation doses from administered radionuclides. Br J Radiol 35:372–387, 1962

7.   Lawrence JH: Nuclear techniques in biomedical research. Nucleonics 23(1):48–49, 1965

8.   Myers WG: Radioiodine-123 for scanning. J Nucl Med 7:390–391, 1966

9.   Rhodes BA, Wagner HN Jr, Gerrard M: Iodine-123: development and usefulness of a new radiopharmaceutical. Isot Radiat Technol 4:275–280, 1967

10. Wellman HN, Anger RT Jr: Radioiodine dosimetry and the use of radioiodines other than ^{131}I in thyroid diagnosis. Semi Nucl Med 1:356–378, 1971

11. Nishiyama H, Sodd VJ, Ashare AB, Berke RA, Saenger EL: Comparison of collimator and clinical value for ^{123}I and ^{131}I for thyroid disease. J Nucl Med 14:434, 1973

12. Fateeva MN: Radioactive isotopes of iodine in the diagnosis and treatment of diseases of the thyroid gland, in Lawrence JH (ed): Progress in Atomic Medicine, vol 1. New York, Grune & Stratton, 1965, Chapter 8, pp 174–218

13. Greenfield MA, Lane RG: Radioisotope dosimetry, in Blahd WH (ed): Nuclear Medicine (ed 2). New York, McGraw-Hill, 1971, Chapter 5, pp 101–128

14. Saenger EL, Kereiakes JG: The safe tracer dose in medical investigation, in Lawrence JH (ed): Recent Advances in Nuclear Medicine, vol 3. New York, Grune & Stratton, 1971, Chapter 5, pp 139–165

15. Wagner HN Jr, Rhodes BA: The radiopharmaceutical, in Wagner HN Jr (ed): Principles of Nuclear Medicine. Philadelphia, Saunders, 1968, Chapter 6, pp 259–301

16. Maynard CD: Clinical Nuclear Medicine. Philadelphia, Lea & Febiger, 1969

17. Fulmer LR: Personal communication, July 1973

18. Myers WG, Anger HO, Lamb JF, Winchell HS: Radioiodine-123 for applications in diagnosis. LBL-1722; IAEA/SM-171/34. Proceedings of a Symposium on New Developments in Radiopharmaceuticals and Labelled Compounds, Copenhagen, Denmark, March 26–30, 1973. Vienna, IAEA, 1973, vol I, pp 249–256

19. Myers WG: Glimpses into some future aspects of nuclear medicine, in Horst W, Pabst HW (eds): Ergebnisse der klinischen Nuklearmedizin, Transactions, 7th Jahrestagung Gesellschaft für Nuklearmedizin, September 25–27, 1969, Zürich. Stuttgart, Schattauer Verlag, 1971, pp 306–319 (in English)

20. Marquez L, Perlman I: Neutron deficient isotopes of iodine. UCRL-555, 1949, 10 pp; Phys Rev 78: 189–190, 1950

21. Lawrence EO: The medical cyclotron of the William H. Crocker Radiation Laboratory. Science 90:407–408, 1939

22. Aebersold PC: The cyclotron: A nuclear transformer. Radiology 39:513–540, 1942

23. Mitchell ACG, Mei JY, Maienschein FC, Peacock CL: Disintegration of I^{124} and I^{126}. Phys Rev 76:1450–1453, 1949

24. Sergolle H, Albouy G, Bouloumié J, Lagrange JM, Marcus L, Pautrat M: Contribution a l'étude de la désintégration de $^{123}_{53}$I. J Phys 28:383–387, 1967

25. Ragaini RC, Walters WB, Gordon GE, Baedecker PA: Decay scheme of 13.3 h ^{123}I. Nucl Phys A115:611–624, 1968

26. Spejewski EH, Hopke PK, Loeser FW Jr: Levels in ^{119,121,123}Te. Nucl Phys A146:182–192, 1970

27. Dillman LT: Personal communication, July 31, 1973

28. Dillman LT, Von der Lage FC: Radionuclide decay schemes and nuclear parameters for use in radiation-dose estimation. J Nucl Med Suppl Pamphlet 10 (in press)

29. Anger HO, Davis DH: Gamma-ray detection efficiency and image resolution in sodium iodide. Rev Sci Instrum 35:693–697, 1964

30. Anger HO, Van Dyke DC, Gottschalk A, Yano Y, Schaer LR: The scintillation camera in diagnosis and research. Nucleonics 23(1):57–62, 1965

31. Powell MR, Anger HO: Blood flow visualization with the scintillation camera. J Nucl Med 7:729–732, 1966

32. Myers WG: A gamma-ray carrier compound useful for clinical physiologic dynamic studies. Int J Appl Radiat 2:158–159, 1957

33. Koons CR: Synthesis of and pharmacological studies on 4-hydroxy-3,5-diiodobenzoic acid labeled with radioiodine-131. MMSc Thesis, The Ohio State University, Columbus, Ohio, 1957

34. Myers WG: Scintillation camera for in vivo studies of dynamic processes. J Nucl Med 4:182, 1963

35. Myers WG, Hunter WW Jr: Radiocarbon-11 for scanning. J Nucl Med 8:305, 1967

36. Matthews CME: Comparison of isotopes for scanning. J Nucl Med 6:155–168, 1965

37. Beck RN, Schuh MW, Cohen TD, Lembares N: Effects of scattered radiation on scintillation detector response, in Medical Radioisotope Scintigraphy, vol 1, Proceedings of a Symposium, IAEA, Salzburg, Austria, August 6–15, 1968. Vienna, IAEA, 1969, pp 595–616

38. Anger HO: Radioisotope Cameras, in Hine GJ (ed): Instrumentation in Nuclear Medicine. New York, Academic Press, 1967, Chapter 19, pp 485–552

39. Myers WG, Vanderleeden JC: Radioiodine-125. J Nucl Med 1:149–164, 1960

40. Dettman PM, Myers WG: Radioiodine-125 for evaluation of thyroid function. Surg Forum 12:17–19, 1961

41. Myers WG: On a new source of x-rays. Ohio State Med J 58:772–773, 1962

42. Winter CC, Myers WG: I-125, a new radioisotope for the labeled hippuran renogram. J Urol 88:100–102, 1962

43. Myers WG: Applications of Radioiodine-125 in Medicine and Biology, 1960–1964, in Deutscher Röntgenkongress 1964. Proceedings Deutschen Röntgengesellschaft, Wiesbaden. Stuttgart, Georg Thieme Verlag, 1965, Part A, pp 61–72

44. Myers WG: Radioiodine-125 radiation sources. J Nucl Med 8:331, 1967

45. Vanderleeden JC: The development of counting techniques for low energy gamma radiation for applications in biology. MSc Thesis, The Ohio State University, Columbus, Ohio, 1959, 91 pp

46. Harper PV, Endlich H, Lathrop KA, Siemens W: Clinical experience with I^{125}. J Nucl Med 2:127, 1961

47. Endlich H, Harper P, Beck R, Siemens W, Lathrop K: The use of I^{125} to increase isotope scanning resolution. Am J Roentgenol Radium Ther Nucl Med 87:148–155, 1962

48. Levy LM, Estrellado TT, Okezie O, Stern HS: The use of I-125 in clinical nuclear medicine. J Nucl Med 3:183–184, 1962

49. Fellinger K, Höffer R, Vetter H: Szintigraphie der Schilddrüse mit Jod-125. Nuclear Medizin 3:20–24, 1962

50. Beronius P, Forberg S, Henrikson C-O, Söremark R: The use of iodine-125 as an x-ray source in roentgen diagnostics. Int J Appl Radiat 13:253–254, 1962

51. Cameron JR, Sorenson J: Measurement of bone mineral in vivo: An improved method. Science 142:230–232, 1963

52. Charkes ND, Sklaroff DM: The use of iodine 125 in thyroid scintiscanning. Am J Roentgenol Radium Ther Nucl Med 90:1052–1058, 1963

53. Ter-Pogossian M, Kastner J, Vest TB: Autofluorography of the thyroid gland by means of image amplification. Radiology 81:984–988, 1963

54. Scheer KE, Zum Winkel K, Georgi M: Compounds labeled with low-energy gamma-ray emitters for medical isotope scanning, in Medical Radioisotope Scanning, vol 2, Proceedings of a Symposium, IAEA, Athens, Greece, April 20–24, 1964. Vienna, IAEA, 1964, pp 47–69

55. Ben-Porath M, Hochman A, Gross J: Scanning with iodine-125, in Medical Radioisotope Scanning, vol 2, Proceedings of a Symposium, IAEA, Athens, Greece, April 20–24, 1964. Vienna, IAEA, 1964, pp 71–77

56. Myers WG: Discussion, in Medical Radioisotope Scanning, vol 1, Proceedings of a Symposium, IAEA, Athens, Greece, April 20–24, 1964. Vienna, IAEA, 1964, pp 417–418

57. Dare JG: Personal communications, 1964–1965

58. Lichtenstein JE: In vivo localization of radioisotopes that emit both gamma-rays and x-rays. MSc Thesis, Ohio State University, Columbus, Ohio, 1966, 110 pp

59. Tauxe WN, Dolan CT: A double-isotope approach to the estimation of depth of source in scintigraphic matrices. J Nucl Med 10:188–191, 1969

60. Lederer CM, Hollander JM, Perlman I: Table of Isotopes (ed 6). New York, Wiley, 1967

61. Myers WG: Radioiodine-121. J Nucl Med 7:390, 1966

62. Myers WG: Adaptations of a physics department cyclotron for generating radionuclides for biomedical applications, in Symposium on the Use of Cyclotrons in Medicine. London, Hammersmith Hospital, 1969

63. Richards P: Personal communication, 1965

64. Hamilton JG, Soley MH: Studies in iodine metabolism by the use of a new radioactive isotope of iodine. Am J Physiol 127:557–572, 1939

65. Hamilton JG, Soley MH: Studies in iodine metabolism of the thyroid gland in situ by the use of radio-iodine in normal subjects and in patients with various types of goiter. Am J Physiol 131:135–143, 1940

66. Livingood JJ, Seaborg GT: Radioactive isotopes of iodine. Phys Rev 54:775–782, 1938

67. Hamilton JG: The use of radioactive tracers in biology and medicine. Radiology 39:541–572, 1942

68. Hevesy G: Radioactive Indicators. New York, Interscience, 1948, 556 pp

69. Winchell HS: Personal communication, March 28, 1973

70. Perlman I: Personal communication, December 8, 1961

71. Sodd VJ, Blue J: Cyclotron generator of high purity ^{123}I. J Nucl Med 9:349, 1968

72. Bureau of Radiological Health, US Department of Health, Education, and Welfare: ^{123}I: new production method. Isot Radiat Technol 7:28, 1969

73. Sodd VJ, Blue JW, Scholz KL: ^{123}I production at energies attainable with the compact cyclotron. J Nucl Med 10:371, 1969

74a. Sodd VJ, Blue JW, Scholz KL: ^{123}I production for pharmaceutical use, in Amphlett CB (ed): Uses of Cyclotrons in Chemistry, Metallurgy, and Biology. London, Butterworths, UKAEA, 1970, pp 125–137

74b. Blue JW, Sodd VJ: ^{123}I production from the β^+ decay of ^{123}Xe, in Amphlett CB (ed): Uses of Cyclotrons in Chemistry, Metallurgy, and Biology. London, Butterworths UKAEA, 1970, pp 138–148

75. Sodd VJ, Scholz KL, Blue JW, Wellman HN: Cyclotron Production of ^{123}I—an Evaluation of the Nuclear Reactions Which Produce This Isotope. US Department of Health, Education, and Welfare BRH/DMRE 70-4. Washington, DC, US Government Printing Office, 1970, 38 pp

76. Wellman HN, Sodd VJ, Mack JF: Production and clinical development of a new ideal radioisotope of iodine—iodine-123, in Horst W (ed): Frontiers of Nuclear Medicine. New York, Springer, 1971, pp 19–30

77. Sodd VJ, Blue JW, Scholz KL: Pure ^{123}I production with a gas-flow target. J Nucl Med 12:395–396, 1971

78. Lambrecht RM, Wolf AP: The ^{122}Te(^{4}He,3n)^{123}Xe $\xrightarrow[2.1\ hr]{\beta^+,EC}$ ^{123}I generator. Radiat Res 52:32–46, 1972

79. Lambrecht RM, Mantescu C, Atkins HL, Wolf AP: Development of new ^{123}I radiopharmaceuticals. Trans Am Nucl Soc 15:131–132, 1972

80. Lambrecht RM, Mantescu C, Redvanly C, Wolf AP: Preparation of high-purity carrier-free ^{123}I-iodine monochloride as iodination reagent for synthesis of radiopharmaceuticals, IV. J Nucl Med 13:266–273, 1972

81. Lambrecht RM, Norton E, Wolf AP: Kit for carrier-free ^{123}I-sodium iodide. VIII. J Nucl Med 14:269–273, 1973

82. Lambrecht RM, Wolf AP: The cyclotron and short-lived halogen isotopes for radiopharmaceutical applications, in Proceedings of a Symposium on New Developments in Radiopharmaceuticals and Labeled Compounds, Copenhagen, Denmark, March, 26–30, 1973. IAEA/SM-171/79. Vienna, IAEA, 1973, vol I, pp 275–290

83. Wolf AP, Christman DR, Fowler JS, Lambrecht RM: Synthesis of radiopharmaceuticals and labeled compounds utilizing short-lived isotopes, in Proceedings of a Symposium on New Developments in Radiopharmaceuticals and Labeled Compounds, Copenhagen, Denmark, March 26–30, 1973. IAEA/SM-171/92. Vienna, IAEA, 1973, vol I, pp 345–381

84. Fusco MA, Peek NF, Jungerman JA, Zielinski FW, DeNardo SJ, DeNardo GL: An inexpensive new method for the cyclotron production of ^{123}I. J Nucl Med 13:430–431, 1972

85. Fusco MA, Peek NF, Jungerman JA, Zielinski FW, DeNardo SJ, DeNardo GL: Production of carrier-free ^{123}I using the ^{127}I(p,5n)^{123}Xe reaction. J Nucl Med 13:729–732, 1972

86. Richards P, Lebowitz E, Stang, LG Jr: The Brookhaven Linac Isotope Producer (BLIP), in Proceedings of a Symposium on New Developments in Radiopharmaceuticals and Labeled Compounds, Copenhagen, Denmark,

March 26–30, 1973. IAEA/SM-171/38. Vienna, IAEA, 1973, vol I, pp 325–341

87. Seaborg GT: Remarks at the dedication of the Biomedical Cyclotron, University of California at Los Angeles, June 30, 1971. Washington, DC, US AEC, pp 1–5

88. Hupf HB: ORNL isotopes development center's cooperative program in new medical radionuclides. J Nucl Med 7:798–799, 1966

89. Rhodes BA, Buddemeyer EU, Stern HS, Wagner HN Jr: The use of iodine-123 in studies of iodine metabolism. J Nucl Med 7:385, 1966

90. Lebowitz E, Greene MW, Richards P: On the production of ^{123}I for medical use. Int J Appl Radiat Isot 22:489–491, 1971

91. O'Brien HA, Ogard A: Investigations of the preparaton of ^{89}Sr, ^{123}I, ^{127}Xe, and ^{129}Cs at LAMPF from spallation reactions in lanthanum and molybdenum. J Nucl Med 14:635–636, 1973

92. Silvester DJ, Sugden J, Watson IA: Preparation of iodine-123 by α-particle bombardment of natural antimony. Radiochem Radioanal Lett 2(1):17–20, 1969

93. Neirinckx R: Purification of cyclotron-produced iodine-123 by liquid-liquid extraction. Radiochem Radioanal Lett 5(4–5):205–208, 1970

94. Lötter MG, Van der Merwe EJ, Van Heerden PDR, Le Roux PLM: The use of ^{123}I in thyroid diagnosis. S Afr Med J 46:186–189, 1972

95. Schwind RA, Rutherford WM: Stable isotope enrichment by thermal diffusion, chemical exchange, and distillation, in Proceedings of a Symposium on New Developments in Radiopharmaceuticals and Labeled Compounds, Copenhagen, Denmark, March 26–30, 1973. IAEA/SM-171/47. Vienna, IAEA, 1973, vol II, pp 255–266

96. Myers WG: Discussion of reference 95, pp 265–266

97. Lamb JF: Radioactivation by ^{3}He bombardment: a practical analytical system. UCRL-18981. PhD Thesis, University of California at Berkeley, 1969

98. Jastram PS: Personal communication, July 24, 1973

99. Blue JW, Sodd VJ, Scholz KL: ^{123}I production from spallation reactions. J Nucl Med 12:417, 1971

100. Blue JW, Sodd VJ, Scholz KL, Roberts WK: ^{123}I production for use in nuclear medicine by spallation of xenon. Int J Nucl Med Biol 1:51–52, 1973

101. Wellman HN, Mack JF: Study of preliminary experience with the use of ^{123}I for thyroid function and scanning compared to ^{131}I. J Nucl Med 9:359, 1968

102. Wellman HN, Mack JF, Saenger EL: Study of the parameters influencing the clinical use of ^{123}I. J Nucl Med 10:381, 1969

103. Sodd VJ, Wellman HN, Branson BM: ^{123}I thyroid measurements with a Ge(Li) detector. J Nucl Med 10:136–139, 1969

104. Crist J, Simmons GH, Wellman HN: Effects of radioisotopic contamination on ^{123}I thyroid scanning. J Nucl Med 10:457–458, 1969

105. Sodd VJ, Scholz KL, Blue JW, Wellman HN: Evaluation of nuclear reactions that produce ^{123}I in the cyclotron. Isot Radiat Technol 9:154–159, 1971–1972

106. Sutton JD, Eister WK: ^{123}I for diagnostic application—cooperative study by PHS, AEC, and clinical investigators. J Nucl Med 10:444, 1969

107. Atkins HL, Klopper JF, Lambrecht R, Wolf A: A comparison of ^{99m}Tc and ^{123}I in thyroid imaging. J Nucl Med 13:411, 1972

108. Atkins HL, Klopper JF, Lambrecht RM, Wolf AP: A comparison of technetium 99m and iodine 123 for thyroid imaging. Am J Roentgenol Radium Ther Nucl Med 117:195–201, 1973

109. DeNardo GL: Private communication, June 14, 1973

110. Verdon TA Jr: Private communication, June 14, 1973

111. Halpern S, Alazraki N, Littenberg R, Hurwitz S, Green J, Kunsa J, Ashburn W: ^{131}I thyroid uptakes: capsules versus liquid. J Nucl Med 14:507–510, 1973

112. Rosenthall L: A fifteen minute test of the rate of thyroid trapping of radioiodine. J Nucl Med 5:657–663, 1964

113. Kohler PO, Wynn J: One-hour thyroid uptake of radioactive iodine. Arch Intern Med 116:177–182, 1965

114. Raventos A, Hale J, Chamberlain RH: Two-hour uptake of iodine 131 by the thyroid. Radiology 75:446–449, 1960

115. Wollman SH: Kinetics of accumulation of radioiodine by thyroid gland: longer time intervals. Am J Physiol 202:189–192, 1962

116. Azevedo MF, Trancoso WL: Use of ^{132}I for diagnostic studies of thyroid gland. Int J Appl Radiat Isotopes 16:41–51, 1965

117. Laughlin JS, Tilbury RS, Dahl JR: The cyclotron: source of short-lived radionuclides and positron emitters for medicine, in Lawrence JH (ed): Recent Advances in Nuclear Medicine, vol 3. New York, Grune & Stratton, 1971, Chapter 3, pp 39–62

118. Laughlin JS, Mamacos JP, Tilbury RS: Isochronous cyclotron installation for radionuclide production. Radiology 93:331–337, 1969

119. Ter-Pogossian MM, Wagner HN Jr: A new look at the cyclotron for making short-lived isotopes. Nucleonics 24(10):50–56, 1966

120. Clark JC, Matthews CME, Silvester DJ, Vonberg DD: Using cyclotron-produced isotopes at Hammersmith Hospital. Nucleonics 25(6):54–62, 1967

121. Proceedings of the Hammersmith Hospital Symposium on the Use of Cyclotrons in Medicine, September 20, 1969, London

122. Gelbard AS, Hara T, Tilbury RS, Laughlin JS: Recent aspects of cyclotron production of medically useful isotopes, in Proceedings of a Symposium on New Developments in Radiopharmaceuticals and Labeled Compounds, Copenhagen, Denmark, March 26–30, 1973. IAEA/SM-171/93. Vienna, IAEA, 1973, vol I, pp 239–247

123. Myers WG: Discussion, in Dynamic Clinical Studies with Radioisotopes, Proceedings of a Symposium at Oak Ridge Institute for Nuclear Studies, October 21–25, 1963. AEC Symposium Series 3, TID-7678. Washington DC, US AEC, pp 431–432

124. Van Middlesworth L, Turner JA, Lipscomb A: Liver function related to thyroxine metabolism. J Nucl Med 4:132–138, 1963

125. Howell GL, Van Middlesworth L: Gastric iodide and chloride clearances in dogs. Proc Soc Exp Biol Med 93:602–605, 1956

126. Czerniak P, Bank H, Sinkower A, Adams R: Usefulness of radionuclides in evaluation of stomach disorders. Semin Nucl Med 2:288–301, 1972

127. Wellman HN, Berke RA, Robbins PJ, Anger RT Jr: Dynamic quantitative renal imaging with ^{123}I-hippuran—a possible salvation of the renogram. J Nucl Med 12:405–406, 1971

128. Myers WG: Personal communication to M. Tubis, June 1957. Discussion in Radioactive Pharmaceuticals, Proceedings of a Symposium at Oak Ridge Institute for Nuclear Studies, November 1–4, 1965. AEC Symposium Series 6. USAEC Conf-651111. p 293

129. Drouet J, Goutheraud R, Amouch P-J, De Vernejoul P, Barritault L, Kellershohn C: Comparaison de l'utilisation de l'albumine et des macroagrégats d'albumine marquée au technétium 99m et a l'iode 123 pour l'étude de la dynamique cardio-pulmonaire. J Biol Med Nucl 4:21–24, 1969

130. Coates G, DeNardo SJ, DeNardo GL: Pharmacokinetics of radioiodinated streptokinase. J Nucl Med 14:623–624, 1973

131. Kirkham KE, Hunter WM (eds): Radioimmunoassay Methods. Baltimore, Williams & Wilkins, 1971.

132. Odell WD, Daughaday WH (eds): Principles of Competitive Protein-Binding Assays. Philadelphia, Lippincott, 1971

133. Welch MJ: Labeling with iodine-123. The reactivity of iodine-123 formed by the decay of xenon-123. J Am Chem Soc 92:408–409, 1970

134. Stone RS: Maximum Permissible Exposure Standards, vol 13, in Proceedings of the International Conference on the Peaceful Uses of Atomic Energy, Geneva, 1955. New York, United Nations, 1956, pp. 132–138

135. Myers WG: Discussion, in Medical Radionuclides: Radiation Dose and Effects, Proceedings of a Symposium, Oak Ridge Associated Universities, December 8–11, 1969. AEC Symposium Series 20, pp 292–293

136a. Feige Y, Gavron A, Lubin E, Lewitus Z, Ben-Porath M, Gross J, Loewinger E: Local energy deposition in thyroid cells due to the incorporation of ^{125}I, in Biophysical Aspects of Radiation Quality. Vienna, IAEA, 1971, pp 383–404

136b. Lewitus Z, Ben-Porath M, Feige Y, Lubin E, Rechnic J, Laor Y: Differences in the radiobiological action of ^{125}I and ^{131}I in the thyroid cell, in Biophysical Aspects of Radiation Quality. Vienna, IAEA, 1971, pp 405–417

136c. Feinendegen LE, Ertl HH, Bond VP: Biological toxicity associated with the Auger effect, in Biophysical Aspects of Radiation Quality. Vienna, IAEA, 1971, pp 419–430

137. Gavron A, Feige Y: Dose distribution and maximum permissible burden of ^{125}I in the thyroid gland. Health Phys 23:491–499, 1972

138. Wrenn ME, Howells GP, Hairr LM, Paschoa AS: Auger electron dosimetry. Health Phys 24:645–653, 1973

139. Berger MJ: Distribution of absorbed dose around point sources of electrons and beta particles in water and other media. J Nucl Med 12:Suppl 5, March 1971 (MIRD Pamphlet 7)

140. Emmons AH: Extraordinary destruction of the catalase molecule by the Auger effect. Health Phys 8:460–461, 1962

141. Report of the United Nations Scientific Committee on the Effects of Atomic Radiation, General Assembly, Official Records: Thirteenth Session, Supplement No. 17 (A/3838). New York, United Nations, 1958, p 41

142. Recommendations of the International Commission on Radiological Protection, National Bureau of Standards, Handbook 47. Washington DC, US Government Printing Office, 1951, p 2

143. Reduction of Radiation Exposure in Nuclear Medicine, in Proceedings of a Symposium, August 7–9, 1967, at Michigan State University. US Department of Health, Education, and Welfare, National Center for Radiological Health, Rockville, Maryland. Washington DC, US Government Printing Office, 1967, 153 pp

144. The Effects on Populations of Exposures to Low Levels of Ionizing Radiation. Division of Medical Sciences, National Academy of Sciences, National Research Council, Washington, DC, 1972, 217 pp

145. Adelstein SJ: The risk:benefit ratio in nuclear medicine. Hosp Pract 8:141–149, 1973
146. Lamerton LF: An examination of the clinical and experimental data relating to the possible hazard to the individual of small doses of radiation. Br J Radiol 31:229–239, 1958
147. Anger HO: Gamma-ray and positron scintillation camera. Nucleonics 21(10):56–59, 1963
148. Myers WG: Dynamic studies with a gamma-ray scintillation camera, in Medical Radioisotope Scanning, vol 1, Proceedings of an IAEA Symposium, Athens, Greece, April 20–24, 1964. Vienna, IAEA, 1964, pp 377–387
149. Lawrence EO: Radioactive sodium produced by deuton bombardment. Phys Rev 46:746, 1934

Rainer Storb

E. Donnall Thomas

4

Irradiation and Marrow Transplantation

INTRODUCTION

Soon after the discovery of x-rays, a number of investigators performed studies on the effect of this new physical agent on the living organism. The studies of Heineke,[1,2] and Benjamin and Sluka[3] were the first to focus attention on the exquisite radiosensitivity of lymphoid and hemopoietic tissues and also the immune response. Susceptibility to infection and hemorrhagic complications were the most prominent features of radiation injury in experimental animals. Probably the first attempts at modifying radiation injury were made by Fabricious-Moeller in 1922.[4] He noticed that shielding the legs of guinea pigs prevented the usual depression of platelet counts and the hemorrhagic picture following total body irradiation (TBI). These studies did not receive widespread attention, and it was only during the development of the atomic bomb that further extensive studies of the effects of irradiation on the hemopoietic system were carried out. An important landmark was the finding of Jacobsen et al[5] in 1949 that mice could be protected from an otherwise lethal exposure to whole-body x-irradiation by exteriorizing and shielding the spleen. Shortly thereafter Lorenz et al[6] obtained impressive irradiation protection by the infusion of syngeneic marrow to mice and guinea pigs immediately after irradiation. These early studies led to the concept that "humoral factors" were present

This investigation was supported by Public Health Service research grant CA 10895 from the National Cancer Institute.

Dr. Thomas is supported by Research Career Award AI 02425 from the National Institute of Allergy and Infectious Diseases, National Institutes of Health.

161

in the shielded spleen or in the infused hemopoietic tissues which induced rapid restoration of the irradiated hemopoietic tissues in the body. Support for the "humoral" hypothesis came from Cole et al,[7] who showed that cell "extracts" of the hemopoietic tissues were also therapeutically effective. These results could not be confirmed by others, and it seems now to be certain that Cole's positive findings were entirely due to the presence of intact living cells in the "extract." By 1955 an increasing number of authors expressed their doubts as to the correctness of the "humoral factor" hypothesis. Three independent groups of investigators using different experimental designs demonstrated irrefutably that the life-saving effect of hemopoietic cell infusions was due to a cellular mechanism.[8–10] Subsequently, a number of other authors confirmed this evidence, and it can now be stated with certainty that the aplastic marrow spaces produced by irradiation can be repopulated by syngeneic, allogeneic, or even xenogeneic cells.

The implications of this discovery reach far beyond the question of modifying irradiation injury. These initial observations were the baseline for further fundamental investigations of the genetics of hemopoietic cells and of the immunologic principles that govern the fate of the transplanted hemopoietic tissue.[11] The demonstration of persistence of transplanted hemopoietic cells in the irradiated host offered a variety of theoretical possibilities not only for the treatment of the patient with marrow failure but also for the replacement of malignant hemopoietic cells by normal ones. In addition, since marrow grafting replaced the host's immunologic system with donor cells, the host was then conditioned to accept grafts of other organs from the same donor.

Stimulated by the studies in inbred rodents, clinical human marrow grafting began in 1957 when the procedure was used to treat a variety of malignant and nonmalignant hemopoietic diseases.[12] This period lasted for approximately 6 years, and on the whole was very disappointing.[13] Most of the 207 reported cases of human marrow grafts failed: only 11 were successful and only 1 patient survived beyond 1 year with sustained engraftment.[14] A careful review of these initial cases showed that most of them were destined to fail from the onset because many of the conditions known from the rodent experiments to be necessary for graft acceptance could not be applied to man. An impressive finding was the recognition that extrapolation from inbred rodents to man can be a very difficult undertaking.

In view of the disappointing clinical experiences, human marrow grafting, except in a few patients with identical twin donors, was almost abandoned over the subsequent years. One of the fundamental advances was the realization that the reactions of two randomly bred animal species, dogs and monkeys, to both irradiation and hemopoietic grafting resemble in many respects those of humans. Advances in marrow grafting in these animal models, as well as new knowledge in the areas of histocompatibility typing, immunosuppressive drug therapy, and in supportive measures for patients with decreased immune mechanisms have led to renewed efforts in clinical marrow grafting. Patients with marrow failure due to nonmalignant causes who have an identical twin or patients with combined immune deficiency diseases have benefited from marrow grafts without conditioning by an immunosuppressive agent. The individual who has achieved immunologic maturity, whether he suffers from aplastic anemia or acute leukemia, requires conditioning by a powerful immunosuppressive agent preceding marrow infusion. More recently, cyclophosphamide (CY), a chemotherapeutic agent, has received investigative attention and has been used as a conditioning agent in experimental and clinical marrow grafting. Other chemical and biological agents such as antilymphocyte serum (ALS) are currently under investigation. The most widely used conditioning agent, however, has been TBI. This chapter discusses studies of irradiation and marrow grafting in animal species and the current status of clinical marrow grafting for marrow failure and hemopoietic malignancy.

IRRADIATION DOSE

Toxicities

Extensive investigations in rodents and primates as well as isolated observations in human beings have shown that three different irradiation syndromes can be distinguished: cerebral, gastrointestinal, and hemopoietic.[15] The cerebral syndrome in animals has been observed following exposures exceeding 12,000 rads. Death occurs within 48 hr of irradiation exposure and is probably due to pyknosis of the granular cell layer of the cerebellum accompanied by widespread vasculitis, encephalitis, and brain edema. The gastrointestinal syndrome, irreversible damage to the intestinal tract, has been observed after exposures of 1500 to 12,000 rads. This syndrome is characterized by anorexia and excessive watery diarrhea leading to protein loss and water and electrolyte imbalance. Animals die between the fourth and sixth day following irradiation exposure. The hemopoietic death has been observed after exposures lower than 1500 rads. The underlying process is an inhibition of hemopoietic cell division with a resulting depletion of the hemopoietic tissues as cells mature and are released into the circulation. The first cell line to disappear from the peripheral blood is the lymphocyte. This occurs within 3 days of irradiation even after exposure to as little as 200 rads. After irradiation exposures in the "supralethal" range (>800 rads), granulocyte and platelet levels fall after exhaustion of the marrow reserve. Profound granulocytopenia occurs after 5 to 6 days and profound thrombocytopenia after 7 to 8 days. After exposures near the LD_{50} (LD is lethal dose) level, the decline in granulocytes and platelet levels is slower, occurring over an interval of 2 to 4 weeks. Due to the long life span of the red blood cell (RBC), anemia becomes prominent only at a later time period after irradiation. As a consequence of the granulocytopenia, the animal's resistance to bacterial infection decreases, setting the stage for life-threatening bacterial sepsis. Thrombocytopenia is accompanied by life-threatening hemorrhage. The exposure dose after which hemopoietic death is observed varies from species to species. For instance, in the dog, the $LD_{50}{}^{30}$ is between 300 and 400 R. In man the exposure is approximately 400 R, in the monkey 550 R, in the mouse 550 R, in the rat 600 R, and in the rabbit and the hamster 800 R. It should be emphasized that most of these data pertain to animals that were not treated with cellular blood elements nor antibiotics and isolation techniques.

CONDITIONING OF RECIPIENTS FOR MARROW TRANSPLANTATION

It is of interest to note that marrow transplantation started as a means for protecting against a lethal marrow syndrome following TBI. Studies in rodent systems as well as in randomly bred animal systems, dogs and monkeys, have shown that this protection could be achieved by infusion of syngeneic or autologous marrow obtained before and returned after irradiation exposure. When allogeneic marrow was infused after barely lethal TBI exposures, an unexpected phenomenon was encountered, the midlethal dose effect.[16] This term refers to the finding that administration of foreign marrow causes an increased mortality when compared with irradiated controls not given marrow. Uphoff[17] and Nouza and Lengerova[18] concluded after extensive studies that this midlethal dose effect is determined mainly by a host-versus-graft reaction which is observed only in a limited number of rodent strain combinations. As a matter of fact, it appears that the midlethal dose effect after allogeneic marrow grafting is the exception rather than the rule. Studies conducted in dogs in this laboratory support this view and also serve to illustrate some other features of TBI.[19] Dogs given 400, 500, or 600 R and allogeneic marrow did not die more quickly than those given irradiation only. Thus, although lethal, this amount of irradiation exposure was not sufficiently immunosuppressive to permit the persistent growth of allogeneic marrow grafts. From these studies it appears that inadequate irradiation exposures may have accounted for many of the failures of human marrow grafting in the past. Consistent and sustained allogeneic marrow grafts in the canine model were achieved only after 1200 to 1800 R midline air exposure which corresponds to a midline tissue exposure of 950 to 1500 rads. After successful engraftment, "reversal" to host type hemopoiesis has been observed in rodents and monkeys after doses up to 800 rads delivered from a single x-ray source.[20] We have not observed "reversal" in the dog.

The TBI exposure currently used in Seattle in man is 1000 rads midpoint tissue exposure delivered from dual ^{60}Co sources at a rate of 5.5 R/min. The irradiation exposure has consistently led to successful engraftment of marrow cells from HL-A (HL-A = human leukocyte antigen) identical siblings. It has been suggested that the use of higher exposure rates might lead to more consistent engraftment.[21] These data have been obtained in mice, and no studies have been carried out to determine whether they apply to larger animals.

In theory it should be possible to condition a recipient for marrow transplantation using internally administered radioactive isotopes. Advantages of this approach include the possibility of very homogeneous TBI or of selective irradiation of certain tissues. For example, Winchell et al[22] used ^{90}Y to prepare dogs for homografts and pointed out that the exposure to lymph nodes was about $2\frac{1}{2}$ times greater than that to the marrow. In practice internally administered isotopes present many problems with radiation safety procedures. Long-lived isotopes cannot be "turned off" at an optimal time for grafting and short-lived isotopes present problems in availability and dosimetry. Even so, it is unfortunate that so little experimental work has been done with this approach.

TIME OF MARROW ADMINISTRATION

Most data dealing with the question as to what interval after irradiation is the most suitable for the infusion of hemopoietic cells have been obtained with syngeneic transplants in rodents. On the basis of these studies and of data concerning the primary antibody response to various antigens in irradiated rodents following lower irradiation exposures, there seems to be general agreement that an interval of 24 hr between irradiation and transplantation is advantageous.[20] Again no studies have been conducted in larger mammals to confirm these rodent observations. In man, as well as in dogs, marrow infusions have been carried out 1 to 4 hr following irradiation with consistent success of the graft. Administration of the marrow immediately following irradiation has the advantage of shortening the period of pancytopenia, thus decreasing the length of time required for supportive care.

THE MARROW GRAFTING TECHNIQUE

The marrow grafting techniques in dogs and monkeys involve aspirations with a long needle from both humori and femora under general anesthesia. In man, multiple aspirations of marrow cells from the sternum and the anterior and posterior iliac crests are carried out.[23] To this purpose approximately 8 holes are made in the skin which then serve to carry out between 100 to 300 aspirations from the marrow cavities. Each aspiration should be kept to a minimal volume (1 to 3 ml) in order to minimize dilution with peripheral blood. The marrow is transferred to a beaker containing tissue culture medium and preservative-free heparin. The suspension is then passed through stainless steel screens of 300 and 200 μ opening. This screening is important to break up particles before intravenous (i.v.) infusion to prevent clinical problems from micropulmonary emboli. The screening results in a suspension of single cells or small clumps of cells, thus permitting accurate cell counts. The number of marrow cells infused in man ranges from 1 to 9×10^8 nucleated cells per kilogram of body weight. The volume of marrow blood suspension ranges from 400 to 800 ml which requires careful monitoring of the recipient during the infusion. In some instances phlebotomy of the recipient is carried out to avoid fluid overload. In a number of patients reported by others, the marrow was injected intraperitoneally (i.p.). It must be remembered, however, that rodent and monkey[24] experiments have shown convincingly that many more marrow cells are required for i.p. as compared to i.v. administration. Since the i.v. route has been shown to be effective in dogs, monkeys, and man, it appears to be the procedure of choice.

The aspiration, under spinal anesthesia or occasionally under general anesthesia, has been carried out in Seattle on more than 100 donors. Without exception, the procedure has been well tolerated without late sequelae.

Procurement of Hemopoietic Precursor Cells from Sources Other Than Marrow

Attempts at hemopoietic grafts in lethally irradiated rodents and dogs have been made using peripheral blood leukocytes instead of marrow or as a supplement to marrow. It was found that hemopoietic stem cells circulate in the blood of rodents[25] and dogs,[26,28] and can be used for autologous and allogeneic marrow engraftment. In vitro tests, using the agar colony technique, have suggested that such hemopoietic precursor cells may be present in human blood.[27] The data in dogs, using peripheral blood leukocytes for allogeneic engraftment, have shown that such grafts are associated with an early and severe graft-versus-host disease (GVHD).[29] In view of this potentially life-threatening complication and in view of the ease with which marrow cells can be obtained from the iliac crest, the use of peripheral blood stem cells must await a more effective separation of stem cells from the lymphocytes or a better control of GVHD.

Preservation of Marrow

Marrow is the only mammalian organ that can be stored for prolonged periods of time. Numerous investigations have been carried out in rodents, dogs, primates, and man with regard to techniques of freezing and storing marrow.[29] The efficacy of marrow graft preservation has been established by testing the capacity of the preserved cells to repopulate the marrow space in otherwise lethally irradiated rodents, dogs, and monkeys, a procedure that cannot be applied in studying human marrow. Although a number of in vitro methods have been alleged to reflect viability, they have been based mainly on the ability of the cells to exclude various dye substances. Such data have not correlated well with the cells' capacity for proliferation in vivo. More recently the viability of stored human marrow was studied using the erythropoietin assay.[30] These studies demonstrated that at least one population of precursor cells, the erythropoietin responsive cell, is functionally preserved by the freezing technique employed.

Canine marrow may be stored for periods measured in years at —169°C in 10 percent dimethyl sulfoxide. It has been possible to set up a bank of canine marrow procured from donors typed for canine histocompatibility antigens.[31] An appropriate unrelated recipient was irradiated and given the thawed marrow. Histoincompatible recipients died early while histocompatible recipients lived significantly longer. Some of these dogs have survived for more than 5 years with normal hemopoietic and immune function. These data indicate the feasibility of storing marrow from living donors or cadavers of various histocompatibility types. From such a "marrow bank" an appropriate donor marrow could be selected on the basis of the recipient's histocompatibility type.

HEMOPOIETIC ENGRAFTMENT

Role of Histocompatibility Typing

There is abundant evidence to implicate an immunologic barrier as the chief impediment to successful organ transplantation. The survival of allogeneic tissue grafts depends on the genetic, i.e., antigenic, differences between donor and recipient. We owe much of the present understanding of the role of transplantation antigens in marrow grafting to work in inbred rodent species. One major histocompatibility locus (H-2) and a number of minor loci have been shown to be the important determinants of the outcome of allogeneic grafts. A major immunogenetic system of histocompatibility has been described for every mammalian species studied so far, including rats, guinea pigs, dogs, chimpanzees, rhesus monkeys, and man.[32] It has been found that the major histocompatibility antigens are genetically determined by a locus on an autosomal chromosome. In man extensive population and family studies have resulted in the identification of at least two segregant series or subloci. A number of antigens are determined by each of these subloci, which are recognized by cytotoxic antisera raised by immunization or found in women during the course of pregnancy. A number of alleles determined by the two subloci probably are still unknown. Despite this polymorphism of the HL-A system one can find HL-A identical individuals among siblings because there are only four possible combinations of the parental haplotypes. HL-A identity can be confirmed by nonreactivity in a one-way mixed leukocyte culture (MLC).[33]

The dog has been used as a model for studies of histocompatibility and marrow grafting in a randomly bred species. Serologic histocompatibility typing and canine MLC are carried out in a manner similar to that in man.[29] MLC reactivity was shown to correlate with serologic histocompatibility typing in littermates, and approximately one-fourth of littermate pairs were nonreactive in MLC.[34] Studies in this laboratory in dogs have shown clearly that histocompatibility is an important factor governing graft rejection, development of lethal GVHD, or eventual survival of the recipient following the marrow graft. When no postgrafting immunosuppression was given, none of the histoincompatible littermates survived beyond day 25 while the survival of the histocompatible littermates was significantly prolonged. Some of the histocompatible dogs have now lived for over 6 years. Encouraging as these results are they also show that matching for DL-A (DL-A = dog leukocyte antigens) alone is not sufficient to guarantee longterm survival. Fatal GVHD was seen in approximately one-half of the DL-A matched dogs, indicating that some important antigenic differences are not detected by either serologic canine histocompatibility testing or the MLC test. The data emphasize the need for postgrafting immunosuppression even in this "compatible" situation.[35] Phenotypic matching for the major dog leukocyte antigen locus significantly prolonged the survival not only of littermate recipients but also of unrelated dogs when recipients were treated with small doses of an immunosuppressive agent postgrafting.

Two-thirds of histoincompatible canine littermates differ by one DL-A haplotype and one-third differ by two. Most unrelated dogs differ by two DL-A haplotypes, on the assumption that the complexity of the DL-A system is similar to that of the HL-A system and that the number of histocompatibility alleles is sufficiently great in the dog population. When comparing the survival of histoincompatible littermates with that of histoincompatible unrelated dogs, most recipients died with GVHD despite the use of postgrafting immunosuppression, but the littermates survived statistically longer than the unrelated recipients.[36] This probably means that the "amount" of DL-A disparity is important in determining the survival of the marrow graft recipient; i.e., cumulative effects of "major" antigen differences hasten the occurrence and increase the incidence of fatal GVHD in unrelated recipients.

Marrow grafting between human siblings differing by one or two HL-A haplotypes has generally resulted either in failure to show evidence of a marrow "take" or in death from GVHD. One patient with leukemia had a successful marrow graft from a sister differing by one HL-A haplotype followed by treatment with methotrexate (MTX) postgrafting.[37] This patient experienced severe GVHD which apparently was controlled by MTX but he died on day 56 postgrafting with a cytomegalovirus (CMV) infection.

At present HL-A identical siblings appear to offer the best possible donor–recipient combinations for marrow grafting in man. Successful grafts with this donor–recipient combination have already been reported in a number of immunodeficient patients, patients with marrow failure and leukemia. The true incidence of fatal GVHD in patients given grafts from HL-A compatible siblings is not known since most patients have been treated with postgrafting immunosuppression. A review of the presently available data suggests that approximately 50 to 75 percent of patients with successful grafts will develop GVHD, and approximately 25 percent will die of GVHD or complications thereof.[38,39]

The situation in respect to phenotypically HL-A identical unrelated individuals is unknown but most such pairs show strong reactivity in MLC, suggesting incompatibility at least for the locus governing the MLC reaction. Successful marrow grafts with such donor–recipient combinations in man have not yet been reported.

The Effect of Preceding Blood Transfusions upon Marrow Grafts

Irradiation is known to be most immunosuppressive when given before antigen administration. Studies at lower irradiation exposures have shown that the secondary immune response is more resistant than the primary response. This characteristic of irradiation is of some concern in view of the fact that most potential human marrow graft recipients have had multiple blood transfusions in the course of their disease. Since histocompatibility antigens are present on platelets and leukocytes, the recipients may be immunized against a subsequent marrow graft. With siblings matched for the major histocompatibility antigens one might not expect immunization to occur. However, recent experiments with DL-A matched littermates have shown that prior transfusions with whole blood may jeopardize the success of a marrow graft even in this "compatible" donor–recipient combination.[40] When recipients were given a single transfusion from their intended marrow donor before irradiation, marrow graft rejection and early death of the recipient with marrow hypoplasia was the rule. To a lesser degree this phenomenon was also observed after random blood transfusions.[41] Presumably, rejection was due to immunity against "minor" histocompatibility antigens that were not detected by the currently employed histocompatibility testing methods. TBI, approximately 3 times the lethal exposure, apparently was not sufficient to destroy the existing immunity. Similar data have been reported in x-irradiated mice and now also in mice treated with CY.[42] By analogy to these data obtained in the inbred mice model and the randomly bred dog model, a human patient who is a candidate for a marrow graft should be managed without blood transfusions from the intended HL-A identical donor or from other family members. The current experience in marrow grafting has justified the concern with respect to the harmful effects of previous blood transfusions. Patients who have been given transfusions from family members have a high incidence of failure of marrow engraftment or of marrow graft rejection.

Studies in dogs given multiple transfusions from unrelated donors followed by marrow grafts from histoincompatible littermates have shown that the majority of dogs rejected the graft. This finding, in combination with the high incidence of fatal GVHD in mismatched canine littermates, indicates that successful marrow transplantation between histoincompatible humans may be very difficult.

More recently studies were carried out in the dog model investigating whether immunization by preceding transfusions can be abrogated by a combination of two immunosuppressive agents, procarbazine and rabbit antidog antithymocyte serum (ATS) preceding TBI.[43] These studies, carried out in DL-A incompatible unrelated dogs, have been encouraging and indicate that immunization can be successfully abrogated by a combination of these two agents while either agent alone is not sufficient. It remains to be seen whether this information can be extrapolated to the human marrow graft situation.

Graft-versus-Host Disease

In randomly bred mammalian species, dogs, monkeys, and man, successful marrow engraftment from randomly selected donors is followed by an early, severe, and usually rapidly fatal GVHD. In rodents, depending somewhat on the strain combination, this syndrome occurs later, takes a milder course, and a variable proportion of the animals recover. GVHD is presumed to be the result of a reaction of the transplanted immunologically competent cells against host histocompatibility antigens. For unknown reasons clinical and pathologic manifestations of GVHD in animals and man primarily occur in lymph nodes, skin, liver, and gut. Detailed descriptions of these changes have been presented elsewhere.[20,44,45] Briefly, the first reaction is usually a skin rash that may progress to severe skin lesions. There is excessive diarrhea and abnormalities of liver function. Histologically, the skin lesions vary from focal or diffuse vacuolar degeneration of epidermal basal cells and acanthocytes to frank loss of epidermis. The changes in the liver involve degeneration and eosinophilic necrosis of parenchymal cells and degeneration and necrosis of the epithelium of small bile ducts. The gastrointestinal tract lesions vary from mild to marked mucosal thinning, edema, and ulceration. Severe lymphoid hypoplasia is usually observed. Lymphoid atrophy may therefore be a consequence of GVHD and may explain the impairment of immunologic defense against pathogens seen in animals with allogeneic marrow grafts. Death in dogs and monkeys given marrow from unrelated donors occurs between 7 and 25 days.[46,20] The average survival in human patients with GVHD is longer, perhaps due to better supportive care.

Prevention or Treatment of Graft-versus-Host Disease

Attempts to prevent or delay the complication of GVHD in randomly bred mammalian species have involved two major approaches. One approach has been the selection of donor and recipient by in vitro methods of histocompatibility testing. However, despite the use of the most compatible donor, an HL-A matched sibling, a wide spectrum of GVHD has been observed ranging from absent to rapidly fatal. Efforts therefore have been concentrated on the use of immunosuppressive agents after transplantation in attempts to prevent GVHD or to treat it when it appears. MTX has been found to be an effective agent to prevent or delay GVHD in mice,[47] dogs,[48] and monkeys[49] when given immediately postgrafting. Studies in dogs have shown that MTX is most effective when continued for a prolonged period of time, and stable long-term chimerism for periods of years was achieved in some DL-A incompatible graft recipients with postgrafting MTX only.[50] Other agents such as CY were beneficial in ameliorating GVHD in mice, rats, and monkeys, but various CY dose schedules used immediately postgrafting have been found ineffective in preventing lethal GVHD in dogs.[51] Studies comparing the usefulness of CY and MTX for achieving long-term survival in species other than the dog have not been carried out. Investigations using other agents, cytosine arabinoside, procarbazine, 6-mercaptopurine, or ATS, in the immediate postgrafting period have on the whole been disappointing.[52]

Based on the dog studies our current routine regimen in human recipients of HL-A matched marrow is MTX 15 mg/m^2 on day 1, and 10 mg/m^2 on days 3, 6, 11, and weekly thereafter for the first 100 days.[53] Other groups have used CY, 7.5 mg/kg for 5 doses on alternate days, beginning on the first day after marrow grafting, followed by CY at irregular intervals.[54] Despite postgrafting immunosuppression, severe and fatal GVHD has been observed in some human marrow graft recipients. This strongly indicates that better immunosuppressive regimens must be found. The treatment of established GVHD following hemopoietic grafting has been evaluated in only a few studies in rodents. More recently the effectiveness of rabbit antidog ATS or prednisone for modifying established GVHD in dogs following hemopoietic grafts from histoincompatible donors was studied.[52] The data were encouraging and showed that established GVHD in dogs with histoincompatible grafts can be affected by ATS with significant prolongation of survival. Prednisone was not effective. Application of this treatment to human marrow graft recipients has also been encouraging, and some patients have recovered from severe GVHD following treatment with antihuman antithymocyte globulin (ATG) raised in rabbits or goats.[55] Controlled studies of the effect of ALS in dogs given DL-A matched marrow or human beings given HL-A matched marrow have not yet been reported.

As described in the clinical section to follow, it is clear that with the use of histocompatibility matching and postgrafting immunosuppression long-term survival can be achieved in patients with leukemia or aplastic anemia. It should be remembered, however, that despite the advances in the identification of histocompatibility antigens and the use of immunosuppressive agents the ultimate goal in this field has not been reached: namely, the specific suppression of the immune response to given antigens while leaving immune responses against other antigens intact. Ultimately this goal may become reality by a more thorough understanding of the immune response and of the phenomenon of immunologic unresponsiveness.

More recently, albumin gradient and velocity sedimentation techniques have been developed in an attempt to eliminate immunocompetent cells from the marrow inoculum. These techniques have been shown to be useful in preventing the acute GVH syndrome in inbred strains of rodents.[56] Proof, however, that this technique is useful in modifying GVHD in a randomly bred species is missing. The technique has been applied in a number of human marrow transplants. The result has been either failure of engraftment or death from GVHD when histoincompatible marrow was employed. This may be due to incomplete separation technique or loss of stem cells due to prolonged exposure of the cells to room temperature during separation. Aside from the technical problems of the separation, a number of theoretical reasons would speak against the efficacy of "stem cell" separation techniques. Even if a perfect separation of lymphoid cells is possible, it is likely that the recipient might still be susceptible to the late form of GVHD which is presumably caused by a subsequent generation of reactive lymphoid cells derived from the "common" stem cell. If there is not a "common" stem cell giving rise to lymphoid cells, then such a separation technique would create a recipient who is severely deficient in immune function and thus might succumb easily to infection. At present, therefore, stem cell separation does not appear to be a promising approach.

The Stable Chimeric State

The definition of a stable chimeric state is based on the persisting presence of a hemopoietic system derived from donor cells and the continued absence of GVHD. As discussed in the previous sections, such stable chimerism can be achieved by proper selection of donor–recipient with histocompatibility matching and transient immunosuppression drug therapy after grafting. Evidence for continued chimerism is provided by appropriate blood genetic markers: sex chromosome markers, RBC antigen markers, white blood cell (WBC) markers, immunoglobulin allotypes, RBC and WBC isoenzymes, or persistence of a skin graft from the marrow donor. Long-term survival may be defined as survival beyond 1 year with continued proof of chimerism. The only two randomly bred mammalian species in which long-term survival has been observed are dog and man. Canine irradiation chimeras have been observed for up to 10 years after marrow transplantation. Analyses of more than 2000 karyotypes of cells in peripheral blood, marrow, and lymph nodes in more than 50 canine recipients up to 10 years after grafting have consistently shown only cells with donor karyotype.[29] Hemopoietic cells with host karyotypes apparently do not persist in irradiation chimeras. In man, also, chimerism seems to be complete. The longest human irradiation chimera is now almost 3 years postmarrow transplantation and continues to show only cells with the female donor karyotype in marrow and peripheral blood.[55]

An important question is whether "tolerance" is due to death of the cell population responding to the host antigens or to changes in the lymphocyte surface structures involved with antigen recognition. Recent experiments focused attention on the possibility that transplantation "tolerance" is really a form of enhancement involving cell-mediated immunity and serum blocking factors. Canine irradiation chimeras were studied 1.0 to 7.5 years after transplantation.[57] The hemopoietic and lymphoid systems in these chimeras were of donor type as determined by cytogenetic and RBC markers. When tested by the in vitro colony inhibition assay against the fibroblasts of the chimera it was found that the chimeric, i.e., donor, lymphocytes were not tolerant but exhibited immunity. They inhibited colony formation by the chimeric fibroblasts while lymphocytes from other chimeras or from normal dogs did not. Serum from the chimera blocked this in vitro inhibition. For the most part the blocking effect of the serum was specific for the lymphocytes and fibroblasts for that particular chimera. Subsequently, these observations were confirmed in murine chimeras.[58,59] These data suggest that the immunologic "tolerance" in the canine chimeras may be mediated in vivo by blocking factors. They are at variance with the hypothesis that those lymphocyte clones that could react against a chimeric animal's own skin fibroblasts have been depleted or inactivated. Currently our human irradiation chimeras are being studied for the presence of cell-mediated immunity and serum blocking factors.

Immunologic Studies with the Irradiation Chimeras

Numerous studies in rodents have pointed out the fact that in the period immediately following irradiation and marrow grafting the chimeras have a very low ability to react to antigenic stimulation. This is observed regardless of whether syngeneic or allogeneic cells are transplanted. The results in rodents vary, depending on the strain combinations used and on the antigenic challenge. For the most part the observations were short term and utilized single antigens. In some instances the chimeric state of the animals has not been confirmed, which greatly limits the value of these experiments. On the whole, it appears that the immune function is more quickly and more completely restored in syngeneic chimeras, while allogeneic chimeras have a more prolonged period of immunoincompetence and sometimes may never recover.[60,61] The only real long-term follow-up studies with observation periods up to 8 years after transplantation were carried out recently in canine irradiation chimeras.[62] Approximately 50 canine marrow graft survivors have been studied. The advantage of the dog is that a single animal can be studied with respect to its humoral and cellular immunity by a battery of tests including injection of sheep RBC antigen, chicken RBC antigen, bacteriophage ØX174, attenuated distemper vaccine, histocompatibility alloantigens, keyhole limpet hemocyanin, analysis of immunoglobulins in the primary and secondary antibody response, PPD and BCG skin tests, third-party skin grafts (first and second set), phytohemagglutinin lymphocyte stimulation, MLC tests, repeated lymph node biopsies, recovery of lymphocyte counts, and other tests. It was observed that although the granulocyte recovery was completed after approximately 25 days postgrafting, the lymphocyte recovery was very much delayed and reached the lower limit of the normal range only after approximately 200 days. In agreement with this parameter, the humoral and cellular immunity in marrow graft recipients in the first 200 to 300 days after marrow grafting was significantly lower than that observed in normal dogs. As a rule, the immune function in canine irradiation chimeras returned to levels in the normal range after that period of time. Long-term canine irradiation chimeras thus represent animals whose lymphoid cells have regained normal or near normal function but have become "tolerant" to the host. In agreement with these rodent and canine studies, human irradiation chimeras were found to be profoundly immunoincompetent with respect to skin reactivity to DNCB and with respect to circulating antibody against bacteriophage ØX174 in the first 100 days after grafting.[63] In contrast to the findings in the canine chimeras, the human recipients of allogeneic marrow grafts made only feeble responses to phage antigen when tested after intervals of up to 2 years. The secondary immune response to phage was IgM rather than the expected IgG. The level of peripheral blood lymphocytes returned to normal after approximately 200 days. Measurements of immunoglobulin levels showed, in general, normal values for IgG, IgM, and IgA. The in vitro response of circulating lymphocytes showed normal reactivity to allogeneic cells and to PHA after MTX therapy was discontinued.

Despite the laboratory evidence of immunologic deficiency with these two tests, most of the patients appear to be doing reasonably well with respect to susceptibility to infection. This again is in agreement with the canine chimera that lives in an unprotected environment without an increased incidence of infection. A possible explanation for the more rapid recovery observed in the dogs is the fact that they received proportionally more marrow (1.6×10^9 marrow cells per kilogram) than the patients (3.3×10^8 marrow cells per kilogram). The studies on immune reconstitution have important clinical implications. Protection against infection and vigilance in early detection and treatment of infections are mandatory. A long-term follow-up of these patients should determine whether or not they will eventually show recovery of immunologic capability as might be predicted on the basis of the canine data. If not, it may be necessary to attempt to hasten the immune reconstitution by measures such as the addition of peripheral blood lymphoid cells to the marrow inoculum, the implantation of thymus, or by nonspecific stimulation of immunity. The ultimate aim of irradiation and marrow grafting in human patients, namely the adoptive immunotherapy of leukemia, may depend on fast and complete immunologic recovery.

CLINICAL MARROW GRAFTING STUDIES

As outlined in the Introduction, marrow grafting started as a means for protecting patients against a lethal marrow syndrome following accidental exposure to TBI. The past experience makes it seem that marrow grafting will not be of practical value for such irradiation accidents. The irradiation exposure would have to be on the order of 800 to 1500 rads to the entire body in order to be in the range in which spontaneous recovery would be unlikely to occur, immunosuppression would be adequate to permit engraftment, and gastrointestinal symptoms would be manageable. As pointed out, in the lower but still lethal exposure range allogeneic marrow grafts would probably not be successful because of inadequate immunosuppression of the host. It is conceivable, however, that progress with additional conditioning regimens may ultimately permit engraftment after such exposures. An example is the recent report by Gengozian et al.[64] They described a patient pretreated with horse antihuman thymocyte globulin for 8 days, and then given 500 R followed by marrow from an HL-A matched sibling. Despite the "low" radiation dose, engraftment was successful. This regimen could not be applied to an irradiation accident victim since pretreatment would obviously not be feasible. Much work needs to be done to develop postirradiation immunosuppressive regimens that might permit successful engraftment of an accident victim, at least for those with an HL-A matched sibling to serve as donor.

The number of patients subjected to marrow grafting following accidental irradiation exposure is very small. The accident victims at Vinca, Yugoslavia were treated in Paris and given allogeneic marrow approximately 21 days following the accident.[65] Although it was thought that some evidence for engraftment was obtained, significant engraftment seems unlikely in view of the "midlethal" irradiation exposure and the absence of subsequent GVHD. In addition, a careful comparison of the clinical course of these patients with the Y-12 accident victims not given marrow led Andrews to conclude that there was no effect of the infused marrow.[66] One irradiation accident victim in Pittsburg, Pennsylvania was fortunate enough to have an identical twin to serve as the marrow donor.[67] This patient was exposed to 600 rads and showed prompt hematopoietic recovery approximately 11 to 14 days following marrow infusion. The patient has since been hematologically well now more than 4 years after marrow transfusion.

Based on the advances made in marrow grafting in randomly bred animal species, in human histocompatibility typing, and in supportive care of patients with decreased defense mechanisms, TBI has now been used as a conditioning agent for marrow grafting in an attempt to cure patients with a variety of otherwise fatal diseases. These attempts, described in the following sections, already have been characterized by frequent successful engraftment and by survival of patients for a time period sufficiently long to evaluate the effect of engraftment on the host and on the disease. A valuable by-product of these studies will be further insight into the basic pathophysiology of diseases such as marrow failure, leukemia, and other diseases of the hematopoietic and lymphoreticular systems. It should be emphasized that the patients described were thought to have had maximum benefit from conventional therapy.

Marrow Grafting in Hematologic Malignancy

ANTILEUKEMIC EFFECT

The possible use of TBI to eradicate malignant hemopoietic cells and condition the individual for restoration of the hemopoietic system by infused normal hemopoietic cells has been very attractive. The first apparent beneficial effects of supralethal irradiation and infusion of marrow from syngeneic mice on mouse leukemia were described by Barnes et al in 1956.[68] A number of their animals became leukemia-free long-term survivors. This was a rather striking finding in view of the radiobiologic studies on the radiosensitivity of tumors showing that complete eradication of mouse leukemia could only be achieved with exposures to several thousand rads.[69] The findings by Barnes and co-workers could only be explained on the basis of further kill of residual leukemic cells by the transplanted cells through a reaction of immunity. Mathe et al[70] used the term "adoptive immunotherapy" to describe the antileukemic effect of the infused immunologically competent marrow. Other investigators reported that the transplantation of foreign hemopoietic cells following lethal TBI in rodents with leukemia could result in a varied prolongation of survival or even permanent cure but only in a small proportion of leukemia-bearing animals. The effect of tumor inhibition appears to be most pronounced when, in addition to the marrow inoculum, lymphoid cells are given.[71]

Nevertheless, based on the findings in the rodent model, attempts at treating end-stage human leukemias with a supralethal dose of TBI and transplantation of marrow from either an allogeneic donor or from a normal identical twin have continued. The rationale is that the transplanted lymphoid cells may develop immunity to a residual minimal population of leukemic cells which survives after 1000 rads radiation exposure. The immunity may be directed against transplantation antigens on the leukemic cells or against leukemia-associated antigens with a resulting "adoptive immunotherapy." Syngeneic cells are incapable of developing an immunotherapeutic effect mediated by histocompatibility antigens but they may have the same potential for adoptive immunotherapy against leukemia-associated antigens as allogeneic cells.

SYNGENEIC GRAFTS

Three patients with acute lymphoblastic leukemia (ALL) were treated with a supralethal dose of TBI and transplantation of marrow from a normal identical twin.[72,73] The patients accepted their graft without difficulty, but showed a return of leukemia within 48 to 84 days. These results, in accord with most mouse studies, suggest that the highest dose of irradiation that can be tolerated without severe intestinal syndromes is not enough to destroy all leukemic cells.

Subsequently an approach to potential immunotherapy[74] was tried based on the assumption that infusion of additional immunologically reactive donor lymphocytes might be beneficial. Secondly, it was thought that the continued exposure of these infused lymphocytes to antigenic leukemia cells [continued subcutaneous (s.c.) administration of previously stored irradiation-killed host leukemia cells following engraftment] might immunize those lymphocytes to hypothetic leukemia-specific antigens. Accordingly, three such transplants in patients with ALL or acute myeloblastic leukemia (AML) were attempted. The patients received buffy-coat lymphocytes from the identical twin 3 times weekly plus weekly s.c. injections of their own leukemia cells stored at —180°C in 10 percent dimethyl sulfoxide and irradiated with 10,000 rads. Although the period of remission in these 3 patients appeared to be longer, leukemia did recur. In an attempt to improve those results it was assumed that the addition of a high dose of chemotherapy to this treatment regimen would be beneficial by decreasing the tumor load to be handled by irradiation and/or immunotherapy. Therefore, 7 patients were given CY, 120 mg/kg, preceding 1000 rads TBI. One patient (AML) did not show disappearance of leukemia. Two patients (CML in blast crisis) showed remissions of 3 and 5 months. Two patients with ALL are in remission at 7 and 17 months, one with AML at 16 months, and one with lymphosarcoma of the marrow at 34 months.

It can be concluded from these studies that the treatment is remarkably well tolerated by the patients and marrow engraftment is not a problem. The fact that a number of patients have now been in remission for up to 34 months is encouraging and suggests that this treatment approach has a definite place in the treatment of patients with hematologic malignancies who are fortunate enough to have an identical twin.

ALLOGENEIC GRAFTS

Thirty-four marrow transplants have been carried out between September 1969 and February 1973 in patients with acute leukemia.[37,53,55] These patients had normal HL-A identical sibling donors confirmed by a nonreactive MLC test. Twenty patients had ALL and 14 had AML. They were given 1000 rads of midpoint tissue exposure from opposing ^{60}Co sources. Twenty-three of these patients also were given CY, 120 mg/kg, preceding irradiation and 1 patient was given daunomycin, 300 mg/m^2.

Patients were given MTX on days 1, 3, 6, 11, and weekly thereafter for 100 days to prevent or ameliorate GVHD. Nine patients were given ATG raised in rabbits or goat to treat established GVHD.

With regard to successful engraftment, 33 of the 34 patients had histologic evidence of a successful "marrow take." In all 19 patients with donors of opposite sex this was confirmed by cytogenetic analyses. Eight patients failed to recover granulocyte and platelet function and died between 11 and 30 days with infectious complications. Twenty-one of the patients developed evidence of GVHD. Thirteen of the 21 died with GVHD which in 11 was accompanied by an interstitial pneumonitis often due to CMV.[75] Eight of the 21 patients recovered from GVHD. Five patients with ALL showed recurrent leukemia.

Eight patients are presently alive and free of disease between 100 to 1080 days postgrafting. These patients received no therapy after day 100 and are leading a relatively normal life without evidence of leukemia.

It is obvious that the overall mortality rate in our series of patients has been very high. Considering, however, that this group of patients had end-stage leukemia with a life expectancy of a matter of a few weeks, the results should not be surprising. We are rather encouraged that marrow grafts between HL-A matched siblings can be consistently achieved in patients with terminal leukemia. Long-term control of leukemia is possible by this procedure, and a few long-term survivors are living normal lives for up to 3 years after grafting. Leukemic relapse or failure to clear blast cells from the marrow has occurred in some patients with ALL and steps to keep this from happening have been taken, as discussed in the next paragraph.

LEUKEMIC RELAPSE

Leukemic relapse has been observed in patients with ALL given 1000 rads TBI followed by marrow from an HL-A matched sibling. The observation that in 2 cases leukemic relapse occured in donor cells has far-reaching implications with respect to the possible etiology of leukemia.[76,77] Therefore, a case report is discussed here in detail. A 7-year-old girl with ALL was given a marrow transplant from her brother. She showed prompt recovery of peripheral blood cell counts following the postirradiation nadir. On day 100, blood counts were normal. Marrow histology was normal. On day 135, a marrow aspiration revealed recurring leukemia and on day 140 peripheral leukemic lymphoblasts began to appear. The marrow on day 153 showed 81 percent lymphoblasts. The patient was unsuccessfully treated with vincristine and prednisone and died on day 168 with pancytopenia. Chromosome analyses of short-term cultures without PHA were carried out. Before grafting, all 65 cells analyzed were female, i.e., host. All 150 cells analyzed after marrow grafting before and after leukemic relapse were male, i.e., donor. Of particular significance was the finding after relapse of 12 male karyotypes in direct preparations of the peripheral blood where the only dividing cells were leukemic lymphoblasts. Fluorescent Y body studies supported the karyotype analyses. The marrow before grafting showed only 4 percent Y body positive cells among 244 cells counted. After the leukemic relapse on days 143 and 154 postgrafting, 350 cells were enumerated and the number of Y body positive cells was approximately 50 percent. Examination of Y body positive peripheral blood cells under phase contrast microscopy showed that the cells were leukemic lymphoblasts; i.e., the lymphoblasts were undoubtedly of male origin. A male ALL control marrow stained in the same batch showed 49 percent Y body positive cells among 134 cells counted.

One possible mechanism to explain the recurrence in donor cells is that leukemia is a disease of regulation in the host so that any grafted marrow would show a leukemic pattern. This cannot be excluded by the data presently available. The possibility of in vivo somatic cell mating followed by diploidization seems unlikely but also cannot be excluded. Another possibility is that antigenic stimulation in the setting of the allogeneic marrow graft produced genetic damage or otherwise promoted the malignant transformation of susceptible clones of donor lymphoid cells. However, we have not as yet seen leukemia in our human marrow transplant recipients whose original disease was marrow failure. Also we have not seen leukemia in normal dogs with allogeneic marrow grafts observed up to 10 years after grafting. Perhaps the most attractive hypothesis is that TBI of the recipient with ALL induced the production of either a fully active oncogenic virus or of a helper virus which collaborated with a defective endogenous virus in the engrafted marrow cells to produce malignant transformation. Experiments in animal model systems have demonstrated the induction of viruses which were either oncogenic or possessed "helper" functions from both normal embryo cells and from nonvirus-producing transformed cells. Such virus induction has been promoted by chemical carcinogens, halogenated pyrimidines, or ultraviolet and x-irradiation.

We are confronted with a situation in which the therapeutic procedure effectively destroyed the host's leukemic cells but the disease recurred in donor cells, possibly due to a residual virus. It appears that our initial concept that irradiation and allogeneic marrow grafting will replace the host leukemic cells by donor type hemopoiesis is valid in most patients. However, the recurrent leukemia in donor cells dictates a change in the therapeutic protocol. Assuming that the observed malignant transformation is due to a virus, additional therapeutic possibilities arise including a delay of several days between irradiation and marrow infusion until virus released from irradiated cells has been cleared, the use of antiviral agents or interferon inducers, and the use of lymphoid cells specifically immunized to virus antigens. Another approach would be to destroy the bulk of the tumor mass before TBI. Therefore, as outlined in the preceding paragraph, we started treating patients with CY, 120 mg/kg body weight, followed in 2 to 4 days by irradiation and allogeneic marrow. So far, we have seen persistence of leukemia in host cells as outlined above,[78] but other patients have survived for periods up to 16 months without evidence of recurrent leukemia.

Marrow Grafting in Aplastic Anemia

Aplastic anemia is a disorder of obscure pathophysiology and high mortality despite introduction of androgen therapy and advances in supportive care. The hope of successful treatment of aplastic anemia by marrow grafting is based on the assumption that the etiology of the disease is a hemopoietic stem cell failure rather than a disorder of the marrow microenvironment. Initial attempts at treating aplastic anemia with syngeneic marrow grafts were encouraging.[67] Based on these observations, the Seattle group has carried out marrow grafting for treatment of this disease using HL-A identical siblings as marrow donors. Most of the presently evaluable cases have been conditioned by the immunosuppressive agent CY.[79,80,81,82] In 6 patients, however, 1000 rads of TBI was used as conditioning agent with the aim of shortening the period of supportive care before the transplant. The duration of marrow aplasia in these patients ranged from 2 to 15 months and all had been successfully treated with conventional therapy. Most of them were infected at the time of admission and some of them were refractory to random donor platelets. One patient died on day 6 with a Pseudomonas septicemia, too early for the graft to be evaluated. One patient, who had received blood transfusions from family members, failed to show marrow engraftment and died on day 24 with infection and an aplastic marrow. Another patient who had only random preceding blood transfusions showed initial engraftment followed by rejection of the marrow graft. A second graft was attempted after conditioning of the patient with 200 mg of CY per kilogram. This graft failed and the patient died on day 41 with infection and an aplastic marrow. Three patients had successful and sustained marrow engraftment. Two of these died on days 45 and 84 with severe GVHD. One patient is alive more than 380 days following hemopoietic transplantation with sustained engraftment. He was returned to normal activities. The present series of cases shows no real difference between patients conditioned by TBI and those conditioned by CY. Although the CY regimen requires a longer period of supportive care, only 1 of 16 patients died too early to demonstrate engraftment. The survival rate of 1 of 6 after the TBI regimen versus 9 of 16 after CY is not significant in view of the uncontrolled major variables of GVHD and prior sensitization.

These data demonstrate that normal stem cells will repopulate the marrow in aplastic anemia patients and show that long-term stable chimerism is possible in man. They suggest that marrow grafting in patients with complete marrow failure and an HL-A matched sibling should be undertaken before major infections and refractoriness to blood transfusions complicate their course.

CONCLUSIONS AND SUMMARY OF OUTSTANDING PROBLEMS IN THE FIELD OF IRRADIATION AND MARROW GRAFTING

1.   After 4 years of intensive clinical activity in this area it has become apparent that many of the principles established in randomly bred mammalian species, dogs and monkeys, can be successfully extrapolated to the clinical situation. A number of human long-term survivors have maintained their stable chimeric state without further therapy. This is particularly encouraging since all of these patients had reached end stages of their disease at the time of marrow grafting.

2.   Important information has been gained about the pathogenesis of hematologic diseases as documented by the successful repopulation of marrow spaces in aplastic anemia or by the recurrence of leukemia in cells of donor type.

3.   GVHD with fatal outcome is still a potential hazard despite matching by currently available histocompatibility typing techniques and the use of postgrafting immunosuppression. Continued research efforts have to be directed to a better understanding of the nature and control of this immunologic reaction.

4.   Recurrent leukemia has been observed in host and in donor cells. Additional research is under way which is designed to prevent recurrent leukemia by more intensive antileukemic therapy before irradiation and marrow grafting or by new therapeutic modalities such as the use of antiviral agents.

5.   A number of patients with successful marrow grafts have died of infection. Decreased immune defenses and increased susceptibility to infection exist for prolonged periods after grafting. Methods for accelerating the immunologic reconstitution of the marrow graft recipients need to be identified. Accelerated immune reconstitution not only may prevent fatal infectious complications but also may provide the graft with a more pronounced antileukemic effect, thus fulfilling the concept of "adoptive immunotherapy."

6.   Sensitization of the intended marrow recipient by preceding blood transfusions remains a serious problem. Earlier transplantation might avoid this problem. Otherwise laboratory efforts must be directed toward recognition and elimination of sensitization.

7.   The nature of the "stable chimeric state" is as yet not fully understood. The studies in canine irradiation chimeras and now also in the human irradiation chimeras have drawn attention to the possible role of "blocking factors" in maintaining the stable chimeric state. The in vivo role of these "blocking factors" has yet to be defined.

8.   It should be pointed out that the recipient of a successful marrow graft will subsequently accept a graft of any other organ from the marrow donor without the necessity of continued immunosuppressive therapy. The role of marrow grafting as a prelude to organ grafting, however, has still to be defined.

9.   In summary, the concept of marrow grafting following TBI has left the experimental stage and has been successfully applied to the treatment of a variety of otherwise fatal diseases. It is conceivable that marrow transplantation may be applicable to other human diseases such as sickle cell disease and thalassemia. It is also possible that further progress might make it possible to graft patients who do not have an HL-A matched sibling. Since marrow can be stored indefinitely at low temperatures, it is possible to establish a marrow bank containing specimens of marrow from donors of known HL-A identity that might be transplanted into unrelated recipients of the same HL-A phenotype after demonstrating nonreactivity in MLC.

REFERENCES

1.   Heineke H: Uber die einwirkung der rontgenstrahlen auf tiere. Munch Med Wochenschr 50:2090–2092, 1903
2.   Heineke, H: Experimentelle untersuchungen uber die einwirkung der rontgenstrahlen auf innere organe. Mitt Grenzg Med Chir 14:21–94, 1905
3.   Benjamin E, Sluka E: Antikorperbildung nach experimenteller schadigung des hamatopoetischen systems durch rontgenstrahlen. Wien Klin Wochenschr 21:311–313, 1908
4.   Fabricious-Moeller J: Experimental Studies of the Hemorrhagic Diathesis from X-Ray Sickness. Copenhagen, Levin & Munksgaards Forlag, 1922
5.   Jacobson LO, Marks EK, Robson MJ, Gaston EO, Zirkle RE: The effect of spleen protection on mortality following x-irradiation. J Lab Clin Med 34:1538–1543, 1949
6.   Lorenz E, Uphoff D, Reid TR, Shelton E: Modification of irradiation injury in mice and guinea pigs by bone marrow injections. J Natl Cancer Inst 12:197–201, 1951
7.   Cole LJ, Fishler MC, Ellis ME, Bond VP: Protection of mice against x-irradiation by spleen homogenates administered after exposure. Proc Soc Exp Biol Med 80:112–117, 1952
8.   Main JM, Prehn RT: Successful skin homografts after the administration of high-dosage radiation and homologous bone marrow. J Natl Cancer Inst 15:1023–1028, 1955

9. Ford, CE, Hamerton JL, Barnes DWH, Loutit JF: Cytological identification of radiation-chimeras. Nature 177:452–454, 1956

10. Nowell PC, Cole LJ, Habermeyer JG, Roan PL: Growth and continued function of rat marrow cells in x-radiated mice. Cancer Res 16:258–261, 1956

11. Trentin JJ: Signposts and landmarks. Exp Hematol 22:18–22, 1972

12. Thomas ED, Lochte HL Jr, Lu WC, Ferrebee JW: Intravenous infusion of bone marrow in patients receiving radiation and chemotherapy. N Engl J Med 257:491–496, 1957

13. Bortin MM: A compendium of reported human bone marrow transplants. Transplantation 9:571–587, 1970

14. Mathe G, Amiel JL, Schwarzenberg L, Cattan A, Schneider M, de Vries MJ, Tubiana M, Lalanne C, Binet JL, Papiernik M, Seman G, Matsukura M, Mery AM, Schwarzmann V, Flaisler A: Successful allogeneic bone marrow transplantation in man: Chimerism, induced specific tolerance and possible anti-leukemic effects. Blood 25:179–196, 1965

15. Cronkite EP, Bond VP: Radiation Injury in Man. Springfield, Illinois, Charles C Thomas, 1960

16. Trentin JJ: Mortality and skin transplantability in x-irradiated mice receiving isologous, homologous, or heterologous bone marrow. Proc Soc Exp Biol Med 92:688–693, 1956

17. Uphoff DE: Genetic factors influencing irradiation protection by bone marrow. III. Midlethal irradiation of inbred mice. J Natl Cancer Inst 30:1115–1151, 1963

18. Nouza K, Lengerova A: Specific features of the outcome of transplantation of foreign haematopoietic and lymphoid cells in the midlethal irradiation range. Folia Biol 11:17–33, 1965

19. Thomas ED, LeBlond R, Graham T, Storb R: Marrow infusions in dogs given midlethal or lethal irradiation. Radiat Res 41:113–124, 1970

20. van Bekkum DW, de Vries MJ: Radiation Chimaeras New York, Academic Press, 1967

21. Gengozian N, Carlson DE, Allen EM: Transplantation of allogeneic and xenogeneic (rat) marrow in irradiated mice as affected by radiation exposure rates. Transplantation 7:259–273, 1969

22. Winchell HS, Pollycove M, Loughman WD, Richards V, Kim L, Lawrence JH: Homotransplantation studies in dogs following selective radioisotopic lymphatic ablation. J Nucl Med 7:416–423, 1966

23. Thomas ED, Storb R: Technique for human marrow grafting. Blood 36:507–515, 1970

24. van Bekkum DW, Vos O, Weyzen WWH: Homo- et heterogreffe tissus hematopoietiques chez la souris. Rev d'Hematol 11:477–485, 1956

25. Goodman JW, Hodgson GS: Evidence for stem cells in the peripheral blood of mice. Blood 19:702–714, 1962

26. Cavins JA, Scheer SC, Thomas ED, Ferrebee JW: The recovery of lethally irradiated dogs given infusions of autologous leukocytes preserved at −80°C. Blood 23:38–43, 1964

27. Chervenick PA, Boggs DR: In vitro growth of granulocytic and mononuclear cell colonies from blood of normal individuals. Blood 37:131–135, 1971

28. Storb R, Epstein RB, Thomas ED: Marrow repopulating ability of peripheral blood cells compared to thoracic duct cells. Blood 32:662–667, 1968

29. Storb R, Thomas ED: Bone marrow transplantation in randomly bred animal species and in man, in Schwarz MR (ed): Proceedings of the Sixth Leucocyte Culture Conference. New York, Academic Press, 1972, pp 805–840

30. Adamson JW, Storb R: The proliferative potential of frozen stored human marrow cells. Transplantation 14:490–494, 1972

31. Storb R, Epstein RB, LeBlond RF, Rudolph RH, Thomas ED: Transplantation of allogeneic canine bone marrow stored at −80°C in dimethyl sulfoxide. Blood 33:918–923, 1969

32. Albert E, Storb R, Erickson V, Graham TC, Parr M, Templeton JM, Mickey M, Thomas ED: Serology and genetics of the DL-A system. I. Establishment of specificities. Tissue Antigens (in press)

33. Bach FH, Amos DB: Hu-1: Major histocompatibility locus in man. Science 156:1506–1508, 1967

34. Templeton JW, Thomas ED: Evidence for a major histocompatibility locus in the dog. Transplantation 11:429–431, 1971

35. Storb R, Rudolph RH, Kolb HJ, Graham TC, Mickelson E, Erickson V, Lerner KG, Kolb H, Thomas ED: Marrow grafts between DL-A matched canine littermates. Transplantation 15:92–100, 1973

36. Storb R, Kolb HJ, Graham TC, LeBlond R, Kolb H, Lerner KG, Thomas ED: Marrow grafts between histoincompatible canine family members. Eur J Clin Biol Res 17:680–685, 1972

37. Buckner CD, Epstein RB, Rudolph RH, Clift RA, Storb R, Thomas ED: Allogeneic marrow engraftment following whole-body irradiation in a patient with leukemia. Blood 35:741–750, 1970

38. Graw RG, Jr, Santos GW: Bone marrow transplantation in patients with leukemia. Transplantation 11:197–199, 1971

39. Buckner CD, Clift RA, Fefer A, Storb R, Thomas ED: Human marrow transplantation—current status, in Brown EB (ed): Progress in Hematology, vol VIII. New York, Grune & Stratton, 1973, pp 299–324

40. Storb R, Epstein RB, Rudolph RH, Thomas ED: The effect of prior transfusion on marrow grafts between histocompatible canine siblings. J Immunol 105:627–633, 1970

41. Storb R, Rudolph RH, Graham TC, Thomas ED: The influence of transfusions from unrelated donors upon marrow grafts between histocompatible canine siblings. J Immunol 107:409–413, 1971

42. Santos GW, Sensenbrenner LL: A sensitive and quantitative assay for non-H-2 histocompatibility antigens. Exp Hematol 21:19–20, 1971

43. Storb R, Floersheim GL, Weiden PL, Graham TC, Kolb HJ, Lerner KG, Schroeder ML, Thomas ED: Effect of prior blood transfusions on marrow grafts: Abrogation of sensitization by procarbazine and antithymocyte serum. J Immunol (in press)

44. de Vries MJ, Crouch BG, van Putten LM, van Bekkum DW: Pathologic changes in irradiated monkeys treated with bone marrow. J Natl Cancer Inst 27:67–97, 1961

45. Lerner KG, Kao GF, Storb R, Buckner CD, Clift RA, Thomas ED: Histopathology of graft-versus-host reaction (GVHR) in human recipients of marrow from HL-A matched sibling donors. Transplant Proc (in press)

46. Kolb HJ, Storb R, Graham TC, Kolb H, Thomas ED: Antithymocyte serum and methotrexate for control of graft-versus-host disease in dogs. Transplantation 16:17–23, 1973

47. Uphoff DE: Alteration of homograft reaction by A-methopterin in lethally irradiated mice treated with homologous marrow. Proc Soc Exp Biol Med 99:651–653, 1958

48. Thomas ED, Collins JA, Herman EC Jr, Ferrebee JW: Marrow transplants in lethally irradiated dogs given methotrexate. Blood 19:217–228, 1962

49. Muller-Berat CN, van Putten LM, van Bekkum DW: Cytostatic drugs in the treatment of secondary disease following homologous bone marrow transplantation: Extrapolation from the mouse to the primate. Ann NY Acad Sci 129:340–354, 1966

50. Storb R, Epstein RB, Graham TC, Thomas ED: Methotrexate regimens for control of graft-versus-host disease in dogs with allogeneic marrow grafts. Transplantation 9:240–246, 1970

51. Storb R, Graham TC, Shiurba R, Thomas ED: Treatment of canine graft-versus-host disease with methotrexate and cyclophosphamide following bone marrow transplantation from histoincompatible donors. Transplantation 10:165–172, 1970

52. Storb R, Kolb HJ, Graham TC, Kolb H, Weiden PL, Thomas ED: Treatment of established graft-versus-host disease in dogs by antithymocyte serum or prednisone. Blood 42:601–609, 1973

53. Thomas ED, Buckner CD, Rudolph RH, Fefer A, Storb R, Neiman PE, Bryant JI, Chard RL, Clift RA, Epstein RB, Fialkow PJ, Funk DD, Giblett ER, Lerner KG, Reynolds FA, Slichter S: Allogeneic marrow grafting for hematologic malignancy using HL-A matched donor-recipient sibling pairs. Blood 38:267–287, 1971

54. Santos GW, Sensenbrenner LL, Burke PJ, Colvin M, Owens AH Jr, Bias WB, Slavin RE: Marrow transplantation in man following cyclophosphamide. Transplant Proc 3:400–404, 1971

55. Thomas ED, Buckner CD, Clift RA, Fass L, Fefer A, Lerner KG, Neiman P, Rowley N, Storb R: Marrow grafting in patients with acute leukemia. Transplant Proc 5:917–922, 1973

56. Dicke KA, van Bekkum DW: Allogeneic bone marrow transplantation after elimination of immunocompetent cells by means of density gradient centrifugation. Transplant Proc 3:666–668, 1971

57. Hellstrom I, Hellstrom KE, Storb R, Thomas ED: Colony inhibition of fibroblasts from chimeric dogs mediated by the dogs' own lymphocytes and specifically abrogated by their serum. Proc Natl Acad Sci 66:65–71, 1970

58. Hellstrom I, Hellstrom KE, Allison AC: Neonatally induced allograft tolerance may be mediated by serum-borne factors. Nature 230:49–50, 1971

59. Hellstrom I, Hellstrom KE, Trentin JJ: Cellular immunity and blocking serum activity in chimeric mice. Cell Immunol 7:73–84, 1972

60. Zaleski M: Effect of host-versus-graft and graft-versus-host reactions on the immune response of mice to sheep red blood cells. Folia Biol 17:111–122, 1971

61. Gengozian N, Congdon CC, Allen EA, Toya RE: Immune status of allogeneic radiation chimeras. Transplant Proc 3:434–436, 1971

62. Ochs HD, Storb R, Graham TC, Rudolph RH, Kolb HJ, Shiurba RA, Thomas ED: Immune status of long-term canine irradiation chimeras. Blood 38:787, 1971

63. Thomas ED, Fass L, Ochs HD, Mickelson EM, Storb R, Fefer A: Immunologic reactivity of human recipients of syngeneic and allogeneic marrow grafts, in Recent Results in Cancer Research (in press)

64. Gengozian N, Edwards CL, Vodopick HA, Hubner KF: Bone marrow transplantation in a leukemic patient following immunosuppression with antithymocyte globulin and total body irradiation. Transplantation 15:446–454, 1973

65. Mathe G, Jammet H, Pendic B, Schwarzenberg L, Duplan JF, Maupin B, Latarjet R, Larrieu MJ, Kalic D, Djukic Z: Transfusions et greffes de moelle

osseuse homologue chez des humains irradies a haute dose accidentellement. Rev Fr d'Etudes Clin Biol 4:226–238, 1959

66. Andrews GA: Criticality accidents in Vinca, Yugoslavia, and Oak Ridge, Tennessee. JAMA 179:191–197, 1962

67. Thomas ED, Rudolph RH, Fefer A, Storb R, Slichter S, Buckner CD: Isogeneic marrow grafting in man. Exp Hematol 21:16–18, 1971

68. Barnes DWH, Corp MJ, Loutit JF, Neal FE: Treatment of murine leukaemia with x-rays and homologous bone marrow. Br Med J 2:626–627, 1956

69. Burchenal JH, Oettgen HF, Holmberg EAD, Hemphill SC, Reppert JA: Effect of total-body irradiation on the transplantability of mouse leukemias. Cancer Res 20:425–430, 1960

70. Mathe G, Amiel JL, Schwarzenberg L, Cattan A, Schneider M: Adoptive immunotherapy of acute leukemia: experimental and clinical results. Cancer Res 25:1525–1531, 1965

71. Fefer A: Adoptive tumor immunotherapy in mice as an adjunct to whole-body x-irradiation or chemotherapy—a review. Is J Med Sci 9:350–365, 1973

72. Thomas ED, Lochte HL Jr, Cannon JH, Sahler OD, Ferrebee JW: Supralethal whole-body irradiation and isologous marrow transplantation in man. J Clin Invest 38:1709–1716, 1959

73. Thomas ED, Herman EC Jr, Greenough WB III, Hager EB, Cannon JH, Sahler OD, Ferrebee JW: Irradiation and marrow infusion in leukemia. Arch Intern Med 107:829–849, 1961

74. Fefer A, Buckner CD, Clift RA, Fass L, Glucksberg H, Mickelson EM, Neiman P, Storb R, Thomas ED: Marrow grafting and immunotherapy in identical twins with hematologic malignancies. Proc Assoc Am Physicians (in press)

75. Neiman P, Wasserman PB, Wentworth BB, Kao GF, Lerner KG, Storb R, Buckner CD, Clift RA, Fefer A, Fass L, Glucksberg H, Thomas ED: Interstitial pneumonia and cytomegalovirus infection as complications of human marrow transplantation. Transplantation 15:478–485, 1973

76. Fialkow PJ, Thomas ED, Bryant JI, Neiman PE: Leukemic transformation of engrafted human marrow cells in vivo. Lancet 1:251–255, 1971

77. Thomas ED, Bryant JI, Buckner CD, Clift RA, Fefer A, Johnson FL, Neiman P, Ramberg RE, Storb R: Leukaemic transformation of engrafted human marrow cells in vivo. II. Lancet 1:1310–1313, 1972

78. Storb R, Bryant JI, Buckner CD, Clift RA, Fefer A, Fialkow PJ, Johnson FL, Neiman P, Thomas ED: Allogeneic marrow grafting for acute lymphoblastic leukemia: leukemic relapse. Transplant Proc 5:923–926, 1973

79. Thomas ED, Buckner CD, Storb R, Neiman PE, Fefer A, Clift RA, Slichter SJ, Funk DD, Bryant JI, Lerner KG: Aplastic anemia treated by marrow transplantation. Lancet 1:284–289, 1972

80. Storb R, Buckner CD, Fefer A, Clift RA, Neiman PE, Glucksberg H, Lerner KG, Thomas ED: Marrow transplantation in aplastic anemia. Transplant Proc (in press)

81. Storb R, Evans RS, Thomas ED, Buckner CD, Clift RA, Fefer A, Neiman P, Wright SE: Paroxysmal nocturnal haemoglobinuria and refractory marrow failure treated by marrow transplantation. Brit J Haematol 24:743–750, 1973

82. Storb R, Thomas ED, Buckner CD, Clift RA, Johnson FL, Fefer A, Glucksberg H, Giblett ER, Lerner KG, Neiman P: Allogeneic marrow grafting for treatment of aplastic anemia. Blood 43:157–180, 1974

James McRae

Hal O. Anger

5

Tomographic Imaging
in Nuclear Medicine

Tomographic imaging results in images of structures within the human body in which details at chosen depths are clearly shown, while those at other depths are either blurred, absent, or identified as to depth. These structures can be organs, lesions, or regions of the body that have been made radioactive by the administration of a radioactive tracer. On occasions, the areas of interest are cold spots surrounded by active tissue. One type of tomography, called *focal-plane tomography* in this chapter (but called *longitudinal tomography* in most of the other literature) may enhance the visibility of structures at a chosen depth in the presence of structures at other depths by blurring all objects off the chosen plane, thereby reducing the confusing effects of the overlying and underlying structures. The blurring of information from the out-of-focus planes improves the visibility of structures on the focal plane. The plane of interest is studied from many directions which produces an average value for overlying and underlying activity.

Another type of tomography, called *section imaging,* is different in that it isolates a cross-sectional layer of the body by examining that layer from its sides and constructing an image that represents distribution of activity as if looking down on that layer from above. The method is particularly valuable when layers above or below the examined layer contain confusing detail or activity. An example is the head where the conventional vertex view is less diagnostic than the section images obtained by Kuhl et al.[1] It is only by applying section imaging techniques that individual transverse layers of the chest or abdomen can be examined.

The most definitive methods, at least in theory, are the *total isolation methods* that completely isolate activity in a given element of tissue from all surrounding activity. *Fluorescent scanning* of heavy stable elements is practical at the present time and the clinical value is being actively explored. *Time-of-flight* methods for positron emitters and *coincident gamma-ray* detection methods for certain gamma-ray emitters have been considered but they do not appear practical at present.

The ultimate aim in tomographic imaging is a complete three-dimensional image with correct location of all activity coupled with a quantitative readout of the distribution of radioactivity. Improved resolution in three dimensions is also an important aim in the further development of radioisotope scanning.

A number of approaches to tomographic scanning have been explored, but to date no single method is in widespread use. In this chapter, the discussion is limited to emissive studies in which isotope has been administered to a patient. We do not discuss fluorescent scanning nor tomographic transmission imaging which takes advantage of small variations in tissue density, nor the details of obtaining tomographic images. Many of these are reviewed in a recent book, Tomographic Imaging in Nuclear Medicine,[2] edited by Gerald Freedman. The emphasis in this chapter is on the clinical advantages of tomographic imaging of radioactive tracers illustrated by examples of our personal experience with the multiplane tomographic scanner.

The aim in any diagnostic method is to provide information which will permit the physician to direct the course of subsequent investigations and to plan the means of treatment. In nuclear medicine imaging, tomograms have been shown to detect new lesions, increase the certainty that a lesion is present, and to better determine the size, shape, position, and depth of lesions. In the cases where conventional images are doubtful a normal tomographic study may allow the study to be placed in the normal category, since a negative tomographic study increases the certainty of the absence of a lesion as a converse of its ability to detect more lesions.

SECTION IMAGING

Kuhl et al[3] have been exploring the potential of tomographic methods in nuclear medicine since 1963. At that time they proposed that discrimination of an image from its background could be improved by separation of images of radioactivity according to their depth in the body. The image of a small tumor is likely to be lost in a confusion of patterns that result when there are sharp images of overlying or underlying radioactivity. Focal-plane tomography, section scanning, and stereoscopic methods were explored using phantoms.

Kuhl and Edwards[4] described the first clinical applications to the brain and liver of focal plane scanning and section scanning. Both methods were shown to have some advantages over routine scans in better characterizing the position and extent of lesions.

Kuhl et al[5] reviewed the value of section scanning of the brain using ^{99m}Tc-pertechnetate in 536 patients. They concluded that section scanning improved accuracy in detecting lesions near the base of the brain. They found that a series of section scans provided a better description of the tumor in three dimensions than did frontal, lateral, and posterior rectilinear scanning views. During this analysis they found that some normal cases had been placed in the abnormal group due to their unfamiliarity with the appearance of normal structures in the section scans at the time of their first report. Experience is obviously needed before results with a technique can be interpreted with maximum accuracy. Kuhl and Edwards[6] analyzed their further clinical experience and described an improved method of constructing the section images using a digital computer. Again, they reported distinct advantages for the tomographic method. Instrument improvements were described in Radiology[7] and the latest method of image construction and analysis was reported in the Journal of Nuclear Medicine.[8] The clinical value of rectilinear vertex scans and section views of the brain was reported in 1970.[1] In other articles the advantages of characterizing the shape and position of brain lesions by section scans[9] and the prognostic significance of deep wedge-shaped areas of abnormality in section scans of cerebral infarctions[10] were described.

The main efforts of Kuhl's group have been concentrated on section scanning of the brain with only limited application to liver and spleen imaging. Section scans are used to complement a basic four-view rectilinear scan in selected patients. In a recent evaluation[9] Kuhl reported that approximately 14 percent of normal patients and 60 percent of abnormal patients underwent section scanning. Ninety-eight percent of normal patients were correctly characterized, and a correct diagnosis was made in 85 percent of tumor patients. Six percent of tumors were detected in the section scan alone. These tumors were located in the difficult basal regions of the brain in which section scanning provides the advantages of image separation and improved statistics, compared with rectilinear scanning. In addition to locating a small fraction of tumors that would have gone unrecognized by conventional imaging techniques, the section scans played an important role in providing additional information about the abnormal area. Additional information included more precise location, clear definition of boundaries, recognition of multiplicity, and information about the homogeneity of the abnormal area. The section defined the medial boundaries, which were often obscured in rectilinear views by radioactivity in overlying structures. Kuhl pointed out that tumors frequently cross the midline and that knowledge of the medial boundary is important since deep involvement often precludes complete excision. In contrast, cerebral infarcts are often shallow, do not cross the midline, and frequently have a sharply defined, center-pointing triangular shape. In addition to assisting in making a distinction between infarct and tumor, the depth of the wedge pattern on the section scan of an infarct is indicative of the severity of the neurologic deficit and distinguishes those patients in whom the prospect for significant recovery is poor. Section scanning has helped to detect deep cerebral contusions beneath superficial subdural or scalp lesions and deep tumor recurrence below craniotomy sites.

In view of the advantages of section views of the brain it is surprising that the equipment and techniques employed by Kuhl et al have not been duplicated by other groups and commercial companies.

Recently there has been increased interest in tomographic methods. Patton, Brill, and King[11,2a] have been exploring different methods of data collection and analysis to obtain better section scans of the brain. They have reduced the data collection time to explore section mapping of cerebral blood flow. They are currently working with an imaging time for a single scan of 2.5 sec, and can reduce this time to approximately 1 sec.

Myers et al[12] gave an analysis of two tomographic systems being developed at the University of Aberdeen in Scotland. This group is working on a scanning system to produce section scans similar to those reported by Kuhl, and on modifications to the scintillation camera so that it will produce focal-plane tomographic scans similar to those produced by the multiplane tomographic scanner designed by Anger.[2b] The authors compare the two instruments on the basis of their physical characteristics and present an analysis of their potential clinical applications. They favor section scanning for the brain but think that the focal plane tomographic scanner is more suited for studying the liver, lungs, kidneys, spleen, and pancreas.

In 1967, Anger[13] reported a method of obtaining section images with a scintillation camera equipped with a special collimator and optical system for data readout. The patient was rotated in a chair as the camera continuously examined a single horizontal slice of tissue through the patient's head. The optical camera recorded each scintillation as a line which corresponded to the path the gamma ray took through the layer of tissue being examined. Areas of high activity were recognized at the intersection of multiple lines. Tumors were satisfactorily delineated in a number of patients, but the method proved too difficult and time-consuming for routine clinical use.

Muehllehner and Wetzel[14] have described a method of obtaining section images using the scintillation camera and computer calculations. They used an unmodified scintillation camera and a chair in which the patient was rotated in front of the camera. Eight views were taken at angles of

45° and section images were constructed by computer. In the first 10 patients studied, structures were visible in some of the section views which could have been due to either artifacts or actual variations in the isotope concentration. These section images were used to aid in the localization of concentrations visible in the standard views used to construct the section images. The methods of constructing the section views are still being explored and the authors report that efforts are underway to include the effect of tissue attenuation in their calculations.

Budinger and others are currently exploring means of obtaining multiple sections by rotating the patient in front of the scintillation camera equipped with a newly designed long collimator using a variety of algorithms to reconstruct the sections.[15]

Arimizu[16] described a method by which radioisotopes at one depth can be exclusively detected to produce section images using a focused collimator and isotopes emitting two distinct gamma rays in cascade. This possibility was previously raised by Hart[17] and seems impractical at present because of the low number of coincident gammas detected.

Three-dimensional imaging of radionuclide distribution by gamma–gamma coincidence detection using two gamma camera detectors at right angles to each other, one with a conventional multihole collimator and the other with a collimator consisting of 13 1.2-cm-wide slots, is being investigated by Monahan and Powell.[2c] The major problem of the technique is its low coincidence counting efficiency. The method employs principles similar to those described by Arimizu[16] and Hart,[17] using a focused collimator, and has the advantage that multiple planes can be read out at once, as opposed to a single plane using a focused collimator. It remains to be seen whether the method will have clinical value.

FOCAL PLANE TOMOGRAPHY

Conventional focused collimator scanners employing large detectors are inherently tomographic. The distribution of isotope on or near the focal plane described by the geometric focus of the collimator and the scanning motion is clearly resolved while structures off the focal plane are blurred. The larger the detector and the shorter the focal length of the collimator the greater is the tomographic effect. Indeed, the tomographic effect is so great with a scanner employing an 8-in-diameter detector and collimator with a $3\frac{1}{2}$-in. focal length that such a scanner is unsatisfactory when used for conventional scanning of thick organs such as the liver, because small lesions off the geometric focal plane can be missed when only a single scan of the organ is taken.[18]

It is possible to perform multiple focal-plane tomography with a large-detector scanner as described above by taking scans with the collimator at various heights above the organ to be scanned. Each scan portrays the isotope distribution at the focal plane of the collimator with better definition than the isotope distribution above or below the focal plane. Naturally, the technique is applicable only to planes superficial to the focal depth of the collimator and a scan of the patient is required for each level.

In 1963, Kuhl and Edwards[3] described a method of reinforcing the tomographic effect of focused collimators by taking four separate scans at different angulations of the focused collimator and then optically superimposing the resulting images to enhance structures lying on the focal plane of the collimator. By employing a scanning system equipped with four detectors, each with focused collimators, Hisada et al[19] reported on a method of performing isosensitive scanning and bilaminoscanning and showed significant reinforcement of structures on two planes. They demonstrated that the system aided in disclosing smaller lesions in thick organs. There was no major application of instruments of this type.

The late Benedict Cassen not only pioneered the mechanical scanner but he also explored the use of a very large solid-angle spherical collimator to obtain focal-plane tomographic scans.[20] The prototype of the instrument produced images with good tomographic effects but there does not appear to have been any continuing clinical evaluation or development of the prototype instrument.

In 1967 Anger developed the multiplane tomographic scanner which is described in a later section. He combined the tomographic features of a large detector scanner with scintillation camera electronics and an optical readout to produce six images simultaneously, each focused at a different depth, from a single scan of the subject.

Muehllehner[21] described the principles of operation of a tomographic scintillation camera which has been marketed by Nuclear Chicago.* By attaching a rotating collimator with parallel holes at an angle of 20° to a scintillation camera, together with a table moving in a circular motion, he obtained four tomographic images simultaneously, each focused on a different plane. He made some specific comparisons between the tomographic camera and the multiplane tomographic scanner developed by Anger. He pointed out that the tomographic camera has 3 times the sensitivity of the tomographic scanner at energies up to 140 keV but that the resolution of the tomographic camera is less than that of the tomographic scanner. He concluded by suggesting that the tomographic camera may prove useful for dynamic studies, which certainly are not possible with the tomographic scanner. He did not discuss the limitations that the time required for rotation of the collimator places on the frame rate, and there have not been any reports of dynamic tomoscans.

* Now known as Searle Radiographic, Inc.

Clinical experience with the tomocamera has been reported by Chamroenngan et al[22] and DeLand et al.[23] James et al[24] more recently described tomographic imaging of the brain, pancreas, and liver. Their results suggested that tomographic scintiphotos may be of help in brain imaging by increasing the diagnostic certainty in doubtful cases and aiding in characterizing the size, shape, and depth of the lesions. Tomography was a useful supplemental tool in about half of their 50 patients when performed in association with either rectilinear scanning or scintillation camera imaging. They stressed that even in negative studies tomography increased the certainty that a lesion was not present.

Their experience in pancreatic imaging was disappointing in that better results were obtained with oblique views; imaging with the patient's pelvis elevated, serial imaging, and studies employing two isotopes to permit subtraction of the liver image.

In their evaluation of tomographic imaging of the liver, they provided guidelines for other investigators who wish to compare different imaging techniques. They proposed that a change in the probability of the final diagnosis of 20 percent or greater should be considered significant. They did not set forward objective criteria on which to judge this greater certainty. However, it is clear from their analysis that tomography was of assistance in establishing a normal anatomical variant in 13 of the 114 patients included in the study. The normal structures that they more readily recognized were the gallbladder fossa, division of the lobes, hepatic veins, a thin left lobe, and the results of extrinsic pressure. Better recognition arose from the ability to recognize the anatomical feature most clearly at the expected depth. In 16 patients they thought the tomoscans significantly confirmed the probability that the patient had a normal liver. Such a decision must lie in the knowledge that tomoscans more clearly delineate abnormalities, and that accordingly the absence of any variability in the tomoscan more certainly excludes the presence of an abnormality.

The authors expressed some concern regarding the value of tomographic imaging in patients with focal or multifocal disease, and yet they classified the tomographic technique as useful in 58 percent of their proven cases of focal disease. In this instance, the better definition of lesions, the recognition of greater numbers of lesions, and the separation of a seemingly large lesion on the routine pictures into a number of discrete lesions in the tomographic readout were the bases of judgment.

It is of interest to note that although artifacts due to the nature of the blur pattern were recognized in some of the scans, no false positive diagnoses were reported.

In their final conclusions they suggested that tomographic scintiphotos are of definite benefit to a small percentage of the total patient workload. This appears to conflict with the relatively high fraction of patient studies in which tomography was deemed helpful. Quite clearly, the additional information from the tomographic images was of little clinical application in their opinion. The basis for this conclusion must be that tomographic imaging with the tomocamera did not often detect lesions which were undetected by conventional techniques using multiple views. We should not be too disappointed in the failure to detect new lesions but should welcome the additional certainty in recognition of lesions which tomography offers in a significant fraction of patients.

In addition, before one can compare a new imaging technique with previously established techniques it is necessary to gain experience in interpreting the new information. Experience in looking at tomographic images certainly increases one's ability to interpret conventional scintigrams. By the time an observer is ready to score the relative merits of the two methods, he is already using the newer information to help him interpret the images provided by the equipment which has been in use for a longer period of time. It is impossible to estimate what bias this introduces in the final analysis of the relative merits of imaging techniques.

Linberg, Larsson, and Roos, at the Monaco meeting,[24] reported a comparison between tomographic and conventional scintiphotos of the liver. From their series of 50 patients they concluded that there is little difference in the efficacy of these two methods, but they had a slight preference for the routine scintillation camera. They preferred the quality of the pictures obtained with the high-resolution scintillation camera and did not like the blurring of normal anatomical borders that was present in some of the tomographic readouts.

Freedman,[25,26,2e] in his evaluation of the clinical results obtained with a scintillation camera digital tomographic system* (similar in principle to the Nuclear Chicago tomocamera but employing a small digital computer† to reconstruct the data from the various planes), concluded that the tomographic images were of assistance in imaging the liver, brain, and bone. In the limited number of cases included in these reports lesions were demonstrated that were not seen during conventional radionuclide imaging and there was improved characterization of the lesions. Freedman did not recommend that patients classified as "normal" in routine studies be reexamined with the tomographic camera in the hope of locating a few additional positive cases. He proposed that it be used to evaluate uncertain cases. Freedman placed emphasis on the advantages of using a digital computer in the reconstructions, in that histograms of particular tomographic readouts and quantitative data could be obtained. In addition, he suggested that once tomographic images of various planes have been determined an iterative process may be possible to selectively remove data arising from

* Atomic Development Corp.
† Nuclear Data, Inc.

planes above and below the plane of interest. Myers, Keyes, and Mallard[12] are exploring methods to achieve this goal.

Another approach to obtaining focal plane tomography has been explored at the Upstate Medical Center, New York, using a modified scintillation camera with an angled parallel-hole collimator and a small digital computer to reconstruct the isotope distribution from various planes as it is collected by rectilinear sweeps centering on a common axis of rotation.[27,2f] The blurring pattern produced by this system consists of a number of spots arranged around the circumference of a circle. No clinical results are reported. The work of this group is currently concentrated on methods of image construction which will allow the distribution of radiation near a single plane to be displayed, whereas radiation from regions not within the selected plane will not be displayed. The advantage of this scanning system over the rotational method is the potential to image large areas.

Arimizu[16] reviewed various methods of obtaining tomographic images using different collimators attached to the scintillation camera. Preliminary results obtained using a pinhole collimator showed better quality images than those produced using an angled parallel-hole collimator. He pointed out that a diverging or converging collimator could also be used to obtain tomographic readouts. A single clinical study was included in the report.

Mathieu from Lyons, France, currently at Donner Laboratory, is using a computer to construct images focused at different depths from multiple views taken with the gamma camera and pinhole collimator.

Cottrall and Flioni-Vyza[28] reported on the design of a scintillation camera tomographic system and preliminary clinical experience at Monte Carlo in 1972. Their system is identical in principle to that described by Muehllehner and Freedman. It uses a rotating collimator with the holes angled at 45°, in comparison with the 20° angulation of the holes in the camera designed by Muehllehner. Their camera, accordingly, has greater tomographic blurring effect. Clinical experience is still limited, but they report that lesions in the brain and liver were located and that plane separations of 1 cm were recognized. They found the images to be blurred and unfamiliar, and artifacts were produced under some conditions. In the brain tomoscans the image of the brain was sometimes obscured by a defocused image of the relatively high activity in the nasal sinuses. The degree of practical application of their method awaits further trial and the authors conclude that further processing of the data will be necessary to suppress information arising outside the plane of interest in the readout of a specific plane.

Image artifacts that result from the nature of the blur pattern produced by tomographic gamma camera systems employing rotating collimators have been described by Goldsmith.[29] Artifacts have been noted by several authors in their review of the clinical applications of such systems and it remains to be seen whether they are indeed limiting factors. Anger[2b] has discussed the merits of different blur patterns.

The tomocamera systems described to date lack resolution in comparison with some other means of tomographic imaging and this may be the reason for their relatively poor clinical acceptance.

Myers et al[12] presented arguments for developing a tomographic scanner from the scintillation camera rather than a rotating collimator tomographic camera; the scanner has better resolution, requires less engineering, produces an ideal disk blurring pattern, and has an unlimited field of view. The main disadvantage is that imaging times are longer. The most exciting proposal in this paper is a potential method for correcting the readouts for counts due to activity in overlying and underlying planes. If this potential can be realized, focal-plane tomography will be markedly improved.

Miraldi and Di Chiro have developed the "Tomoscanner"[2g] and have reported their early clinical experience.[2h] This instrument employs a line detector with an angled collimator and makes many passes over the body in different directions. The information acquired on each pass is digitized and stored on magnetic tape. To obtain the tomoscan for a given level the images from all passes are replayed and appropriately superimposed on an oscilloscope screen one layer at a time. Each reconstructed image contains the same amount of information with different spatial arrangements. The blur pattern for out-of-focus planes is ring-shaped, and artifacts have been noted.

Clinical experience with the "Tomoscanner"[2h] is still limited. In their original design the inclination of the scanning probe was 45°, which gave a strong tomographic effect but also created obscuring blur patterns. The scanner has been modified to have a variable angle of inclination; an angle of 30° is being used. Only further experience will determine the clinical value of this instrument. Possibly a change of radiopharmaceutical for brain imaging from ^{99m}Tc-pertechnetate to ^{99m}Tc-DTPA, which does not concentrate in the salivary glands, will give better results, since interference from the blur pattern of these high-activity structures would then be absent.

A Fresnel zone plate can be used as a "coded aperture" to image gamma rays.[31] The theory and details of this method of imaging are beyond the scope of this chapter, and the purpose of mentioning it here is to draw attention to its prospects. Barrett et al[2i] have been exploring the use of Fresnel zone plates in phantom studies and in clinical applications. They have shown that it is possible to obtain high-resolution images focused on specific planes. They point out that a number of questions still need to be resolved about this system: What is the best way to process and display the images? Can a true three-dimensional image be obtained? When do artifacts occur and how may they be recognized? Can the artifacts be eliminated? It will be interesting to follow the developments in Fresnel zone plate imaging and to learn the answers to these questions.

POSITRON IMAGING SYSTEMS

The positron camera as developed by Anger at Donner Laboratory[32] has significant tomographic capability. The plane of best focus can be varied electronically to any desired depth and multiple levels can be read out simultaneously by pulse stretching techniques. Such positron cameras, however, are subject to electronic overload. An upper limit of 50 μCi can be in their field of view, with a coincidence detection rate of around 20,000 events per minute. If tracers labeled with positron-emitting isotopes are developed for small organs such as the parathyroid gland, the excellent resolution provided by the positron camera may be valuable.

The Massachusetts General Hospital positron camera[2j] is designed to obtain rapid sequential images of positron-emitting radionuclides and has a high data-rate capacity. The instrument uses two identical detector arrays, each containing 127 small crystals. The use of discrete detectors introduces a problem with distinct patterns of detectors being apparent in the readouts unless motion is used to interpolate between detectors. Tomography is an integral part of the MGH camera, where a focal plane must be selected before an image can be constructed. To date the full tomographic capability of the instrument has not been pursued. The future clinical applications of this instrument as a practical means of imaging positron-emitting tracers in rapid sequence studies together with high-resolution tomographic readout will be of great interest.

In theory it is possible to locate the site of annihilation of positrons in tissue from the difference in time between the detection of the two 0.51-MeV gamma rays in two fast gamma-ray counters placed on opposite sides of the subject. Data coming from just one site in the patient are selected, an example of a true isolation technique. A relatively small number of detected counts from a region should be sufficient. The time differences involved in these time-of-flight measurements are extremely small and further improvement in time resolution is required over that reported by Lynch[33] before we will have an instrument with sufficient spatial resolution to be of clinical value.

CLINICAL EXPERIENCE WITH THE MULTIPLANE TOMOGRAPHIC SCANNER

Anger summarized the characteristics of the multiplane tomographic scanner and compared its performance with that of a conventional 5-in. rectilinear scanner and the tomocamera system.[2b] The multiplane tomoscanner, with its 8½-in.-diameter crystal, has about twice the sensitivity of the conventional scanner, and it gives high resolution at all depths from zero to 6 in. from the collimator, whereas the 5-in. conventional scanner gives high resolution only at depths near the geometric focal plane. The multiplane tomoscanner has better resolution than the tomocamera, but imaging time is longer. The scanner can image any size field up to the limits of its mechanical design, and its field is inherently uniform. Each readout contains the same number of dots; those arising from the structures in the readout plane are accurately placed while scintillations coming from out-of-focus structures are spread over an area of film which increases with distance from the structure to the readout plane. The scanner has no blur pattern artifact in its readouts because it produces a disk-shaped blur pattern, whereas the tomocamera produces a ring pattern, which can cause artifacts.[29,2k]

The total clinical experience with 448 patient studies using the Donner Laboratory multiplane tomographic scanner[2b] was last reviewed in November 1972.[21] In that analysis it was reported that the six-plane tomoscans provided better images of all organs except the kidney, pancreas, thyroid, and adrenal glands in comparison with conventional scintiphotos. The pancreatic images have been reappraised. In 21 studies in which technically satisfactory scintiphotos and tomoscans of the pancreas were obtained, the tomographic images were superior in 13, equal in quality in 6, and inferior in 2. The tomoscans of the pancreas were suboptimal, but it is clear that further clinical evaluation is needed. In other respects the conclusions remain unchanged. In a number of cases, lesions have been detected in tomoscans that were not recognized in scintiphotos of the lung and liver. In ^{67}Ga tumor surveys and in bone scans using ^{18}F and ^{99m}Tc-labeled bone tracers the multiple readouts have helped to differentiate between anatomical structures and pathology. The tomoscans have provided a practical guide to the depth of lesions and small organs and we use them to determine the depth of the adrenal glands when calculating the fractional uptake of 19-iodocholesterol (Fig. 5-1).

Figure 5-1 shows a six-plane tomoscan and a conventional scintiphoto taken with the Donner Laboratory 16-in. scintillation camera (below) of the adrenal area 7 days after injection of 1 mCi of ^{131}I-19-iodocholesterol. The adrenal glands are best seen in the sixth readout of the tomoscan, which is focused on a plane 6 in. from the collimator face. The depth of the organ, as determined from the readout in best focus, is used to determine the tissue absorption correction in calculating the fraction of the injected tracer which accumulates in each adrenal gland. Uptake is about twice normal in this patient with bilateral adrenal hyperplasia.

It has proved of significant help to see a questionable area going out of focus in the readout planes above and below the readout in which a

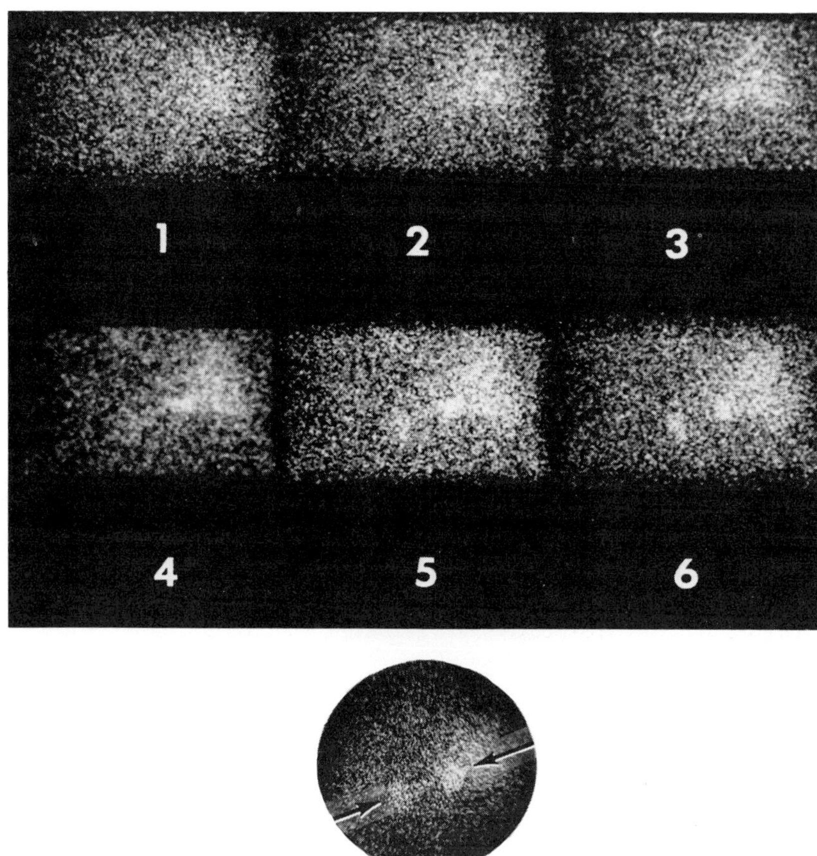

Fig. 5-1. A six-plane tomoscan and a scintiphoto of the adrenal area 7 days after injection of 1 mCi of ^{131}I-19-iodocholesterol.

questionable area is recognized. With the multiplane tomograhic scanner there is still a need for multiple views, such as frontal, lateral, posterior, etc., because the readouts of deeper planes lack the information density of superficial planes due to the absorption of gamma rays. In addition there is a moderate loss of resolution for the deeper planes because of increased distance from the collimator face.

During 1973 the major clinical application of the multiplane tomographic scanner has been in bone scintigraphy using Tc-labeled polyphosphate and EHDP. The skeleton has a varied distribution of isotope at different depths which the tomoscanner shows particularly clearly since the surrounding tissue contains a relatively low level of tracer. As we noted in

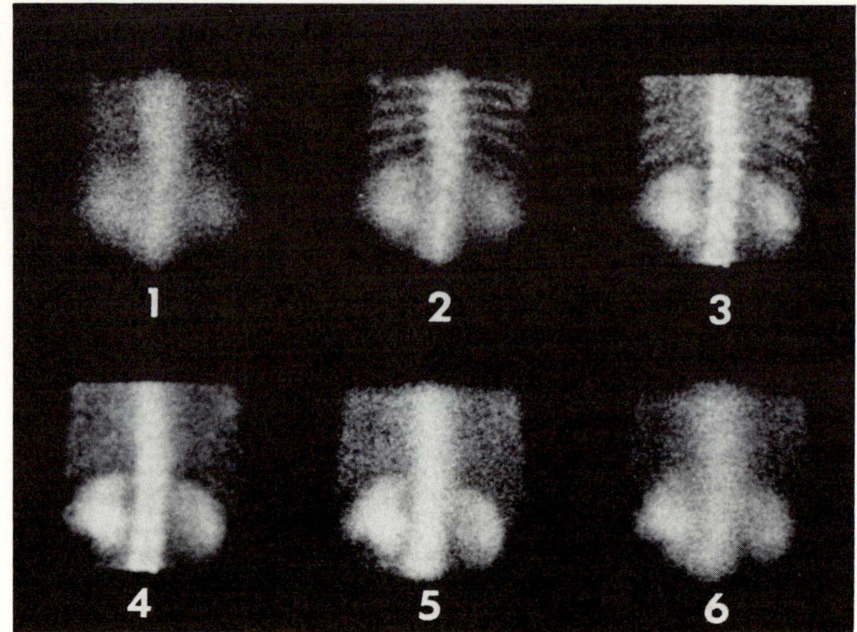

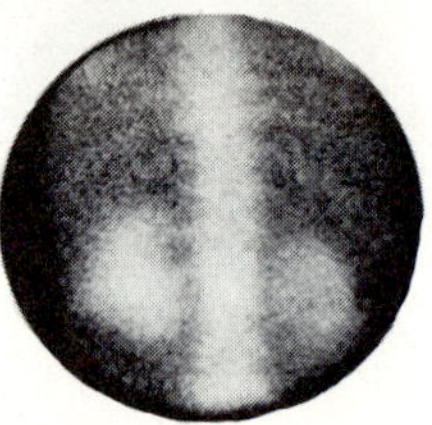

Fig. 5-2.   A six-plane tomoscan and a scintiphoto of the lower thoracic and upper lumbar area after injection of 10 mCi ^{99m}Tc bone scanning agent.

an earlier report,[2k] much anatomical detail can be recognized. In the posterior view of the spine, two rows of discrete paired spots of high uptake are apparent in a significant fraction of patients. These foci almost certainly represent uptake into the articular processes. This appearance is illustrated in Figure 5-2. The numbers on the six-plane tomogram indicate the distance in inches from the collimator face to the readout focal plane. For bone studies an area of 18×16 in. is scanned in approximately 15 min, and 200,000 to 300,000 dots are recorded 3 to 5 hr following the injection of 10 mCi of ^{99m}Tc-labeled tracer.

The images cover the lower thoracic and upper lumbar area. In readout 2 the tips of the scapulae and the ribs are in focus and the spinous

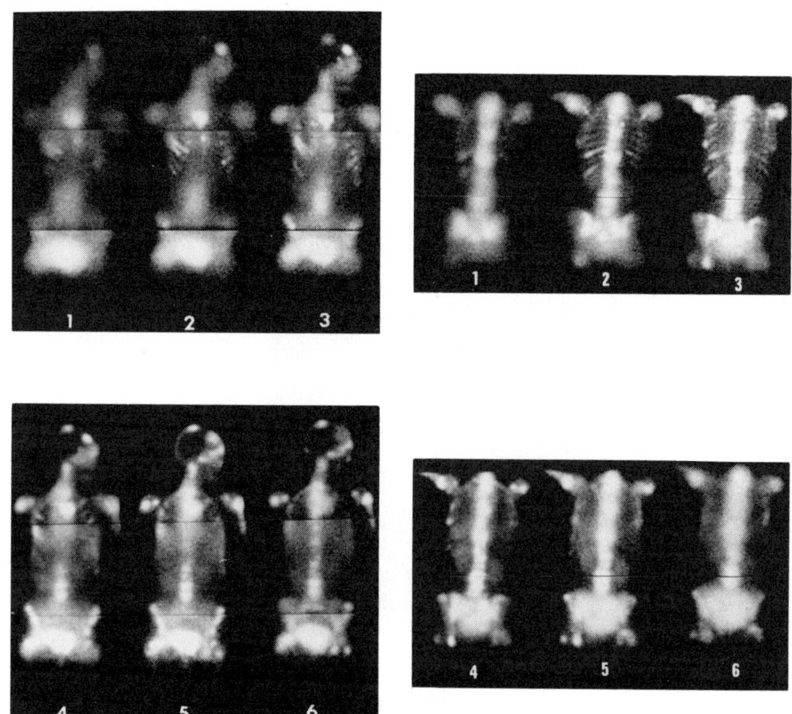

Fig. 5-3.   Composite anterior and posterior tomoscans of a patient with multiple bone metastases.

processes of the lower thoracic and lumbar vertebrae can be distinguished. In readout 3 the rows of paired articular processes are clearly seen and have an ordered degree of labeling. In readouts 4 and 5 the kidneys are in focus; this patient has a renal abnormality with a dilated renal pelvis containing tracer on the left side. The scintiphoto of the same region is not as clear as the tomograms.

In a number of patients being scanned to exclude metastatic disease, the articular processes do not have an ordered progression of labeling and one pair may appear more active than adjacent pairs. When the study is otherwise normal, we attribute the findings to increased strain on these particular joints. More important than considerations of the mechanisms of higher labeling in a single pair of joints or a single joint is the possible error that may arise in the interpretation of bone studies. If these small structures are not seen with high resolution, but are blurred by lying above or below the focal plane of a conventional scanner or are seen with less resolution in a scintiphoto, it is possible to interpret them as local abnor-

SIX-PLANE TOMOSCANS OF PATIENT WITH BRAIN TUMOR

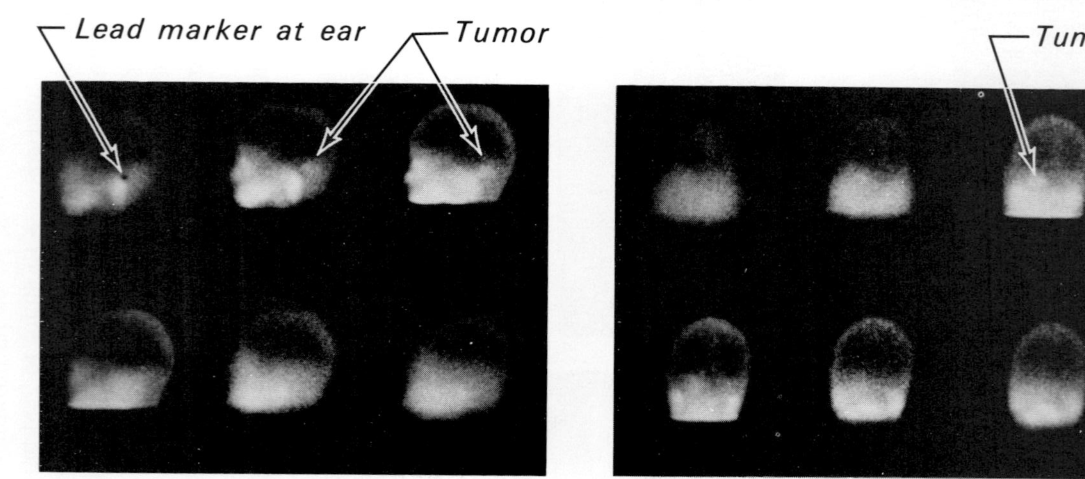

Fig. 5-4.   Left lateral and posterior tomoscans of a patient with a posterior fossa tumor.

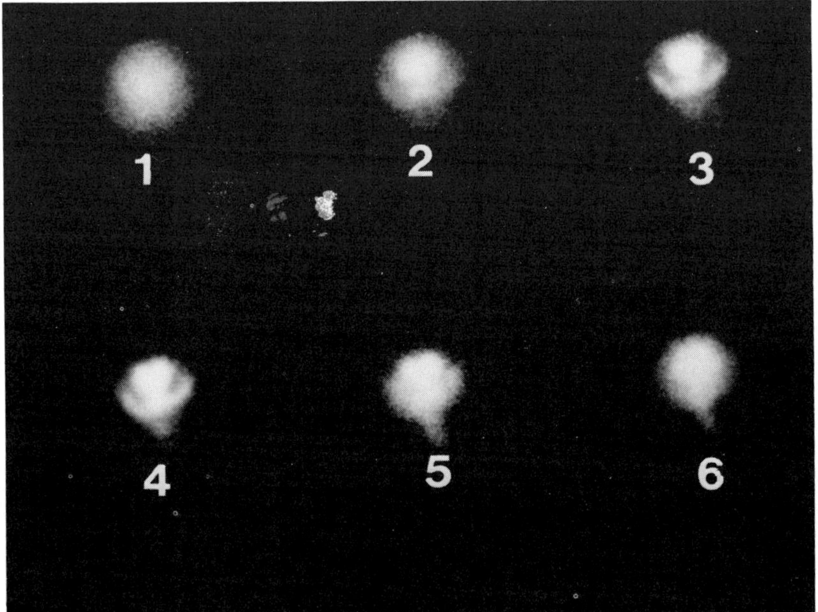

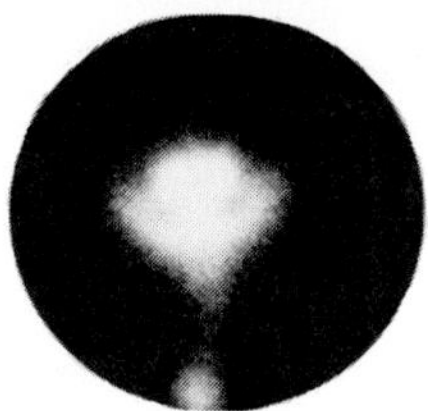

Fig. 5-5.   Anterior tomoscan and scintiphoto taken 4 hr after injection of 1.5 mCi ^{169}Yb-DTPA into the lumbar thecal space. Tracer is apparent within the lateral ventricles.

malities such as metastatic disease. In some patients with widespread metastatic disease, high uptake has been seen in pairs of articular processes (Fig. 5-3). These may well be common sites of metastases and pose a problem in interpretation which only further experience will solve.

Figure 5-3 is a composite of anterior and posterior tomoscans of a patient with widespread metastatic bone disease from the breast. Numerous metastases can be seen in and out of focus in the readouts focused at progressively deeper levels. Involvement of the bodies of the vertebra are probably best appreciated in anterior tomoscans (left); in this patient there is high uptake in the bodies of several lumbar vertebrae (readout 5). Note that in the posterior tomoscan of the spine (right) high uptake is apparent in several pairs of articular processes.

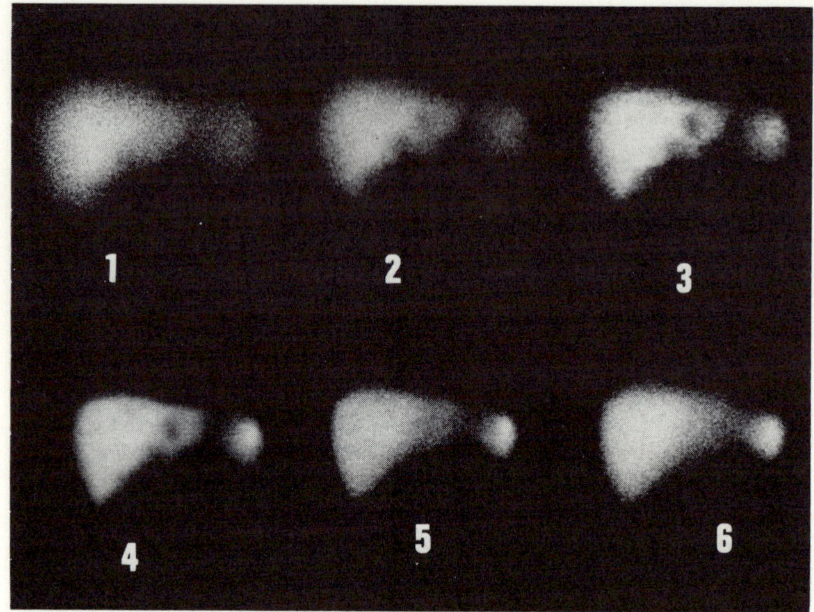

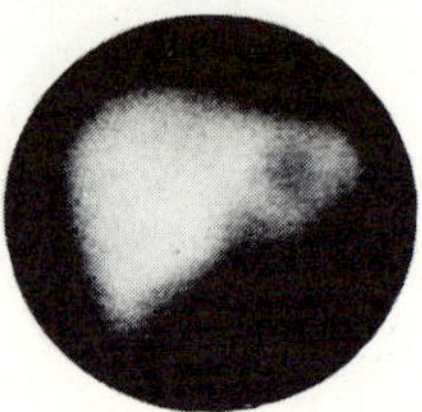

Fig. 5-6. Anterior tomoscan and scintiphoto of the liver with multiple metastases.

Over 50 patients have had bone studies performed, using ^{99m}Tc-poly-phosphate and EHDP, in which tomoscans have been included in the study. In almost every instance the high resolution of the six-plane tomoscans and the appreciation of depth have proved of significant value in interpreting the study and better defining the site of bone lesions. It is clear that whole-body tomographic images will be excellent for metastatic bone surveys and tumor localization with tumor-specific agents.

Applications of the multiplane tomographic scanner for other organs are illustrated by the following clinical examples. Tomoscans have proved useful in brain imaging; the sharp definition that can be obtained is apparent in Figure 5-4, which includes the left lateral and posterior tomoscans of a patient with a posterior fossa tumor. These tomoscans were taken 1 hr following the injection of 10 mCi of ^{99m}Tc-pertechnetate and each

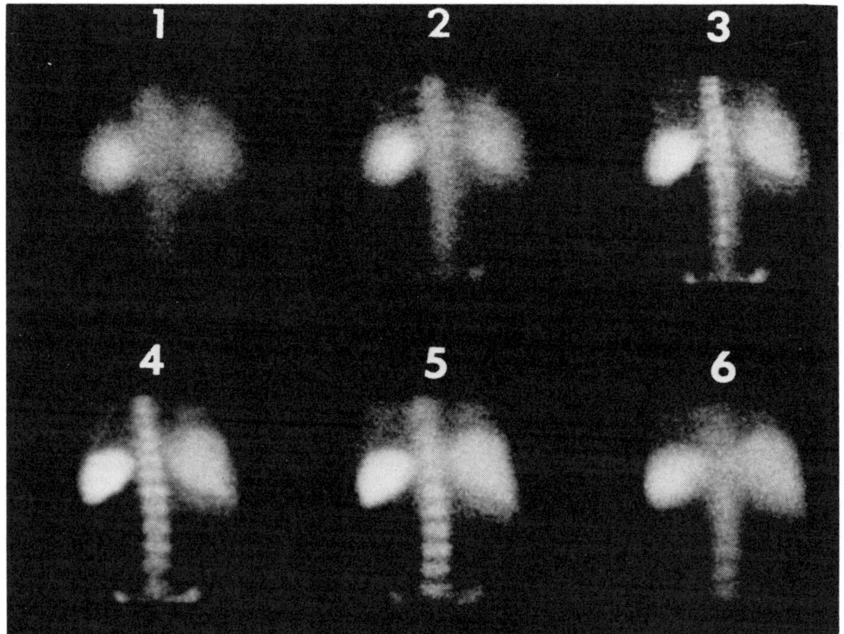

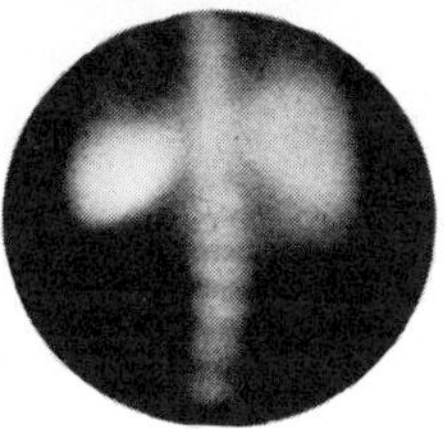

Fig. 5-7. Posterior tomoscan and scintiphoto of a patient with cirrhosis with increased ^{99m}Tc colloid uptake in the bone marrow.

scan took 7 min. A small lead marker has been placed over the tragus of the ear, and is clearly seen in the first readout in the lateral view. The parotid gland is in sharp focus in readout 2, the nasal structures in readout 3. The tumor is equally well seen in readouts 2 and 3. In the posterior view the tumor is in sharp focus in readout 3 and the parotid glands can be seen in readout 4.

Tomoscans have been performed using both ^{169}Yb-DTPA and ^{111}In-DTPA for cisternography studies. Figure 5-5 shows an anterior tomoscan and scintiphoto taken 4 hr following the injection of 1.5 mCi of ^{169}Yb-DTPA into the lumbar thecal space. Tracer is clearly apparent within the lateral ventricles. No further progression over the surfaces of the hemispheres was noted at later times.

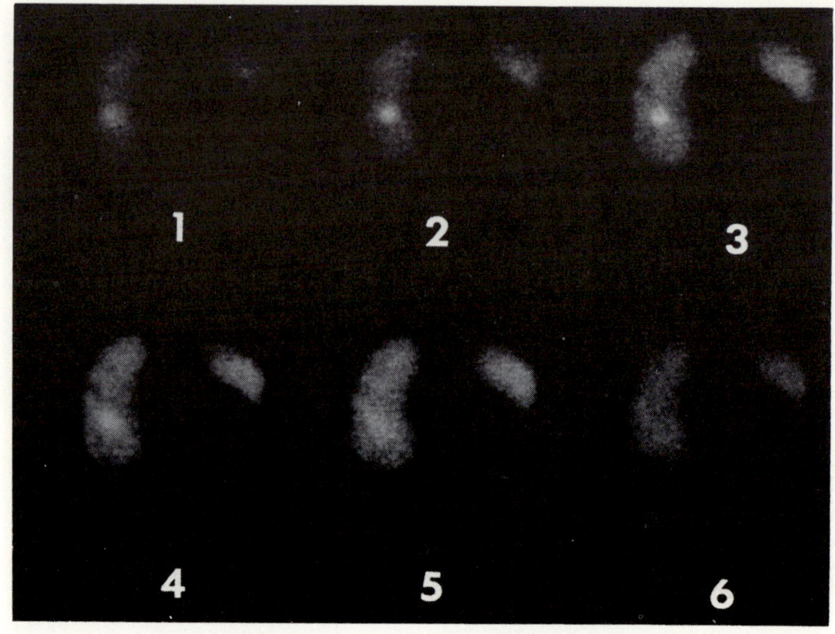

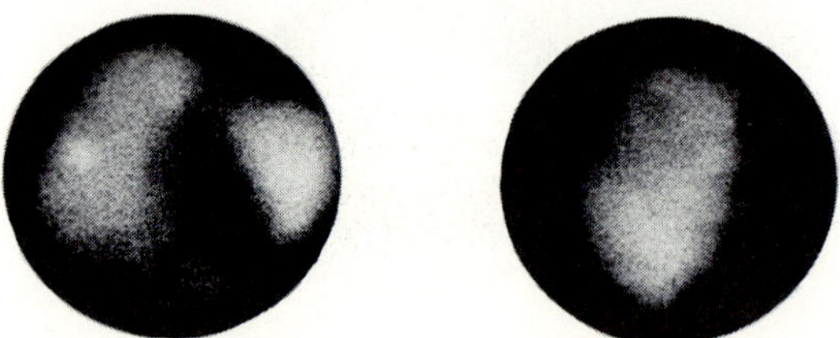

Fig. 5-8.   Posterior tomoscan and posterior and left lateral scintiphotos of a patient with an enlarged spleen and small posteriorly situated splenuncle.

Interpretation of liver studies is easier when they include tomoscans. Figure 5-6 includes an anterior tomoscan and scintiphoto of the liver of a patient with multiple metastases from carcinoma of the breast. The tomoscan was obtained using 2 mCi of ^{99m}Tc colloid and a plane spacing of 1 in. Metastases are in focus in readouts 2, 3, and 4. The smaller lesions within the right lobe apparent in readout 4 cannot be distinguished in the scintiphoto.

The number of occasions on which metastases were detected only in the tomoscans and not in scintiphotos was small, but the better definition in the tomoscans was an advantage. In instances where the radioactive colloid was within the bone marrow (Fig. 5-7) or other extraneous sites

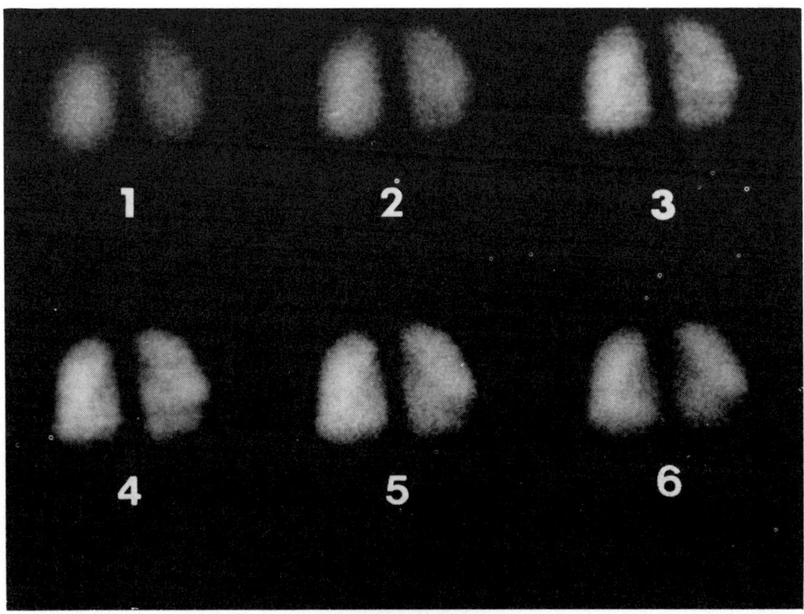

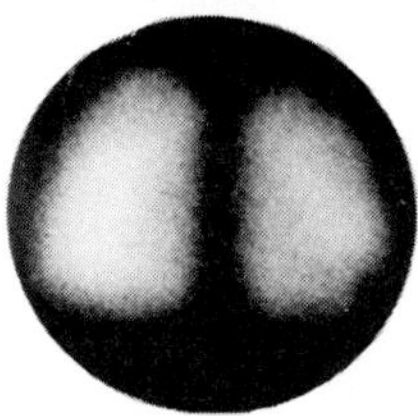

Fig. 5-9. Posterior tomoscan and scintiphoto of the lungs with a wedge-shaped defect in the right lower lobe.

such as in a splenuncle (Fig. 5-8), the tomoscans provided superior definition.

Figure 5-7 shows a posterior tomoscan and scintiphoto of a patient with cirrhosis of the liver. Colloid is apparent in the ribs (readout 2), spinous processes (readout 3), articular processes (readout 4), and vertebral bodies (readout 5). It is of interest to note that the intervertebral spaces can be more clearly distinguished when the tracer is within the marrow rather than in the bone itself (see Fig. 5-2).

Figure 5-8 shows a posterior tomoscan of the liver and spleen of a patient with lymphoma with a very enlarged spleen and a small posterior placed splenuncle. The small splenuncle can be seen sharply in readouts 2 and 3. Posterior and left lateral scintiphotos below also show the size and position of the splenuncle quite clearly.

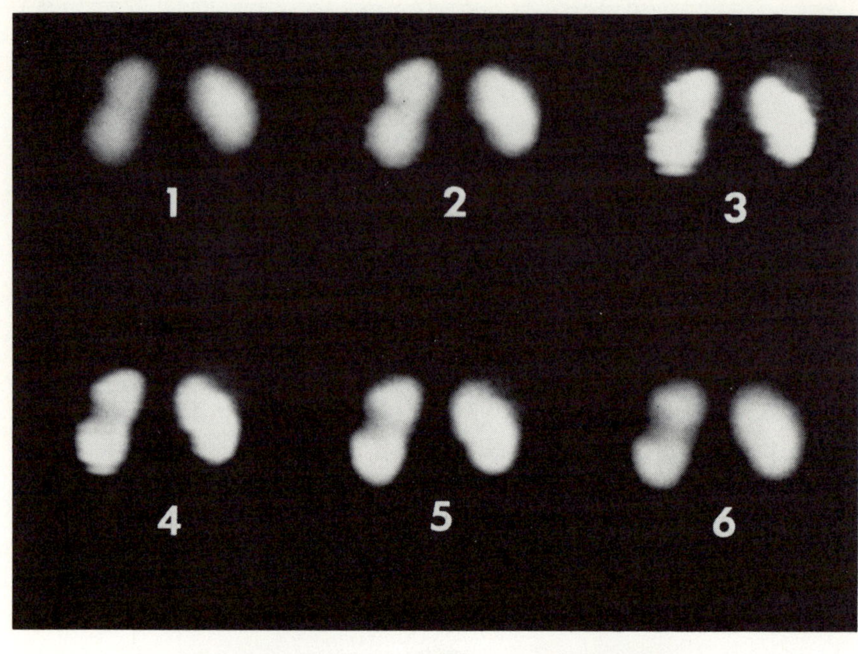

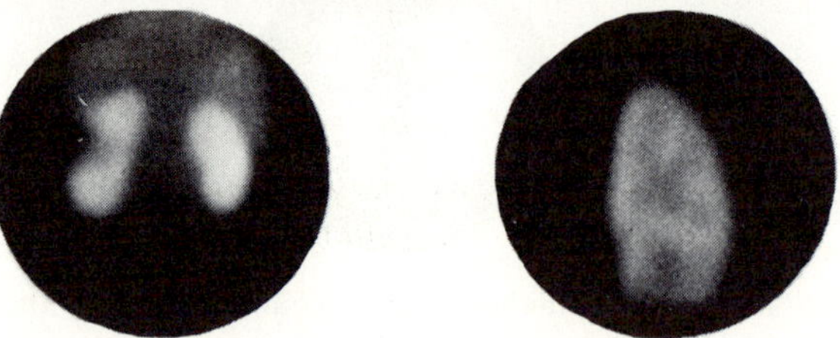

Fig. 5-10. Tomoscan and scintiphotos of the kidneys. The left kidney contains a cyst. Note the detail in the pinhole scintiphoto of the upper half of the right kidney.

Our experience with lung imaging is limited because we are not part of a clinical facility and relatively few patients are referred for lung scanning on an outpatient basis. An example of the better definition that we have obtained in one patient with a pulmonary embolism is given in Figure 5-9, which shows a posterior tomoscan and scintiphoto of the lungs following the injection of 2 mCi of ^{99m}Tc-labeled microspheres. Note the clear definition of the wedge-shaped defect in the right lower lobe, best seen in readouts 5 and 6.

Renal imaging is best performed with a scintillation camera using a pinhole collimator if sharp anatomical detail is desired. However, to appreciate the depth of the kidneys, the tomoscan is valuable and could prove useful prior to biopsy.

Figure 5-10 shows tomoscans and scintiphotos of a patient with a cyst in the left kidney. The plane spacing on this occasion was set at $\frac{1}{2}$ in. with the first readout focused at 2.2 in., and the sixth readout at 4.7 in. Five millicuries of ^{99m}Tc-caseidin were used and the scan time was 5 min. The details shown in the tomoscan are equivalent to those in the parallel-hole scintiphoto shown on the left below. However, a close-up study of the upper pole of the right kidney taken with a pinhole collimator contains much more detail; the rim of cortex and columns of Bertin are seen. Such fine anatomical detail can only be achieved with the pinhole collimator and is not seen in tomoscans using our present collimators, even with close plane spacing.

CONCLUSIONS

The present methods of tomography function best for imaging areas of relatively high concentration of isotope rather than for displaying areas of decreased uptake. Section images of the brain provide valuable information that cannot be gained from conventional rectilinear scans or scintiphotos. Focal-plane tomography with multiple readouts focused at different depths appears particularly promising in bone imaging and tumor surveys using tumor-specific agents.

There is a continuing need in nuclear medicine for better methods for imaging the distribution of radioactive tracers within the body. Progress is being made. As new radiopharmaceuticals are developed which trace the diverse functions of the different organs of the body we will gain additional valuable distribution of the tracer. This three-dimensional information is important for both static and dynamic studies.

REFERENCES

1. Kuhl DE, Sanders TP: Comparison of rectilinear vertex and transverse section views in brain scanning. J Nucl Med 11:2–8, 1970
2. Freedman GS, (ed): Tomographic Imaging in Nuclear Medicine. New York, The Society of Nuclear Medicine, 1973
2a. Patton SA, Brill AB, King PH: Transverse section brain scanning with a multicrystal cylindrical imaging device, in Freedman GS (ed): Tomographic Imaging in Nuclear Medicine. New York, The Society of Nuclear Medicine, 1973
2b. Anger HO: Multiplane tomographic scanner, in Freedman GS (ed): Tomographic Imaging in Nuclear Medicine. New York, The Society of Nuclear Medicine, 1973

2c. Monahan WA, Powell MD: Three-dimensional imaging of radionuclide distributions by gamma-gamma coincidence detection, in Freedman GS (ed): Tomographic Imaging in Nuclear Medicine. New York, The Society of Nuclear Medicine, 1973

2d. Everette JA Jr, Langan JK, Fisher KA, et al: Clinical experience in tomographic imaging with a tomocamera, in Freedman GS (ed): Tomographic Imaging in Nuclear Medicine. New York, The Society of Nuclear Medicine, 1973

2e. Freedman GS: Clinical experience with a digital gamma camera tomography system, in Freedman GS (ed): Tomographic Imaging in Nuclear Medicine. New York, The Society of Nuclear Medicine, 1973

2f. Stabler EP: Nuclear medicine tomography at Upstate Medical Center, NY, in Freedman GS (ed): Tomographic Imaging in Nuclear Medicine. New York, The Society of Nuclear Medicine, 1973

2g. Miraldi F, Yon ET, Di Chiro G: Tomoscanner: theory and prototype, in Freedman GS (ed): Tomographic Imaging in Nuclear Medicine. New York, The Society of Nuclear Medicine, 1973

2h. Di Chiro G, Johnston GS, Miraldi F, et al: The tomoscanner; clinical experience, in Freedman GS (ed): Tomographic Imaging in Nuclear Medicine. New York, The Society of Nuclear Medicine, 1973

2i. Barrett HH, De Meetser AD, Wilson DT, et al: Tomographic imaging with a Fresnel zone plate system, in Freedman GS (ed): Tomographic Imaging in Nuclear Medicine. New York, The Society of Nuclear Medicine, 1973

2j. Brownell GL, Burnham CA: MGH positron camera, in Freedman GS (ed): Tomographic Imaging in Nuclear Medicine. New York, The Society of Nuclear Medicine, 1973

2k. Goldsmith SJ: Clinical artifacts encountered using circular tomography, in Freedman GS (ed): Tomographic Imaging in Nuclear Medicine. New York, The Society of Nuclear Medicine, 1973

2l. McRae J, Anger HO: Clinical results from the multiplane tomographic scanner, in Freedman GS (ed): Tomographic Imaging in Nuclear Medicine. New York, The Society of Nuclear Medicine, 1973

3. Kuhl DE, Edwards RQ: Image separation radioisotope scanning. Radiology 80:653–661, 1963

4. Kuhl DE, Edwards RQ: Cylindrical and section radioisotope scanning of the liver and brain. Radiology 83:926–935, 1964

5. Kuhl DE, Pitts FW, Sanders TP, Mishkin MM: Transverse section and rectilinear brain scanning with ^{99m}Tc pertechnetate. Radiology 86:822–829, 1966

6. Kuhl DE, Edwards RQ: Reorganizing data from transverse section scans of the brain using digital processing. Radiology 91:975–983, 1968

7. Kuhl DE, Edwards RQ: The Mark III scanner: a compact device for multiple-view and section scanning of the brain. Radiology 96:563–570, 1970

8. Kuhl DE, Edwards RQ, Ricci AR, Reivich M: Quantitative section scanning using orthogonal tangent correction. J Nucl Med 14:196–200, 1973

9. Kuhl DE, Sanders TP: Characterizing brain lesions with use of transverse section scanning. Radiology 98:317–328, 1971

10. Manlio FL, Masland WS, Kuhl DE, Staum MM: The prognostic significance of a deep-wedge pattern in transverse section scanning of cerebral infarctions. Radiology 103:135–137, 1972

11. Patton JA, Brill AB, King PH: A new mode of collection and display of three-dimensional data for static and dynamic radiotracer studies. Symposium on Medical Radioisotope Scintigraphy, Monte Carlo, 1972

12. Myers MJ, Keyes WI, Mallard JR: An analysis of tomographic scanning systems. Symposium on Medical Radioisotope Scintigraphy, Monte Carlo, 1972
13. Anger HO, Price DC, Yost PE: Transverse-section tomography with the scintillation camera. J Nucl Med 8:314, 1967
14. Muehllehner G, Wetzel RA: Section imaging by computer calculation. J Nucl Med 12:76–84, 1970
15. Budinger TF: Chapter 2, this volume
16. Arimizu, N: Methods of tomographic imagings in preference of collimator. Symposium on Medical Radioisotope Scintigraphy, Monte Carlo, 1972
17. Hart, HE: Focusing collimator coincidence scanning. Radiology 84:126, 1965
18. McAfee JG, Mozley JM, Natarajan TK, Fueger GF, Wagner HN Jr: Scintillation scanning with an eight-inch-diameter sodium iodide (T1) crystal. J Nucl Med 7:521–547, 1966
19. Hisada K-I, Hiraki T, Ohba S, Matsudaira M: Simultaneous performance of isosensitive scanning and bilaminoscanning. Radiology 88:129–134, 1967
20. Gottschalk A, Beck, RN (eds): Fundamental problems in Scanning. Springfield, Illinois, Charles C Thomas, 1968
21. Muehllehner G: A tomographic scintillation camera. Phys Med Biol 16:87–96, 1971
22. Chamroenngan S, Langan JK, Tratter JM, Muehllenhner G, Wagner HN Jr: Tomographic imaging with the scintillation camera in the detection and characterization of brain lesions. Radiology 98:445–448, 1971
23. DeLand FH, James AE, Muehllehner G, Wagner HN Jr: The value of tomography in liver scanning. Radiology 102:429–432, 1972
24. Lindberg RS, Larsson GAB, Roos BO: A comparison between tomography and conventional scintigraphy of the liver with a scintillation camera. Symposium on Medical Radioisotope Scintigraphy, Monte Carlo, 1972
25. Freedman GS: Tomography with a gamma camera. J Nucl Med 11:602–604, 1970
26. Freedman GS: Gamma camera tomography. Radiology 102:365–369, 1972
27. McAfee JG, Mozley JM: Longitudinal tomographic radioisotopic imaging with a scintillation camera: theoretical considerations of a new method. J Nucl Med 10:654–659, 1969
28. Cottrall MF, Flioni-Vyza A: The design of a scintillation camera tomographic system and investigations of its performance. Symposium on Medical Radioisotope Scintigraphy, Monte Carlo, 1972
29. Goldsmith SJ: Image artifacts in tomographic gamma camera systems. J Nucl Med 14:103–106, 1973
30. Miraldi F, Di Chiro G: Tomographic techniques in radioisotope imaging with a proposal of a new device: the tomoscanner. Radiology 94:513–520, 1970
31. Barrett HH: Fresnel zone plate imaging in nuclear medicine. J Nucl Med 13:382–385, 1972
32. Anger HO: Radioisotope cameras, in Hine GJ (ed): Instrumentation in Nuclear Medicine. New York, Academic Press, 1967, pp 485–552
33. Lynch FJ: Improved timing with NaI (T1). IEEE Transactions on Nuclear Science. NS-13. New York, Institute of Electrical and Electronic Engineers, 1966, pp 140–147

Martin A. Winston

James H. Pritchard

William H. Blahd

6

The Correlation of Ultrasonic and Nuclear Medicine Techniques

The rapid strides made during the past few years in ultrasonic instrumentation and technique have resulted in an extremely useful new diagnostic tool. Like radioisotope nuclear scanning, ultrasonography is well adapted to the study of solid organs. The nuclear medicine physician, therefore, should be aware of the many areas in which the two techniques are complementary, as well as those in which the newer modality seems likely to replace the older one.

Vibration in the frequency range of 1 to 5 mHz is termed "ultrasound." By comparison, audible sound is in the range of 25 to 15,000 Hz. Special crystals can be made to vibrate in the ultrasonic range by the passage of electrical impulses that cause rapid rearrangements of the crystal lattice, resulting in expansion and contraction, thereby generating bursts of ultrasound. This conversion of electrical to mechanical energy—termed the piezoelectric effect—occurs in reverse as well, sound vibrations returning to the crystal being converted into electrical impulses.[1,2]

When such a crystal transducer is suitably coupled to the skin, the ultrasound waves may be propagated in a straight but slightly diverging path through the body. Reflection of a portion of the sound wave energy occurs when the wave encounters a transition plane, or interface, between conducting media of different characteristic impedance (a factor combining tissue density and the velocity of sound within the tissue). When this interface is roughly perpendicular to the path of the sound beam, the reflection eventually returns to the crystal transducer. Since the latter emits 10-μsec bursts of ultrasound waves about 1000 times per second, it is in a nontransmitting mode some 99 percent of the time, thus capable of receiving returning echoes.

The echoes may be displayed in several ways. The amplitude mode (A) consists conventionally of a horizontal baseline calibrated in centimeters corresponding to distance from the transducer. Returning echoes are displayed as deflections from the baseline. The depth of the echo-producing interface is automatically calculated from the time taken for the echo to return and the mean speed of sound in the body. In the brightness mode (B), echoes are displayed not as vertical lines but as dots of an intensity corresponding to the strength of the echo returned. In the scanning mode (Compound B), the baseline moves through 360° to correspond to the movements of a scanning transducer. When a persistence oscilloscope or time-exposure photography is used, the dots can be integrated into an image representing a cross section—either transverse or longitudinal—through the body.[3]

The time/motion mode (T/M) is basically an adaptation of the B mode for the study of oscillating structures, such as the heart wall or valves. When these structures move within the sound beam toward or away from the transducer, the dot corresponding to their reflecting surface moves back or forward along the baseline. If the baseline is moved across the oscilloscope from bottom to top, the dot describes a modified sine wave pattern. This too is recorded using either time-exposure photography or a persistence oscilloscope.

Attenuation of the sound beam in the more distal structures can be compensated for by an increase in gain on the returning echoes—the time–gain compensation, or TGC. In addition, near-gain controls are used to dampen heavy echoes at the transducer–skin interface. Finally, the overall gain may be varied to bring out echoes from relatively minor interfaces, such as the blood and other tissues within a solid organ. Even at high gain settings a fluid-filled structure, such as a cyst or an abscess, is too homogeneous to generate internal echoes.

The conductance of air and bone is sufficiently different from that of soft tissue that an interface between them reflects a very large amount of sound energy. For this reason, a coupling medium such as mineral oil is spread over the body to eliminate air at the skin–transducer junction. Similarly, air-filled loops of bowel effectively block transmission and thus interfere with the study of portions of the abdominal contents. Barium within bowel loops further degrades imaging.[4] The heart can only be studied through a relatively small window where it is not overlain by lung. In emphysematous individuals, even this window may disappear.

The lungs themselves cannot be studied, although one report describes a technique for detecting areas of consolidation near the pleural surface, such as those caused by thromboemboli.[5]

Water, on the other hand, is an excellent conducting medium. The filled bladder thus provides an ideal window for studying the pelvic contents. Not only does the bladder conduct sound well, but as it expands, bowel loops are pushed out of the way.

LIVER

This organ is well suited to study by both nuclear and ultrasonic imaging, and several investigations have illustrated the advantages of each technique.[6,7] For surveying the organ as a whole, nuclear imaging is clearly more suitable. It is tedious to study such a large organ by performing successive cross-sectional cuts, as required in ultrasonic studies. When a specific area is called into question by a radioisotopic scan, it may then be evaluated ultrasonically. A questionable abnormality, such as may occur in the porta hepatis region or left lobe where the anatomy is particularly variable, may thus be confirmed[6] (Fig. 6-1A–C). A distinct focal abnormality may be classified as either solid—and therefore presumably a neoplasm—or cystic—a cyst, hematoma, or abscess.[7] Further information can be gained from scanning with gallium 67, so that the nature of a mass lesion can be accurately pinpointed (Fig. 6-1D–K).

The resolution limits of a discrete lesion are essentially the same for both techniques—approximately 2 cm.[8] Unfortunately, in diffuse hepatic disease, ultrasonography is not more accurate than radioisotope scanning, and distinguishing between cirrhosis and carcinomatosis is still quite difficult.[9]

A transducer with a central canal has been adapted for accurate guidance of liver biopsy. A Menghini needle may be passed through this canal precisely in the plane and to precisely the depth desired.[10]

SPLEEN

Acoustically, the spleen is much like the liver. Because it is in contact with the abdominal wall over a considerable portion of its length, it can be thoroughly explored. Positioning the patient in the right lateral decubitus position exposes the entire left flank and allows manipulation of the probe over a considerable portion of the splenic circumference. Again, abnormalities noted on scanning may be classified either as anatomic peculiarities, or solid or cystic masses.

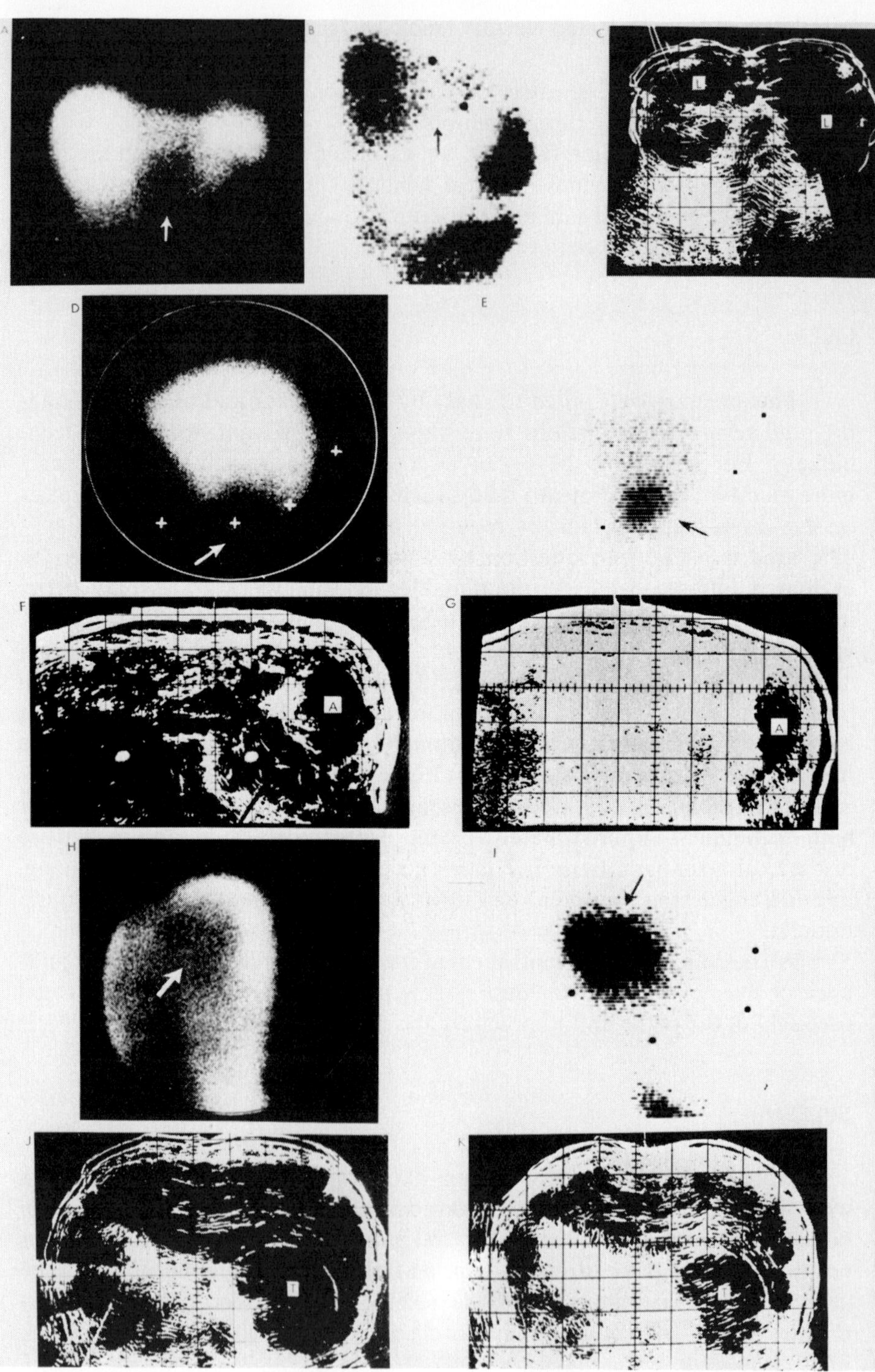

See legend on opposite page.

ASCITES

Ascites can be accurately detected and even quantified using ultrasonography. The picture of dense echoes arising from bowel loops floating in the center of an echo-free pool of ascitic fluid is quite distinctive.[11,12] As little as 100 ml may be detected.

GALLBLADDER

Ultrasonography, along with radioiodinated rose bengal excretion studies, can be of great aid in the diagnosis of obstructive jaundice, and may even give significant clues as to the etiology of the obstruction. A dilated gallbladder is basically a fluid-filled, homogeneous, cystic structure of the type easily delineated by Compound B scanning (Fig. 6-2). This is not always pathologic, since under fasting conditions a normal gallbladder may be dilated. However, after administration of a stimulus to contraction, such as a fatty meal or cholecystokinin, the normal gallbladder demonstrably decreases in size while the obstructed one does not. Such measurements can be made very accurately. Because they do not depend

---

Fig. 6-1. Combined radioisotope and ultrasound studies can often improve the accuracy with which the etiology of focal hepatic lesions is delineated.

(A–C) Diagnosis—normal anatomical variant. The anterior ^{99m}Tc-sulfur colloid scan (A) is abnormal and demonstrates decreased tracer concentration in the porta hepatis. The ^{67}Ga scan (B) is normal and demonstrates decreased volume of liver tissue in the left lobe. The ultrasound B scan (C) explains the thinning in the porta hepatis as secondary to the aorta (arrow), which lies less than 4 cm from the surface of the anterior abdominal wall. L = liver. The right lobe is to the reader's right, the left lobe to his left.

(D–G) Diagnosis—intrahepatic abscess. A large intrahepatic lesion in the inferior posterior position of the right hepatic lobe is seen clearly in both the right lateral ^{99m}Tc-sulfur colloid (D) and the ^{67}Ga (E) studies. The transverse ultrasound study demonstrates that the same area is transsonic at both low (F) and high (G) gains. The combined findings are most consistent with a pyogenic intrahepatic abscess. A = abscess.

(H–K) Diagnosis—metastatic carcinoma involving the right adrenal gland. The posterior ^{99m}Tc-sulfur colloid (H) and ^{67}Ga (I) views demonstrate a large lesion involving the posterior superior aspect of the right hepatic lobe. The echogram outlines the tumor well at low gain (J), but at high gain (K) numerous internal echoes are seen. The combined findings are most consistent with a solid malignant mass involving the posterior superior position of the right hepatic lobe. T = tumor.

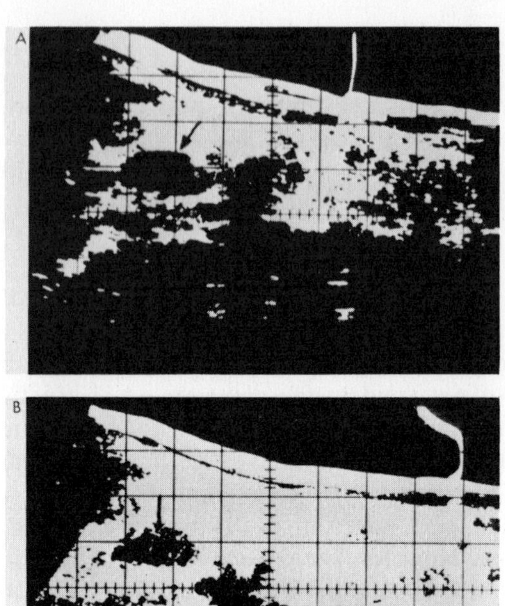

Fig. 6-2. (A) This longitudinal echogram demonstrates the ultrasonic appearance of a normal gallbladder
(arrow) at low gain settings. Note the strong posterior
echoes characteristic of cystic structures. (B) At high gain
the gallbladder remains transsonic relative to the surrounding tissues and is smaller in all diameters. These are characteristic changes produced by cystic structures. The vertical line above the skin surface indicates the position of the
umbilicus.

on hepatic excretion or biliary concentration of contrast media, they can
be made easily on patients with a nonvisualizing gallbladder. The technique
is less rewarding in attempts to visualize gallstones, perhaps because the
stones are frequently too small to produce significant echoes.[13]

PANCREAS

The diagnosis of pancreatic pseudocyst is probably best made by ultrasonography[14] (Fig. 6-3A). A sonolucent region (one that remains free
of internal echoes even at high gain settings and that has a clearly deline-

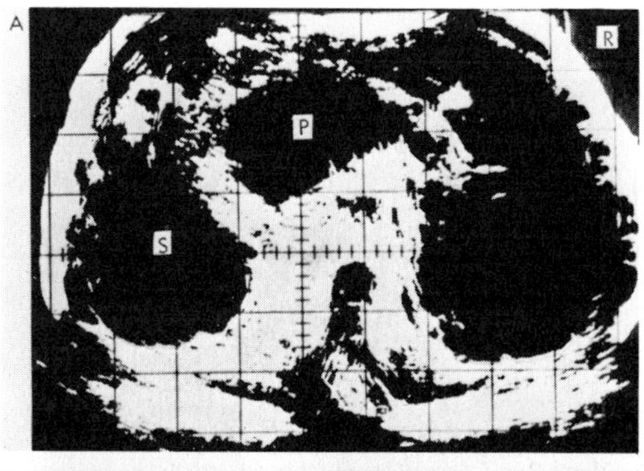

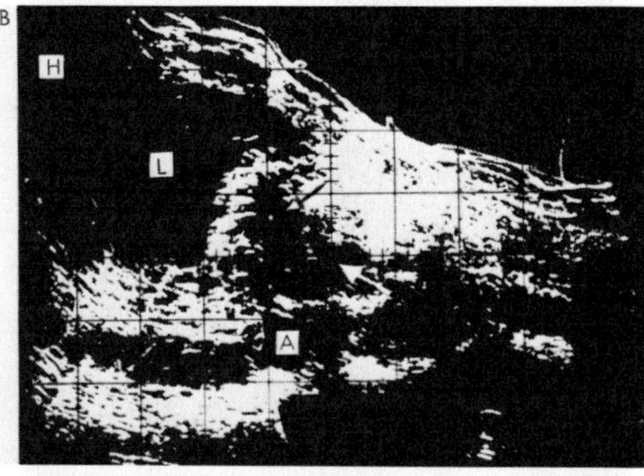

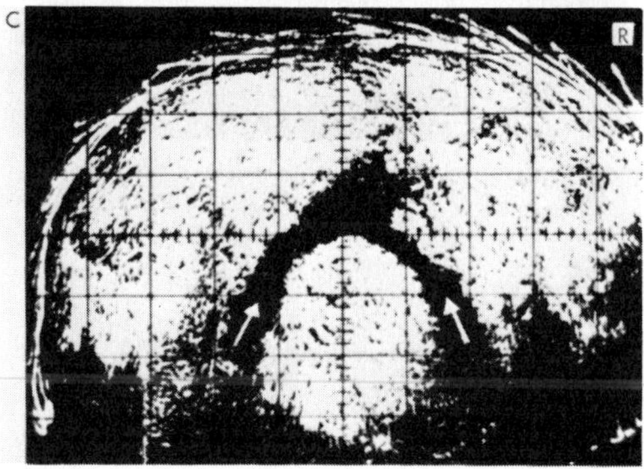

Fig. 6-3. (A) This transverse echogram delineates a large epigastric pancreatic pseudocyst (P) just anterior to and to the left of the spine and aorta. It remains sonolucent at higher gains and displays the typical sonographic characteristics of cystic lesions.

(B) A longitudinal echogram 2 cm to the left of the midline demonstrates a large mass (arrow) containing internal echoes representing a pancreatic carcinoma located inferior to the liver (L) and anterior to the aorta (A). H = direction of head.

(C) A transverse echogram of a patient with acute pancreatitis. The edematous pancreas has become sonolucent and is well outlined lying over the spine. The normal pancreas is not sonolucent and cannot be differentiated from surrounding structures.

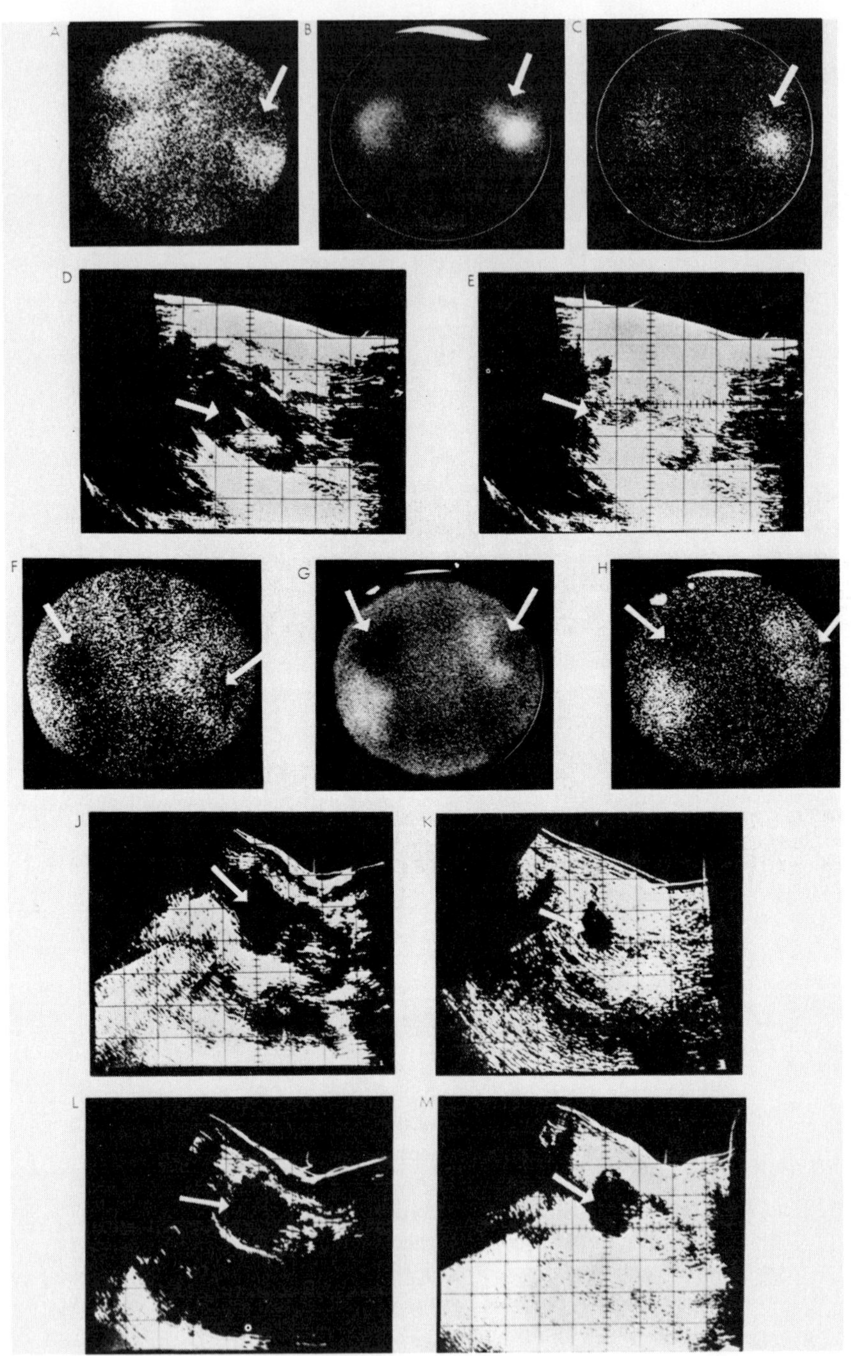

See legend on opposite page.

ated distal margin owing to good through transmission of sound) in the appropriate anatomic place is quickly spotted; changes in size or even spontaneous drainage are easily followed.[15]

Other pancreatic lesions are more problematic. Visualization depends on a pathologic process that makes the normally sono-opaque pancreas more sonolucent than the adjacent retroperitoneal structures. Freimanis has shown that this occurs in acute pancreatitis, probably because of the presence of edematous swelling of the organ[16] (Fig. 6-3C). Pancreatic tumors may occasionally be recognized as a retroperitoneal mass, echo free at lower gain settings but filling in at higher gain.[17] In the authors' experience, such tumors are best visualized in longitudinal view along the course of the aorta, owing to the contrast provided by this structure (Fig. 6-3B). However, this procedure is not at present considered likely to replace the pancreas radioisotope scan.

KIDNEYS

Again, the ability to distinguish cystic from solid masses makes ultrasonography of immense value to renographic work[18] (Fig. 6-4). Nuclear medicine and conventional radiographic contrast studies can do no more than identify the presence of a mass. Radioisotope perfusion or angiographic studies can demonstrate the vascularity of the mass, but even this is not always wholly reliable.[19]

Ultrasonic identification of a cyst may be combined with a guided needle aspiration for cytologic studies to eliminate the small percentage of cysts harboring neoplasms.

Fig. 6-4. Combined radioisotope and ultrasound scanning can accurately detect and differentiate renal cysts and neoplasms.

(A–E) Diagnosis—hypernephroma. The ^{99m}Tc-DTPA (B) and ^{131}I-hippuran studies demonstrate a defect in the upper pole of the right kidney. The ^{99m}Tc-DTPA perfusion study (A) shows this area to be relatively avascular, suggesting a cyst. Although the low gain echogram (D) shows the mass to be transsonic, at high gain (E) numerous internal echoes are seen. By ultrasound criteria, the mass is composed of solid tissue and is therefore consistent with a renal tumor.

(F–M) Diagnosis—bilateral renal cysts. Again, the ^{99m}Tc-DTPA (G) and ^{131}I-hippuran (H) studies demonstrate defects in the left upper pole and right lower pole. The ^{99m}Tc-DTPA perfusion study (F) demonstrates both areas to be avascular. The longitudinal echograms show them to be transsonic at both low (J,L) and high (K–M) gain, characteristic of cystic lesions.

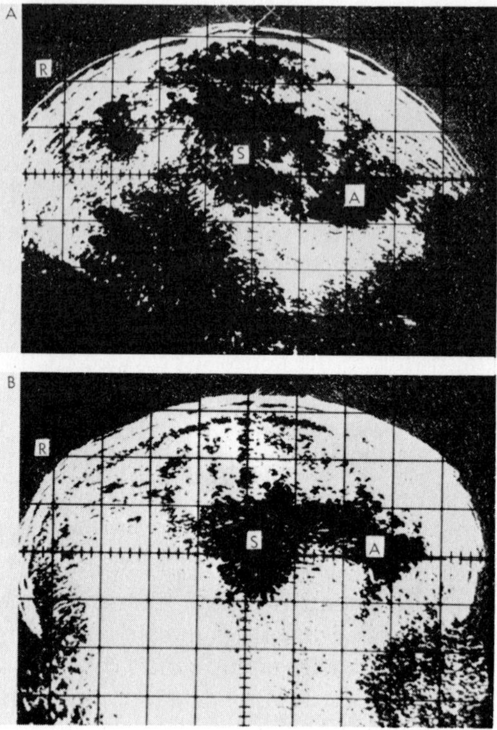

Fig. 6-5.   Diagnosis—left psoas abscess. Transverse
echograms with the patient in the prone position demonstrates a retroperitoneal transsonic area (A) just lateral
to the spine (S) at both low (A) and high gains (B).
These are typical ultrasonic findings produced by
abscesses.

Ultrasonography is clearly capable of other renal diagnostic work,
such as identifying ureteral obstructions by the distortion of pelvic-calyceal
echoes or stones by the sonic shadow they cast, or following the size of
renal transplants for early clues to rejection,[20-22] but in these areas it does
not possess a clear advantage over more established procedures.

When study is extended to the perirenal retroperitoneal spaces, however, advantages do emerge, primarily because other methods of studying
these spaces (such as pneumography and angiography) are fraught with
hazards and difficulties. Leopold, in particular, has described the ultrasonic
anatomy of the region and demonstrated the distortions caused by perine-
phric hematomas and abscesses, and psoas abscesses[23] (Fig. 6-5).

The technique may be applied advantageously even in infants, but
a special water bath must be used as a coupling medium.[24]

AORTA

Aneurysms are easily diagnosed and their diameters accurately measured[25] (Fig. 6-6). In contrast to angiographic studies, which can only show that portion of the lumen not obstructed by clot, ultrasound can depict the external diameters of the aortic wall. At low gain settings the wall, which is often at least partially calcified, creates strong echoes; clots, which are nearly as transsonic as blood, are found at higher gain settings. Thus, one avoids the danger of underestimating the size or extent of a large aneurysm, while one may easily and atraumatically follow small aneurysms at frequent intervals for changes in size.[26]

The measurement can be made in either the A or the B mode. However, it is usually of value to perform longitudinal B scanning first. This allows the detection of deviations in the course of the aorta which might otherwise result in measurements of transverse diameter being made in a plane transverse to the body but not to the aorta. Such measurements would appear spuriously enlarged.[27]

Similar measurements may be made in the vessels of the neck,[28] and occasionally the anteroposterior diameter of the thoracic aorta may be measured where it enlarges or bends sufficiently to come into direct contact with the posterior chest wall.[29]

The lucency of the aorta may be used to advantage in detecting enlarged para-aortic nodes, which may be of much the same characteristic impedance as the nearby aortic wall. The anterior aortic wall thus appears to merge into the overlying mass, while echoes from the posterior aortic wall, lodged against the spine, are well maintained.[30] In contrast, while

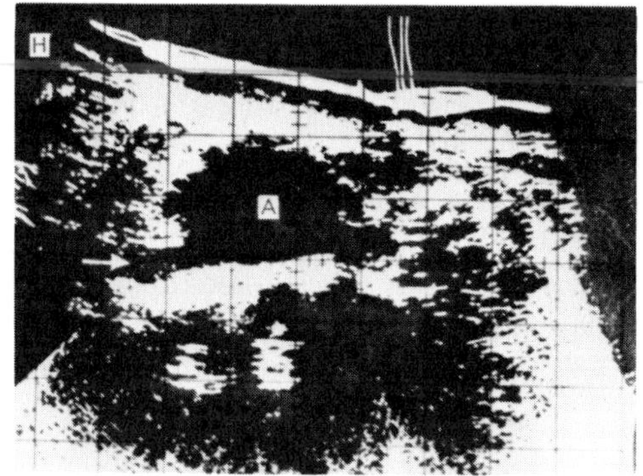

Fig. 6-6. A longitudinal echogram of a large aortic aneurysm (A) measuring 6 cm at its widest point. (Each square is 3 × 3 cm.) The normal aorta can be seen proximally (arrow).

the anterior wall echo may also be lost in the shadow of an overlying bowel loop, in this case the posterior wall and spine echoes will be lost as well. In combination with ^{67}Ga studies, this midline node-bearing area may be extensively evaluated by ultrasonography, thus obviating the need for potentially hazardous lymphangiographic or surgical procedures in the staging of lymphomas, at least when the results are positive. The accuracy of negative studies is more doubtful.

OBSTETRICS-GYNECOLOGY

In studies of the pelvis, ultrasonography and nuclear procedures compete in placental localization. The placenta is identified ultrasonically by the chorionic plate along the fetal surface and by characteristic internal echoes produced at higher gain settings. Several investigators have shown the two techniques to be approximately equally effective in full-term pregnancy.[31-34] However, the placenta may be identified and localized ultrasonically at a much earlier stage in pregnancy, often from the 10th week.[35] This is clearly of value when amniocentesis is contemplated well before term and in the diagnosis of hydatidiform mole.

In addition, many obstetrical and gynecological conditions that can be diagnosed ultrasonically are not amenable to nuclear medicine techniques. Studies of such conditions include early identification of multiple pregnancy, measurement of fetal biparietal diameter to assess gestational age, identification of various ovarian cysts and tumors, identification of uterine fibroids, and location of intrauterine contraceptive devices that may no longer be intrauterine [36,37] (Fig. 6-7).

CARDIAC

Echocardiography is beginning to emerge as a separate subspecialty. The motion of the mitral valve has been the longest and best studied, but the motion of other valves may be studied to advantage,[38-40] as well as that of the ventricular wall; thus cardiac chamber size and ejection fractions may be determined.[41,42] This work is preliminary, as are nuclear medicine techniques for the same purposes, and comparisons of the two methods are yet to be made.

In comparisons of ultrasonic and nuclear medicine techniques for the detection of pericardial effusion, the edge for sensitivity appears to belong to ultrasonography. The technique consists in positioning the transducer in the fourth or fifth interspaces, slightly to the left of the sternum, and directing the ultrasound beam slightly to the left of and below the anterior leaflet of the mitral valve, where it will traverse, in order, the chest wall, anterior heart wall, right ventricle, interventricular septum, left ventricle, posterior heart wall, and pericardium. In the absence of effusion, the anterior heart wall and chest wall echoes blend together. The posterior pericardial–lung interface, a strong echo owing to the air in the lung just beyond, blends with the posterior heart wall. When effusion is present, a nonmoving pericardial–lung echo becomes separated from the moving left ventricular wall echo (Fig. 6-8). Occasionally, an anterior separation of chest wall and anterior heart wall echo is also noted.[43-45]

Christensen and Bonte[46] produced experimental effusions in dogs, so that the size was accurately known. Seventy-five milliliters could be detected by ultrasonography, compared with a minimum of 200 ml using ^{99m}Tc-albumin as a blood-pool scanning agent. Use of intravenous carbon dioxide and x-ray was intermediate in sensitivity, requiring about 100-ml effusions for detection.

THYROID

In the continuing search for a means of distinguishing benign from malignant thyroid nodules, Blum et al[47] reported ultrasonic studies of a large series of solitary nonfunctional (by ^{131}I scanning) thyroid nodules. In the size range of 1 to 3 cm, cystic nodules could be separated ultrasonically from solid nodules. (Smaller nodules could not be classified, and larger ones generally presented a nonspecific ultrasonic appearance owing to degenerative changes.)

Since cysts have a low malignant potential, a small but substantial portion of nodules that would otherwise require surgical removal and pathologic diagnosis can be separated out for conservative management. Solid nodules cannot be further distinguished ultrasonically as to type.

It is of interest that with relatively superficial structures such as the thyroid, the use of transducers of higher frequency (e.g., 5 mHz) than those normally employed has been suggested. Their greater resolution (attributable to their shorter wavelength) is offset in other areas by poor penetration. This is of less consequence in the neck, where they can be used to advantage.[48] Either the Compound B scanning mode or the A amplitude mode of transmission may be used.

Ultrasonography allows precise measurement of the third dimension of thyroid size, depth. In conjunction with the two-dimensional nuclear scan, thyroid size may be more exactly measured for calculation of a thera-

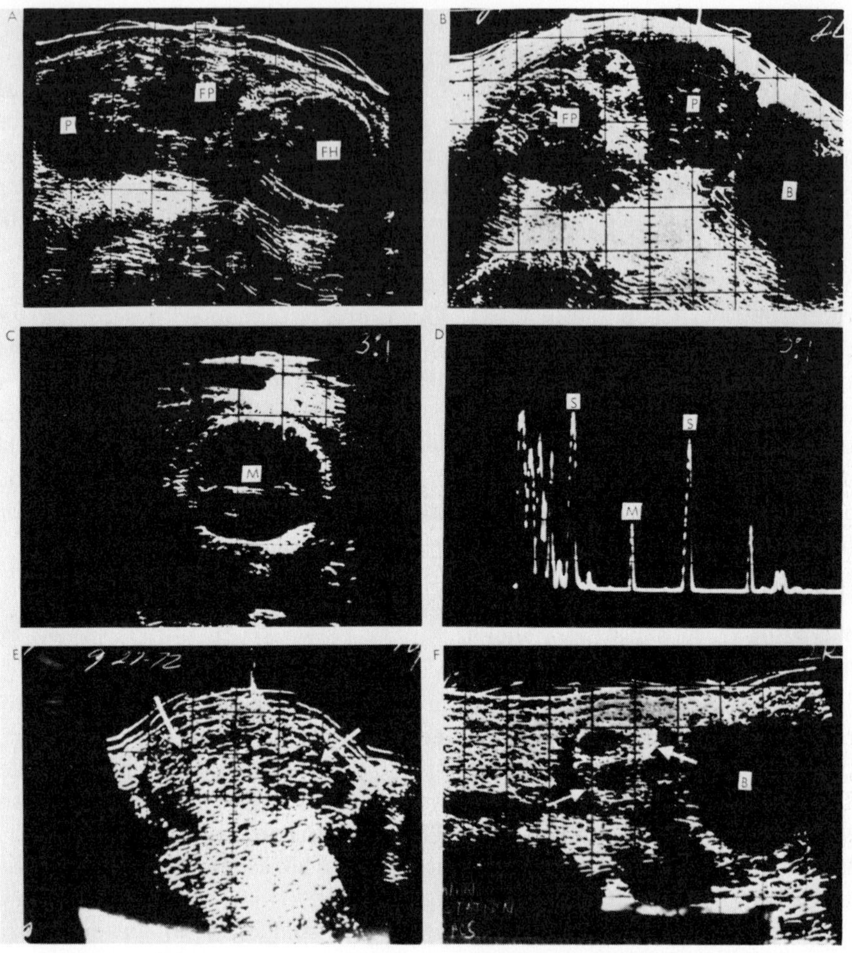

Fig. 6-7. Ultrasound B scanning is helpful in diagnosing a wide variety of obstetrical problems. Illustrative examples of only a few are shown.

(A) A longitudinal echogram of a normal near-term pregnancy. The placenta (P) is well outlined in the superior posterior portion of the uterus. Fetal parts (FP) and head (FH) are easily identified.

(B) Diagnosis—placenta praevia. A longitudinal echogram outlines the placenta (P) in the inferior portion of the uterus separating the fetus (FP) from the bladder (B) and cervix (not visualized in this section).

(C) An echogram of the fetal head with the midline echo (M). Demonstration of the midline echo assures the examiner that the beam is directed in the biparietal plane. Head size can then be measured, correlating well with fetal size and age.

(D) A-mode representation of the same fetal skull, the skull echoes (S), and midline echo (M). This method of representation is felt by some to permit more accurate measurement of the fetal head size.

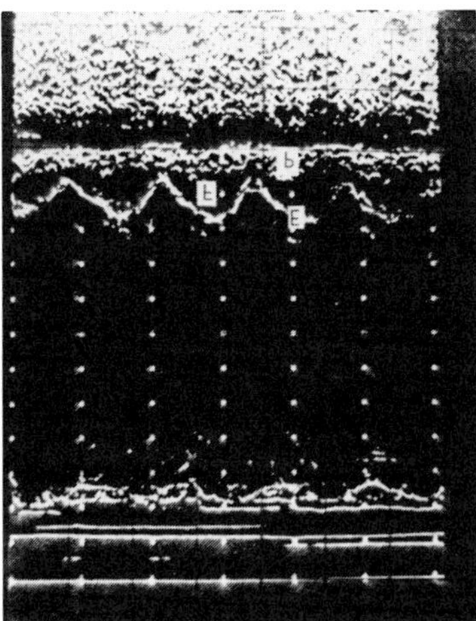

Fig. 6-8.   An echocardiogram of a pericardial effusion. The effusion (F) is represented as an echo-free space
separating the to-and-fro movement of the epicardium
(E) from the now immobile pericardium (P). Normally,
the epicardium and pericardium move together without
an intervening clear space.

peutic dose of ^{131}I; or thyroid size may be followed without the need for
repeated scans, which necessitate interruptions of suppression therapy.[49]

OTHER APPLICATIONS

Preliminary work has been done on B-mode scanning of the *breast*
using a multiple receiver crystal array grouped about a transmitter crystal.
This arrangement permits the use of a narrow-diameter transmitter, which
produces a sound beam with less spread and better lateral resolution. At
the same time there is no sacrifice of surface area for the reception of
returning echoes. Palpable masses are classified as benign or malignant

---

(E)   Diagnosis—hydatidiform mole. The transverse echogram shows
the "snowflake" distribution of echoes throughout the whole uterus, which is
characteristically seen with this disorder.

(F)   Diagnosis—twin gestation at 5 weeks. The filled bladder (B) effectively lifts the uterus out of the pelvis. This is mandatory for consistently good
studies. The gestational sac for each twin (arrows) is well outlined. (Figures
6-7B–F were kindly supplied by Dr. Milo Webber, Nuclear Medicine Division,
UCLA Center for the Health Sciences, Los Angeles, California.)

on the basis of echo patterns showing either smooth walls without internal echoes (benign), or irregular margins with internal echoes (malignant). Unfortunately, the medullary type of carcinoma is sufficiently homogeneous to present a benign pattern.[50,51]

In the extremities, *Baker's cysts* located behind the knee and in the upper calf can be ultrasonically imaged. The clinical distinction of this condition from thrombophlebitis is sometimes difficult, but it can be made ultrasonically without the need for contrast media studies.[52]

The detection of *arterial flow* is based on measurement of the Doppler shift—the change in frequency between transmitted and returning sound waves that occurs when they are reflected from a moving medium. This technique is beyond the scope of the present chapter, which is intended to cover imaging applications—except to note that in one instance the two techniques have been combined. A Doppler-shift detector was coupled to a Compound B scanning system so that wherever a shift was detected, a mark was made in the corresponding area on a persistence oscilloscope. As the probe was moved transversely across a leg, an image was constructed of the cross section of the major blood vessel at that level. Cross sections were made at successively lower levels until the point of narrowing or obstruction was located.[53]

Movement of the lateral *pharyngeal wall* during speech may be monitored and recorded in much the same way as movements of the cardiac walls. This has been found to be of prognostic value in patients requiring surgical correction for velopharyngeal insufficiency.[54]

The ability to measure a mass in three dimensions is made use of in planning *radiation therapy ports*; the measurements may be repeated and the ports changed as often as necessary in response to changes in target size during therapy.[55]

No somatic damage has been attributed to diagnostic ultrasound, and most investigators have failed to find evidence of chromosomal damage when blood or lymphocyte cultures were exposed for long periods.[56,57,58]

Ultrasonography is thus a safe and in some areas a uniquely effective diagnostic method that naturally complements many nuclear medicine imaging procedures. Not unexpectedly, a considerable knowledge of cross-sectional anatomy and experience with variations that may be induced by different methods of probe handling and gain settings are required for adequate performance and interpretation of studies. We, like many others, have found that the one who interprets the study should ideally be the one who performed it. No doubt technicians can be adequately trained, but not in a matter of weeks nor as a collateral duty.

Nevertheless, the time is rapidly approaching when ultrasonography will be a common and even an expected and required hospital diagnostic service.[59] While it will no doubt be handled in many different ways, in our experience ultrasonic B scanning fits in quite naturally and conveniently with the work of a nuclear medicine department.

REFERENCES

1. Wells PNT (ed): Ultrasonics in Clinical Diagnosis. Baltimore, Williams & Wilkins, 1972
2. Brown B, Gordon D (eds): Ultrasonic Techniques in Biology and Medicine. Springfield, Illinois, Charles C Thomas, 1967
3. Scheifer W, Kazner E, Kunze S: Clinical Echo—Encephalography, New York, Springer-Verlag, 1968
4. Leopold G, Asher W: Deleterious effects of gastrointestinal contrast material on abdominal echography. Radiology 98:637–640, 1971
5. Collins L, Myhill J: Radioisotopic vs ultrasonic testing for pulmonary embolism. Am J Roentgenol 106:766–769, 1969
6. Leyton B, Halpern S, Leopold G, Hagen S: Correlation of ultrasound and colloid scintiscan studies of the normal and diseased liver. J Nucl Med 14:27–33, 1973
7. Wells P, McCarthy C, Ross F, Read A: Comparison of A scan and compound B scan ultrasonography in the diagnosis of liver disease. Br J Radiol 42:818–823, 1969
8. Fuchs W, Vogeli E, Schwegler N, Hunig R, Rosler H: Angiography, scintigraphy, and ultrasound tomography of liver. Schweiz Med Wochenschr 101:1180–1186, 1971
9. McCarthy C, Davies E, Wells P, Ross F, Follett D, Muir K, Read A: Comparison of ultrasonic and isotopic scanning in liver disease. Br J Radiol 43:100–109, 1970
10. Rasmussen S, Holm H, Kristensen J, Barlebo H: Ultrasonically guided liver biopsy. Br Med J 2:500–502, 1972
11. Goldberg B, Clearfield H, Goodman G, Morales J: Ultrasonic determination of ascites. Arch Intern Med 131:217–220, 1973
12. McCarthy C, Wells P, Ross F, Read A: Ultrasound in diagnosis of cystic lesions of liver and upper abdomen and in detection of ascites. Gut 10:904–912, 1969
13. Hublitz U, Kahn P, Sell L: Cholecystosonography: an approach to the nonvisualized gallbladder. Radiology 103:645–649, 1972
14. Ferrucci J, Eaton S: Current concepts—radiology of the pancreas. N Engl J Med 288:506–510, 1973
15. Templeton A, Stuber J: Abdominal and retroperitoneal sonography. Am J Roentgenol 113:741–748, 1973
16. Freimanis A, Filly R: Echographic diagnosis of pancreatic lesions. Radiology 96:575–582, 1970
17. Engelhart G, Blauenstein U: Ultrasound diagnosis of malignant pancreatic tumors. Gut 11:443–449, 1970
18. Schrech W, Holmes J: Ultrasound as a diagnostic aid for renal neoplasms and cysts. J Urol 103:281–285, 1970
19. Leitner W, Anderson E, Weber C, Grimes J, Johnsrude S: Limitations of arteriography in renal mass evaluation. Arch Intern Med 130:868–873, 1972
20. Barnett E, Morley P: Diagnostic ultrasound in renal disease. Br Med Bull 28:196–199, 1972

21. King D: Renal ultrasonography. Radiology 105:633–637, 1972
22. Leopold G: Renal transplant size measured by reflected ultrasound. Radiology 95:687–689, 1970
23. Leopold G, Asher W: Diagnosis of extraorgan retroperitoneal space lesions by B-scan ultrasonography. Radiology 104:133–138, 1972
24. Lyons E, Fleming J, Arneil G, Murphy A, Sweet E, Donald I: Nephrosonography in infants and children: a new technique. Br Med J 2:689–691, 1972
25. Nusbaum J, Freimanis A, Thomford N: Echography in the diagnosis of abdominal aortic aneurysm. Arch Surg 102:385–388, 1971
26. Leopold G: Ultrasonic abdominal aortography. Radiology 96:9–14, 1970
27. Holm H, Rasmussen S, Kristensen J: Errors and pitfalls in ultrasonic scanning of the abdomen. Br J Radiol 45:835–840, 1972
28. Olinger C: Ultrasonic carotid echoarteriography. Radiology 106:282–285, 1969
29. Goldberg B, Lehman J: Aortosonography: Ultrasound measurement of the abdominal and thoracic aorta. Arch Surg 100:652–655, 1970
30. Asher W, Freimanis A: Echographic diagnosis of retroperitoneal lymph node enlargement. Am J Roentgenol 105:438–445, 1969
31. Kohorn E, Secker Walker R, Morrison J, Campbell S: Placental localization. A comparison between ultrasound compound B scanning and radioisotope scanning. Am J Obstet Gynecol 103:868–877, 1969
32. Robinson D, Garrett W: Ultrasonic visualization of placenta. Med J Aust 2:1062–1064, 1970
33. Niehoff R, Hendee W, Brown J: Placenta scanning with [113m]In. J Nucl Med 11:15–18, 1970
34. Wood J, Jones L, Maisey M: Placental localization using [113m]In and a portable scintillation detector: comparison with Doppler ultrasound. J Obstet Gynaecol Br Comm 77:139–144, 1970
35. Kobayashi M, Hellman L, Cromb E: Atlas of Ultrasonography in Obstetrics and Gynecology. New York, Appleton-Century-Crofts, 1972, p 53
36. Morley P, Barnett E: Use of ultrasound in diagnosis of pelvic masses. Br J Radiol 43:602–616, 1970
37. Cochrane W, Thomas M: Use of ultrasound B-mode scanning in the localization of intrauterine contraceptive devices. Radiology 104:623–627, 1972
38. Edler I: Ultrasoundcardiography in mitral valve stenosis. Am J Cardiol 19:18–31, 1967
39. Kerber R, Isaeff D, Hancock E: Echocardiographic patterns in patients with the syndrome of systolic click and late systolic murmur. N Engl J Med 284:691–693, 1971
40. Gramiack R, Shah P: Echocardiography of the normal and diseased aortic valve. Radiology 96:1–8, 1970
41. Feigenbaum H, Popp R, Wolfe S, Troy B, Pombo J, Haine C, Dodge H: Ultrasound measurements of the left ventricle. Arch Intern Med 129:461–467, 1972
42. Wharton C, Smithen C, Sowton E: Changes in left ventricular wall movement after acute myocardial infarction measured by reflected ultrasound. Br Med J 4:75–77, 1971
43. Moss A, Bruhn F: The echocardiogram—an ultrasound technique for the detection of pericardial fluid. N Engl J Med 274:380–384, 1966
44. Feigenbaum H: Echocardiographic diagnosis of pericardial effusion. Am J Cardiol 26:475–479, 1970

45. Casarella W, Schneider B: Pitfalls in the ultrasonic diagnosis of pericardial effusion. Am J Roentgenol 90:760–767, 1970
46. Christensen E, Bonte F: The relative accuracy of echocardiography, intravenous CO_2 studies, and blood-pool scanning in detecting pericardial effusions in dogs. Radiology 91:265–270, 1968
47. Blum M, Goldman A, Herskovic A, Hernberg J: Clinical applications of thyroid echography. N Engl J Med 287:1164–1168, 1972
48. Blum M, Weiss B, Hernberg J: Evaluation of thyroid nodule by A-mode echography. Radiology 101:651–656, 1971
49. Thÿs L: Diagnostic ultrasound in clinical thyroid investigation. J Clin Endocrinol 32:709–716, 1971
50. DeLand F: Ultrasound diagnosis of tumors of breast. Roentgenblaetter 23:237–246, 1970
51. DeLand F: A modified technique of ultrasonography for the detection and differential diagnosis of breast lesions. Radiology 105:446–452, 1969
52. McDonald G, Leopold G: Ultrasound B-scanning in the differentiation of Baker's cyst and thrombophlebitis. Br J Radiol 45:729–732, 1972
53. Fish P, Corrigan T, Kakkar V, Nicolaides A: Arteriography using ultrasound. Lancet I:1269–1270, June 10, 1972
54. Kelsey C, Ewanowski A, Crummy A, Bless I: Lateral pharyngeal wall motion as a predictor of surgical success in velopharyngeal insufficiency. N Engl J Med 287:64–68, 1972
55. Cohen W, Hass A: Application of ultrasound B scan in planning of radiation therapy treatment ports. Am J Roentgenol 111:184–188, 1971
56. Boyd E, Abdulla U, Donald S, Fleming J, Hall A, Ferguson-Smith M: Chromosome breakage and ultrasound. Br Med J 2:501–502, 1971
57. Abdulla U, Talbert D, Lucas M, Mullarkey M: Effect of ultrasound on chromosomes of lymphocyte cultures. Br Med J 3:797–799, 1972
58. US Department of Health, Education, and Welfare, Food and Drug Administration. Interaction of ultrasound and biological tissues; Workshop Proceedings, 1972
59. Lele P: Application of ultrasound in medicine (editorial). N Engl J Med 286:1317–1318, 1972

Richard P. Spencer

7

Radioisotopic Studies of Growth, Development, and Regeneration

Nuclear medicine is concerned with the estimation of structure and function, during life, in individual patients. This concern with the individual, at one point in time, has obscured the fact that such studies can be used (a) sequentially, to follow growth, development, and regeneration, and (b) to provide epidemiological data as to the distribution of organ size, shape, and function. In this chapter we discuss the experience of one laboratory with quantitative sequential studies for following organ and tumor growth, and only briefly touch on epidemiological data.

A PERSPECTIVE

The principal reason for pursuing this subject is the restricted number of techniques for studying the size and functioning of internal organs during life. Indeed we can list the principal methodologies for quantifying in vivo organ or tumor size as follows:

1. Direct observation for superficial and ocular lesions.
2. Ultrasound.
3. Radiography (with or without contrast media).
4. Organ scanning.

It can be recognized that limitations of the first three procedures (often their inability to follow changes of, or within, soft tissue structures) necessi-

Supported by ET-44C from the American Cancer Society, by USPHS HE 14179 (Lung Research Center), and by USPHS CA 14969.

235

tate scrutiny of the procedures of nuclear medicine. A number of cautions must be sounded before proceeding further.

1. Organ scanning, by means of radionuclides, has a spatial resolution that is much coarser than radiographic techniques.
2. If actual sizes are to be reported, then great care must be exercised so that adequate consideration is given to such factors as angulation, magnification, and respiratory motion.
3. For serial studies to have validity, the same scanning technique must be utilized each time.
4. Often multiple views (different positions) and tomographic sections must be obtained in order to define the organ or lesion of interest.
5. On occasion, multiple radiotracers will have to be utilized to define the extent of an organ or lesion. A few examples may suffice.
    (a) "Hepatic" tissue extending into the left upper quadrant on ^{99m}Tc-sulfur colloid scans may have to be further studied by means of ^{131}I-rose bengal or ^{75}Se-selenomethionine, in order to distinguish the liver from the spleen.
    (b) A hepatic "filling defect" on a ^{99m}Tc-sulfur colloid scan, located near the upper medial surface of the organ, may represent (in part) thinning caused by the inferior vena cava. Hence a repeat scan with a radiotracer that localizes within the blood pool (such as ^{113m}Intransferrin) should be considered.
6. Organ scans represent the distribution of a radionuclide at some particular point in time. Scans are, in essence, a map of the organ, whose functioning or blood flow allowed the radiotracer to be accumulated. There may or may not be a one-to-one correspondence between this function and a gross anatomic structure. For example, most tumors within the thyroid gland do not possess the ability to accumulate radio-iodide or its analogs; there is a correspondence between the iodide transport system and the scan result.

PRENATAL DEVELOPMENT

The developing fetus is part of a multicompartment system.

Maternal circulation	Placenta	Fetal circulation	Amniotic fluid

We have indicated some major pools by blocks, rather than by conventional compartmental notation, as the interrelationships can be complex and (in many cases) uncertain. A considerable literature has grown up around animal studies on the passage of materials from the maternal circulation to the fetus. Since use of radiotracers is usually contraindicated in human pregnancy, such investigations have been limited to cases of therapeutic abortion, or to the use of stable nuclides. For example, passage of D_2O from the mother to both the fetus and amniotic fluid can be studied. Stable nuclides, followed by sample removal and activation analysis, may provide a promising technique for investigating the kinetics of maternal–fetal transport.

Some years ago we noted that it was possible to directly introduce gamma-ray-emitting radionuclides into the amniotic fluid.[1] With the present availability of short-lived radionuclides, this topic deserves restudy as a potential tool for investigating fetal size, position, amniotic fluid volume, and the rate of removal of the radioactive material. It is probable that radiographic studies[2] and ultrasonic fetal cephalometry[3,4] can yield more definitive data as to fetal size. However, if the radiation exposure can be kept low, radioisotopic studies may find a role in looking at the volume and dynamics of amniotic fluid (particularly when polyhydramnios or other problems are suspected). [99m]Tc (as pertechnetate) avidly concentrates in the mouse fetus after introduction into the mother,[5] but comparable human data on fetus and amniotic fluid are of course not available.

The topic of placental function is of key importance, since it is believed that insufficiency of the organ may underly some cases of fetal mortality. ^{14}C-amino acids are incorporated into the placenta of animals.[6] However, to allow external detection, an amino acid with a gamma-ray emission would be required. Garrow[7,8] has proposed utilizing placental uptake of ^{75}Se-selenomethionine as a functional index. The principal problems with this involve (a) separating the placental contribution from that of other tissues, and (b) the radiation exposure due to the long half-life of [75]Se. The radiation dose to human beings has been estimated at 0.03 rads/μCi in the liver;[9] if the placenta or fetus concentrated the radionuclide, the radiation exposure could be quite real.

Imaging the placenta by means of agents that remain within the vascular tree (such as [113m]In) is a well-recognized procedure (although it has been largely replaced by ultrasonic techniques in some centers). The fetal radiation dose from placental imaging appears to be of reasonable magnitude.[10] Of special interest is the observation that [113m]In ($T_{1/2} = 1.7$ hr, 390-keV gamma rays) can actually accumulate in the placenta of animals.[11] Whether this means that the longer lived [111]In ($T_{1/2} = 2.8$ days, 247-keV gamma rays) can be used to follow the placenta over a period of time, in problem cases, is uncertain. We have been particularly interested in utilizing [113m]In dynamic studies in an effort to separate placental and myometrial blood flow.[12] The procedure appears relatively easier for use during life, than methods which depend on the washout of [133]Xe.[13] The ability to perfuse the placenta in vitro[14] should provide a system for following uptake by that organ, and possibly for gauging metabolic alteration of radiolabeled nutrients.

It will likely be of key importance to relate the movement of nutrients and radionuclides to the size of the fetus, amniotic fluid, and placenta. In addition to improved techniques for measuring these quantities during life, sound theoretical approaches are needed for examining their interrelationships and dependence on the time of gestation. For example, by use of Haase's[15] observation (that the length of the human fetus could be given as a linear function of the gestational age from lunar months 5 to 10), and the assumption of a spherical model, we were able to derive a simple relationship[16] for fetal weight W as a function of the sitting height H:

$$W = a \cdot H^3 \tag{1}$$

and fetal weight as a function of the duration of gestation (T = time of gestation, M = constant)

$$W = (MT + Q)^3. \tag{2}$$

The term Q was then shown to be related to the weight percentile P of the fetus.[17] Hence

$$W = (MT + A \cdot P + B)^3. \tag{3}$$

where A and B are constants. Such attempts to consider developmental percentiles in growth parameters have to be further extended. We have used such an approach in describing placental development.[18]

Payne and Wheeler[19] noted that if nutrients were supplied to the fetus at a constant rate per unit surface area of the surrounding membranes, then (c = a constant)

$$dW/dt = c \cdot W^{2/3} \tag{4}$$

(since for an approximately spherical fetus, the surface area would be proportional to the two-thirds power of weight).
Haase's law immediately follows from Eq. (4) by an analysis of the dimensions involved:[20]

$$L^3/t = c \cdot L^2 \tag{5}$$

where L is length and t is time. Upon solving, we obtain

$$L = c \cdot t. \tag{6}$$

This is Haase's law, which had been observed empirically nearly 100 years ago. The surface across which nutrients are supplied to the fetus may thus be of primary interest in understanding fetal growth and development. Radiotracers can be of importance in examining fluxes across this surface, and in determining the rate of accumulation of materials into the fetus.

POSTNATAL DEVELOPMENT

Birth brings with it the change from an aqueous to an air-breathing environment. In addition, there is a redirected circulatory system and multiple other adjustments. Despite this, the growth equations which describe the prenatal situation can occasionally be extended into the postnatal period. For example, Laird[21] showed that a single expression described both the prenatal and the immediate postnatal specific growth rate of the guinea pig. We have noted that a single expression can be used to describe sternal ossification from about the middle of gestation until approximately age 7 years.[22] From the viewpoint of nuclear medicine, are the organ sizes and physiological processes (which form the basis of the clinical procedures) following birth continuously variable, or not? We obviously cannot yet provide an answer, but will assume that monotonic functions can be used to describe the size of the major organs. There are obviously a limited number of studies performed on normal individuals in the 0 to 19 year age bracket. Care must then be taken in interpreting investigations on the functional length of an organ as a property of age.

Thyroid scans with ^{131}I or ^{99m}Tc were used to estimate the size of the thyroid gland in children.[13] The right thyroid lobe length, R was very slightly larger than the left, X (further asymmetry might develop later in life):

$$R = 1.031X + 0.05. \tag{7}$$

The correlation coefficient was 0.87, with a sample size of 39 cases. The relationship between the mean length L of the thyroid in centimeters, and the age in years A was

$$L = 0.177A + 1.58 \tag{8}$$

with a correlation coefficient of 0.79. In 29 cases it was possible to relate thyroid length to the height H of the youngster:

$$L = 0.034H - 0.98. \tag{9}$$

The correlation coefficient was 0.75. A plot of thyroid length versus body weight W revealed a bend at about 30 kg. There appeared to be an approach to an asymptote, as though a rectangular hyperbola was involved. A plot of $1/L$ versus $1/W$ revealed

$$\frac{1}{L} = 4 \cdot \frac{1}{W} + 0.15 \tag{10}$$

with a correlation coefficient of 0.77. Efforts should also be made to relate thyroid length to the calculated body surface area. Of interest was the observation that for the normal thyroid in these youngsters, there was a close relationship between the scan surface area of the thyroid S and the mean length of the gland:

$$L = 0.254S + 1.13. \tag{11}$$

The correlation coefficient was 0.84. Kay and co-workers[24] described the weight W of the thyroid gland of children as a function of age; their data can be cast into the following form:

$$W = 1.48 + 0.65A. \tag{12}$$

Using this and Eq. (8), we can arrive at an approximate expression for thyroid weight in children as a function of the mean length of the gland:

$$W = 3.66L - 4.30. \tag{13}$$

Each of these expressions will have to be carefully reexamined as data on larger series of cases are obtained.

For the liver, a similar analysis was carried out, based on radioisotopic scan data.[25] The length L, width W, and surface area Z of the liver scans were related to age as follows (66 cases):

	Correlation coefficient	
$L = 8.79 + 0.458A$	0.89	(14)
$W = 9.89 + 0.406A$	0.83	(15)
$Z = 55.4 + 6.66A$	0.88	(16)

Expressions were also described for liver scan length, width, and surface area as a function of height, weight (up to 30 kg), and body surface area. The general uniformity of configuration of the normal liver scan in these children, despite some variations, was shown by the close relationship of liver width to liver length

$$W = 2.90 + 0.82L \tag{17}$$

with a correlation coefficient of 0.84. There was an especially close relationship between liver scan surface area and length (correlation coefficient 0.95):

$$S = 66.6 + 14.1L. \tag{18}$$

The spleen has also been analyzed in terms of scan length as a function of age.[26] In 45 children, splenic length (in centimeters) was related to the age in years by (correlation coefficient 0.87)

$$L = 5.7 + 0.31A. \tag{19}$$

The prediction was slightly high at birth (true value of about 5.0 cm), but gave a good description for other ages. These data could be combined with the report by Seltzer and co-workers.[27] These workers provided figures that showed that splenic weight (grams) could be approximated by

$$W = 24 + 7A. \tag{20}$$

Combining Eqs. (19) and (20) yields

$$W = 22.6L - 104. \tag{21}$$

This is a description of normal splenic weight in terms of spleen length in children. Scan length of the spleen was closely related to the height of the child (correlation coefficient 0.90) in 23 cases:

$$L = 2.3 + 0.05H. \tag{22}$$

From birth to 30-kg body weight B, splenic length was approximated by

$$L = 4 + 0.22B. \tag{23}$$

Above this weight, splenic length began to approach an asymptotic value.

RELATIONSHIP OF SCAN DIMENSIONS TO ORGAN SIZE

We may attempt to relate the length, width, or surface area of an organ to two distinct quantities:

A. The volume or weight of the organ being scanned.
B. More general properties such as the age, height, body weight, or surface area of the host.

We examine item A first. There have been five approaches to relating scan measurements to organ size.

1. A widely used method has been to plot the weight of the organ (obtained at autopsy or surgery) as a function of the scan length (or of width, or of the product of length times width, or of the scan surface area). A typical result might be as follows:

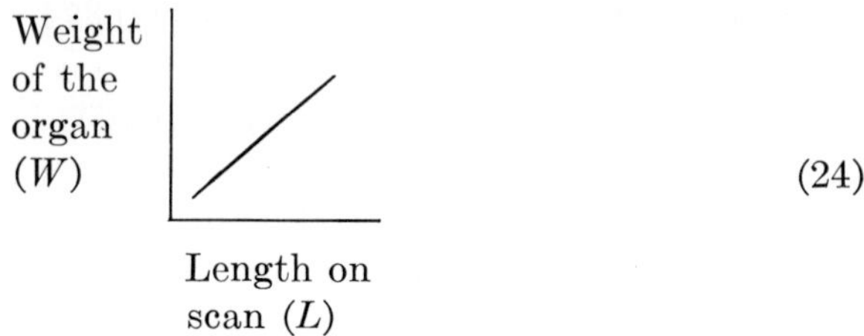

$$(24)$$

The difficulty with such proposals is that, although they work well over the normal range of organ size, they do not allow (see for example reference 28):

(a)   Extension to very large or very small organs.

(b)   A smooth transition from the growth phase to the adult range.

2. Empirical equations have been tried in describing organ weights as a function of scan dimensions. This has been particularly applied to estimates of thyroid weight.[29,30] The descriptions assume a constant relationship between the depth of the thyroid and such measurable quantities as scan surface area and length. A widely used variant is

$$\text{thyroid weight} = [\text{average scan length}][\text{scan surface area}](0.3). \quad (25)$$

For the diffusely enlarged thyroid, this appears to hold (± 20 percent) in most cases. When irregular growth, or a multinodular goiter, is present, the description tends to lose validity.

3. Attempts have been made to relate scan dimensions to organ weight by use of models. An example would be that the distended bladder approximates a sphere; in reality, a spherical segment of one or two bases is a more realistic model.[31] The kidneys can often be related to ellipsoids of revolution. The liver[32] and spleen[33] have both been related to geometric figures, whose equations are known. The validity of such approaches, during the period of growth, and when the organs are distorted by intrinsic disease or external pressure, has still to be determined.

4. Another approach is to recognize that scans are a planar representation of the organ being imaged. If scanning were carried out in the

anteroposterior and lateral views, the volume would (dimensionally) be given by the following:[31]

$$V = K(A_1 \cdot A_2)^{3/4} \tag{26}$$

where A_1 and A_2 represent the areas on the two scans. From a scan in a single plane, the area would (dimensionally) be related to the volume by[34]

$$V = K \cdot S^{3/2} \tag{27}$$

where S is the surface area. A more general expression would be of the form

$$V = K \cdot S^n \tag{28}$$

or

$$\log V = n \log S + \log K. \tag{29}$$

We have shown that this holds for a number of organs.[34]

Such an approach is of interest for another reason: it bears a resemblance to the equations relating organ size to body weight. Huxley[35] noted that an organ may increase in relative weight W so that there is a linear relationship to the relative increase in the weight of the body B. That is,

$$\frac{dW}{W} = q \cdot \frac{dB}{B}. \tag{30}$$

This integrates to

$$\log W = q \log B + \log c \tag{31}$$

or

$$W = cB^q. \tag{32}$$

This is the allometric equation. In addition to having fairly wide applicability to describing the growth of organs, Stahl[36] has pointed out that the equation also often describes the relationship of organ weight to body weight in the adult animal. We have shown, for example,[37] that for human males (based on autopsy data), the relationship of spleen weight S (in grams) to body weight B was

$$S = (3.5 \times 10^{-3})B^{0.97}. \tag{33}$$

5. A further technique, which awaits full exploration, is the use of gamma-ray tomography to determine cross-sectional areas through an

organ. Then, upon summing the sections, the volume of the organ could be calculated:

$$V = \Sigma T_i A_i. \tag{34}$$

Here T_i is the thickness of the ith section, and A_i is its area. It will be of interest to compare hepatic volumes, determined this way, with those determined by use of the ultrasonic technique,[38] or by biplanar radiographs,[39] or through use of radionuclide scanning with "multiple cuts."[40] It is of note that in the description of the ultrasonic procedure for determining liver weights,[38] the values were compared with those calculated by using the allometric equation for the liver proposed by Spencer.[41] In 15 males, using a specific gravity of 1.04 for the liver, the mean value for the ultrasonically determined liver volume agreed almost exactly (1771 versus 1777) with that predicted by the allometric equation.

EFFECTS OF THERAPY ON THE THYROID

Estimates of organ size can be extended from the normal population to the abnormal. In such cases we must be aware of the fact that the descriptive equations might be of limited use. Hence, a reporting of organ length or surface area might be of as much value as estimates of organ weights. For the population we are seeing, we have described the size of the normal thyroid gland on the scan.[42] A description was also given of the probable wide range of thyroid weights in the hyperthyroid population.[43] There were two extensions of this work. First, thyroid scan length after therapy with radioiodide (L_A) was compared with that before (L_B) treatment:[44]

$$L_A = 0.25 + 0.78L_B \tag{35}$$

(35 cases, correlation coefficient 0.80). For the scan surface area, the relationship was

$$S_A = 1.18 + 0.62L_B. \tag{36}$$

The correlation coefficient was 0.87. It was pointed out that biochemical changes were also occurring, in addition to the loss of tissue volume. Further quantification of the response of the thyroid to therapy has also been achieved.[45] This was accomplished by noting that, after use of radioiodide therapy, the individuals could be divided into two groups: those uncured of their hyperthyroidism (H), and those cured (C, whether euthyroid or hypothyroid).[45] Patients were then followed from one treatment ("drink") to the next. With H_0 representing the original number of hyperthyroid individuals, the response to therapy was described by

$$H = H_0 e^{-\lambda D} \qquad (37)$$

where D was the number of drinks required to cure hyperthyroidism, and λ was the rate constant describing the event. The number of cured individuals was thus

$$C = H_0 - H. \qquad (38)$$

The analysis then pointed out that this was an adequate description of the results of radioiodide therapy of hyperthyroidism, in series of cases where an effort was made to administer a certain quantity of radioactivity per unit weight of the thyroid (microcuries per gram). The rate constant λ was also shown to be directly related to the concentration (μ, in microcuries per gram) of radioiodide in the thyroid gland:

$$\lambda = \mu \cdot Z \qquad (39)$$

where Z is a constant. Hence the rate of cure of hyperthyroidism depended on the radiation delivered to the thyroid.

What could be considered the second development of these studies was an attempt to gauge the functional capacity of a unit of thyroid tissue. This was done by using the concept of percent uptake per weight of functioning thyroid tissue.[46] This index was shown to separate euthyroid, hyperthyroid, and hyperthyroid but partially thyroidectomized cases; it also pointed out the advantage of early radioiodide uptake studies.

EXTENSION OF THE CONCEPT OF FUNCTIONAL INDICES

The use of a "functional image" has been developed by the Hopkins group.[47] An organ or region is visualized by the magnitude of the rate constant, for the event under study, at various locales in the region. Another variant has been used in studies of the lungs. The quantity of radioactivity (for example, of a radioactive gas or of ^{99m}Tc-macroaggregated albumin) in multiple points of the lung image can be corrected by the estimated thickness of the lung (determined radiographically) at each point, to yield a value of activity per thickness or volume.

We have pointed out, during studies of splenic function,[48] that estimates of both function and size are necessary for an understanding of the organ. The proposal was made to compare the scan estimated organ volume with that predicted from the allometric equation (see the previous discussion on the ultrasonic estimation of liver weight and its comparison with the prediction of the allometric equation). The ratio of functional indices in two organs can be compared with the estimate of their volume relationships. In some cases, the equations simplify considerably. Consider the case of the liver (L) and the spleen (S). The ratio of the allometric expressions for their weights is given as follows (B = body weight):

$$\frac{S}{L} = \frac{0.0042B^{0.85}}{0.052B^{0.93}} \tag{40}$$

or

$$S/L = 0.081B^{-0.08}. \tag{41}$$

For all intents, the residual exponent (0.08) is indistinguishable from zero. Hence the prediction is that the ratio of the weight of the spleen to that of the liver is practically a constant. Various disorders may be characterized by a deviation of this relationship toward one of the organs or the other. It will be of immense interest to attempt to extend this concept in terms of the functional capacity of each of the organs.

GROWTH AND HEALING OF LESIONS IN THE LIVER

The size of the liver, the availability of agents which localize in the organ, and the ability to obtain multiple views have allowed studies to proceed on the production of intrahepatic lesions, and the regression of established defects. For example, we have described 2 cases where irradiation of tumors (compromising the liver) was followed by the reappearance of functional hepatic tissue in the region.[49] At the other extreme, radiation can transiently or permanently impair hepatic function.

We have attempted to quantify the rate of healing of hepatic amebic abscesses, by use of serial scan measurements.[50] Chemotherapy of these abscesses leads to healing, presumably occurring at the interface of the abscess and normal tissue. Thus, the volume (V) change with time t might be proportional to the surface area S of the interface:

$$dV/dt = -f \cdot S. \tag{42}$$

The minus sign indicates that the lesion is decreasing in size. The radius of the lesion is introduced by noting that the volume of a sphere is $4\pi R^3/3$, while its surface area is $4\pi R^2$. Upon substituting into Eq. (42) and integrating, we obtain

$$R = Q - ft. \tag{43}$$

That is, the radius decreases linearly with time from its original value Q. The analogy to the previously mentioned Haase's rule is apparent.

A more general formulation is obtained by setting the rate of change of the volume of the lesion equal to a power function of the lesion (again a minus sign is present, since the lesion is decreasing in size):

$$dV/dt = -cV^P. \tag{44}$$

This integrates to $(P \neq 1)$

$$V^{1-P}/(1 - P) = K - ct. \tag{45}$$

When the power term (P) is equal to $\frac{2}{3}$, Eq. (45) reduces to a form resembling Eq. (43). The healing of the abscesses, in terms of the decrease of the radius, was on the order of 0.011 to 0.048 cm/day. The calculated change in mass per unit surface area of the lesions was shown to be quite large, approximating that of fetal growth.[50]

On the opposite side of the coin, studies are presently under way to determine the rate of growth of intrahepatic tumors.[51] The study of 5 cases of metastatic tumors in the liver revealed changes in the diameter of the lesions of 100×10^{-3} to 400×10^{-3} mm/day. This is comparable to radiographically reported changes in lung tumors.

BLOOD SUPPLY AND GROWTH

Nutrients are supplied by the blood and lymphatic vessels in a tissue. The magnitude of this supply is of importance, and it will be recalled that the equations of fetal growth could be derived on the assumption of a surface which limited their availability. We can also inquire as to the extent of blood supply to a region, particularly to rapidly growing tissue (tumor). We approached this problem by equating the specific growth rate of the tumor (W = weight) to the specific rate of change of blood flow (all blood flow estimates, made by radioisotopic means, were taken from the literature):[52]

$$\frac{dF}{F} = m\,\frac{dW}{W} \tag{46}$$

or

$$F = cW^m \tag{47}$$

$$\log F = \log c + m \log W. \tag{48}$$

The exponent m was shown to vary from 0.52 to 1.24 in various types of tumors. In the "ideal" case of delivery of a nutrient across the surface of a sphere, the exponent would be $\frac{2}{3}$ (area $= W^{2/3}$). Values more or less than this represent either varying geometries or that the exponent is an interaction parameter (perhaps crudely similar to a nuclear cross section, which measures an interaction, but is given in units of a geometric plane figure). With the variety of radioisotopic techniques presently available for examining blood flow, this could be an area of increasing importance.

SOME ADDITIONAL AREAS OF STUDY

Studies of body composition by means of radioisotopic dilution have been a part of nuclear medicine for many years. In some cases the total quantity of a material can be measured, while in other instances only the "exchargeable" amount can be assayed. There are, however, other techniques of use.

1. Body potassium measurements (^{40}K assayed by whole-body counting) have been related to body parameters in adults[53] and in children.
2. Studies utilizing the absorption of monoenergetic photons to estimate the mineral in bone[54] have applications to surveying large populations during growth.
3. Activation analysis, for determining body composition, also has applications to following changes in an individual or in a population.[55]

SUMMARY

Some radioisotopic approaches for following aspects of growth, development, and regeneration during life have been outlined. Despite their limitations, these techniques might provide fresh insights as to the rate and control of key biological events.

REFERENCES

1. Spencer RP, Fishbone G, Davis CD: Amniotic fluid studies by isotope dilution and scanning. J Nucl Med 7:629–632, 1966
2. Harrison RF: The use of amniography in the estimation of fetal maturity. J Ir Coll Phys Surg 2:18–20, 1972
3. Flamme P: Ultrasonic fetal cephalometry: percentiles curve. Br Med J 3:384–385, 1972
4. Sabbagha RE, Turner JH: Methodology of B-scan sonar cephalometry with electronic calipers and correlation with fetal birth weight. Obstet Gynecol 40:74–81, 1972
5. Lathrop KA, Gloria IV, Taylor C, Harper PV: Localization of ^{99m}Tc in the mouse fetus from Na ^{99m}TcO$_4^-$ administered intravenously to the mother. J Nucl Med 12:375, 1971

6. Tarachand U, Eapen J: Incorporation of leucine-^{14}C into proteins of the placenta and liver of mice. Am J Obstet Gynecol 114:62–64, 1972

7. Garrow JS, Douglas CP: A rapid method for assessing intrauterine growth by radioactive selenomethionine uptake. J Obstet Gynaecol Br Commonw 75:1034–1039, 1968

8. Lee P, Garrow JS: A clinical evaluation of the selenomethionine uptake test. J Obstet Gynaecol Br Commonw 77:982–986, 1970

9. Lathop KA, Johnston RE, Blau M: Radiation dose to human beings from ^{75}Se-L-selenomethionine. J Nucl Med 11:374, 1970

10. Lathrop KA, Gloria IV, Harper PV: Fetal radiation absorbed doses from placental imaging. J Nucl Med 11:341–342, 1970

11. Graber SE, McIntyre PA, Heyssel RM: Comparison of the kinetics of [113m]In and ^{59}Fe-lebeled transferrin in pregnant rats. J Nucl Med 10:338, 1969

12. Antar MA, Spencer RP: Dynamics of placental and uterine blood flow: a functional index using [113m]In. Obstet Gynecol 40:385–390, 1972

13. Janson J: [133]Xe clearance in the myometrium of pregnant and nonpregnant women. Acta Obstet Gynecol Scand 48:302–321, 1969

14. Schneider H, Panigel M, Dancis J: Transfer across the perfused human placenta of antipyrine, sodium, and leucine. Am J Obstet Gynecol 114:822–828, 1972

15. Haase; Entbindungs-Anstalt. Jahresbericht pro 1875. Charite–Annalen 2:669–696, 1875

16. Spencer RP: Relationship of fetal weight to the lunar month of pregnancy. Growth 28:91–96, 1964

17. Spencer RP, Coulombe MJ: Observations on fetal weight and gestational age. Growth 28:243–247, 1964

18. Spencer RP: Placental growth: semiquantitative approaches. Biol Neonate 12:180–185, 1968

19. Payne PR, Wheeler EF: Growth of the fetus. Nature 215–849–850, 1967

20. Spencer RP: Physical basis for Haase's law of fetal growth. J Theor Biol 26:507–508, 1970

21. Laird AK: Dynamics of growth in tumors and in normal organisms. Natl Cancer Inst Monogr 30:15–28, 1969

22. Spencer RP: Radiographically determined sternal ossification: an approach to skeletal maturity. Biol Neonate 14:341–343, 1969

23. Spencer RP, Banever C: Human thyroid growth: a scan study. Invest Radiol 5:111–116, 1970

24. Kay C, Abrahams S, McClain P: The weight of the normal thyroid glands in children. Arch Pathol 82:349–352, 1966

25. Spencer RP, Banever C: Growth of the human liver: a preliminary scan study. J Nucl Med 11:660–662, 1970

26. Spencer RP, Pearson HA, Lange RC: Human spleen: scan studies on growth and response to medications. J Nucl Med 12:466–467, 1971

27. Seltzer RA, Kereiakes JG, Saenger EL: Radiation exposure from radioisotopes in pediatrics. N Engl J Med 271:84–90, 1964

28. Larson SM, Tueli SH, Moores KD, Nelp WB: Dimensions of the normal spleen and prediction of spleen weight. J Nucl Med 11:341, 1970

29. Libby RL: Empirical formulae for the estimation of thyroid weight. J Clin Endocrinol 14:1265–1268, 1954

30. Myhill J, Reeve TS, Figgis PM: Measurement of the mass of the thyroid gland in vivo. Am J Roentgenol 94:828–836, 1965

31. Spencer RP: Determination of organ volumes by scintillation scanning. J Nucl Med 5:444–452, 1964

32. Rollo FD, DeLand FH: The determination of liver mass from radionuclide images. Radiology 91:1191–1194, 1968

33. Rollo FD, DeLand FH: The determination of spleen mass from radionuclide images. Radiology 97:583–587, 1970

34. Spencer RP: Relationship of surface area on roentgenograms and radioisotopic scans to organ volumes. J Nucl Med 8:785–791, 1967

35. Huxley JS: Problems of Relative Growth. New York, Dial Press, 1932

36. Stahl WR: Organ weights in primates and other mammals. Science 150:1039–1042, 1965

37. Spencer RP, Chaudhuri TK: Quantitative estimates of changes in splenic size during life. Yale J Biol Med 41:333–339, 1969

38. Rasmussen SN: Liver volume determination by ultrasonic scanning. Br J Radiol 45:579–585, 1972

39. Walk L: Roentgenologic determination of the liver volume. Acta Radiol Diag 6:369–371, 1967

40. Yagan R, MacIntyre WJ, Christie JH: Estimation of liver size by the multiple cutoff scintillation scanning technique. Am J Roentgenol 88:289–295, 1962

41. Spencer RP: Quantitative radioisotope approaches to hepatic size and function. Am J Dig Dis 12:515–521, 1967

42. Spencer RP, Waldman R: Size and positional relationships between thyroid lobes in the adult as determined by scintillation scanning. J Nucl Med 6:53–58, 1965

43. Gallaher WH, Spencer RP: Preliminary estimation of functional thyroid weights in a selected hyperthyroid population. J Nucl Med 5:649–650, 1964

44. Antar MA, Antar A, Spencer RP: Effect of initial radioiodide therapy on thyroid scan length, surface area, and uptake. J Nucl Med 11:381, 1970

45. Spencer RP: Response of the overactive thyroid to radioiodine therapy. J Nucl Med 12:610–615, 1971

46. Spencer RP, Montana G: Percent uptake per gram: a parameter in following thyroid function. Invest Radiol 3:382–383, 1968

47. Kaihara S, Natarajan TK, Wagner HN Jr, Maynard CD: Construction of a functional image from regional rate constants. J Nucl Med 10:347, 1969

48. Spencer RP, Rockoff ML, Spector H: Studies on quantitation of the ^{51}Cr-erythrocyte spleen-to-liver ratio. J Nucl Med 9:51–57, 1968

49. Spencer RP, Kligerman MM: Scan evidence of hepatic "refunction" after tumor irradiation. J Nucl Med 11:140–141, 1970

50. Spencer RP, Johnston GS: Healing rate of hepatic amebic abscesses: theory and scan measurements. J Nucl Med 11:452–454, 1970

51. Spencer RP, Witek JT: Radionuclide studies on the growth of intrahepatic tumors and of the infiltrated liver. Cancer 32:838–842, 1973

52. Spencer RP: Blood flow in transplanted tumors: quantitative approaches to radioisotopic studies. Yale J Biol Med 43:22–30, 1970

53. Boddy K, King PC, Hume R, Weyers E: The relation of total body potassium to height, weight, and age in normal adults. J Clin Pathol 25:512–517, 1972

54. Cameron JR, Sorenson J: Measurement of bone mineral in vivo: an improved method. Science 142:230–232, 1963

55. Murano R, Pailthorp KG, Palmer EH, Hinn GM, Rich CR, Rudd TG, Williams JL, Nelp WB: Total-body neutron activation analysis system for measuring total-body calcium. J Nucl Med 10:360, 1969

Index

Index